LC Gupta's
Practical Nursing Procedures

LC Gupta's
Practical Nursing Procedures

Fourth Edition

Alisha Talwar
MSN Medical Surgical (Gastroenterology) Nursing
RNRM BSc (H) Nursing
New Delhi, India

Teresa Lamniang
MSN Mental Health Nursing
RNRM BSc (H) Nursing
New Delhi, India

Priya Verma Gupta
BDS, MDS, PhD, FPFA
Specialist Pediatric Dentist
Dr Joy Dental Clinic
Dubai, UAE

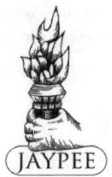

JAYPEE BROTHERS MEDICAL PUBLISHERS
The Health Sciences Publisher
New Delhi | London

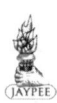 **Jaypee Brothers Medical Publishers (P) Ltd**

Headquarters
Jaypee Brothers Medical Publishers (P) Ltd
EMCA House, 23/23-B
Ansari Road, Daryaganj
New Delhi 110 002, India
Landline: +91-11-23272143, +91-11-23272703
+91-11-23282021, +91-11-23245672
Email: jaypee@jaypeebrothers.com

Corporate Office
Jaypee Brothers Medical Publishers (P) Ltd
4838/24, Ansari Road, Daryaganj
New Delhi 110 002, India
Phone: +91-11-43574357
Fax: +91-11-43574314
Email: jaypee@jaypeebrothers.com

Overseas Office
J.P. Medical Ltd
83 Victoria Street, London
SW1H 0HW (UK)
Phone: +44 20 3170 8910
Fax: +44 (0)20 3008 6180
Email: info@jpmedpub.com

Website: www.jaypeebrothers.com
Website: www.jaypeedigital.com

© 2024, Jaypee Brothers Medical Publishers

The views and opinions expressed in this book are solely those of the original contributor(s)/author(s) and do not necessarily represent those of editor(s) and Publisher of the book.

All rights reserved. No part of this publication may be reproduced, stored or transmitted in any form or by any means, electronic, mechanical, photocopying, recording or otherwise, without the prior permission in writing of the publishers.

All brand names and product names used in this book are trade names, service marks, trademarks or registered trademarks of their respective owners. The publisher is not associated with any product or vendor mentioned in this book.

Medical knowledge and practice change constantly. This book is designed to provide accurate, authoritative information about the subject matter in question. However, readers are advised to check the most current information available on procedures included and check information from the manufacturer of each product to be administered, to verify the recommended dose, formula, method and duration of administration, adverse effects and contraindications. It is the responsibility of the practitioner to take all appropriate safety precautions. Neither the publisher nor the author(s)/editor(s) assume any liability for any injury and/or damage to persons or property arising from or related to use of material in this book.

This book is sold on the understanding that the publisher is not engaged in providing professional medical services. If such advice or services are required, the services of a competent medical professional should be sought.

Every effort has been made where necessary to contact holders of copyright to obtain permission to reproduce copyright material. If any have been inadvertently overlooked, the publisher will be pleased to make the necessary arrangements at the first opportunity.

Inquiries for bulk sales may be solicited at: jaypee@jaypeebrothers.com

Practical Nursing Procedures

First Edition: 1987
Second Edition: 1991
Reprint: 2003, 2004
Third Edition: 2007
Fourth Edition: **2024**

ISBN: 978-93-5696-361-0

Printed at: Sterling Graphics Pvt. Ltd. India

The art of nursing is based on a deep understanding of the human condition, a willingness to serve, and an unwavering dedication to making a difference in the lives of others."

—**Florence Nightingale**

Tribute

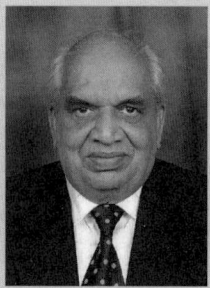

Late Dr LC Gupta

Dr LC Gupta was a pioneer in the field of medicine and a true inspiration to all those who were fortunate enough to have known him. He dedicated his life to the betterment of the medical field, tirelessly working to find new ways to improve patient care, research, and education.

Dr Gupta was more than a renowned medical professional; he was a gifted writer and communicator, seamlessly blending his profound expertise in healthcare with the art of storytelling. His book, "Practical Nursing Procedures," stands as a testament to his brilliance, encapsulating a wealth of knowledge and wisdom that has empowered nurses and healthcare professionals across the globe.

With clarity and precision, Dr Gupta demystifies the intricate procedures, providing step-by-step instructions and invaluable tips. His expertise not only educates but instills confidence in the hearts of nurses, assuring them that they possess the skills to make a significant difference in the lives of their patients. Through his work, he has nurtured a generation of competent and compassionate caregivers, leaving an indelible mark on the nursing community.

Through his unwavering commitment to lifelong learning, Dr Gupta sets an example for others to follow. He reminds us that the pursuit of knowledge is an ongoing endeavor, and by continuously seeking to improve our skills and understanding, we can elevate the standard of care for patients around the world.

May his work continue to guide and inspire us as we carry forth his legacy of compassion and dedication to the art and science of healing.

Rest in eternal peace, Dr Gupta.

Preface

Nursing is not merely a profession, but a vocation driven by compassion, empathy, humanity and a dedication to healing. With a great profound sense of purpose and dedication to the nursing profession, we would like to introduce the fourth edition of *LC Gupta's Practical Nursing Procedures*. The aim of this book is to serve as a practical and reliable compassion for nurses, bridging the gap between theoretical knowledge and hands-on application. In these pages, you will find a detailed compendium of essential nursing procedures, each precisely outlined and illustrated with step-by-step instructions.

Since the first edition of this book, nursing has evolved significantly, with technologies, innovations, evidence-based practices, and an unwavering commitment to patient-centered care shaping the landscape of healthcare. This fourth edition reflects the culmination of years of progress and growth, mirroring the dynamic nature of the nursing profession.

In this edition, you will find a comprehensive array of nursing procedures presented in 50 chapters, carefully curated according to the new revised INC syllabus to encompass both fundamental skills and cutting-edge techniques. The contents are meticulously reviewed and updated to align with the latest evidence-based practices in the field of nursing.

To all nurses, we hope that this edition will reinforce your skills, spark curiosity, and open to new avenues for exploration in your practice. Never forget the profound impact you have on the lives of your patients and their families.

Alisha Talwar
Teresa Lamniang
Priya Verma Gupta

Acknowledgments

"Amidst the boundless intricacies of nursing care, we find ourselves humbly acknowledging the hands that have guided and uplifted us along this arduous yet rewarding path. To those whose expertise and compassion have graced these pages, we owe a debt of gratitude beyond words. This book stands as a testament to the power of collective wisdom and serves as a beacon, guiding caregivers to embrace the art and science of nursing with unwavering dedication and kindness."

First and foremost, we extend our deepest thanks to our families for their unwavering love and understanding throughout this endeavor. Their patience and belief in our abilities have been the driving force behind our commitment to see this project through.

We are immensely grateful to Shri Jitendar P Vij (Group Chairman), Mr Ankit Vij (Managing Director), Mr MS Mani (Group President) who are the continual source of inspiration throughout this journey.

We would like to express our heartfelt gratitude to Dr Madhu Choudhary (Director–Educational Publishing) whose guidance and expertise have been instrumental in shaping the content of this book. Her valuable insights and constructive feedback have elevated the quality of our work.

We are extremely blessed to have friends like Ms Jitika and Dr Aditya who offered their encouragement and support along the way. Their words of wisdom, brainstorming, and moral support have been crucial in keeping us motivated in this journey.

A special acknowledgment goes to our dedicated team at Jaypee Brothers Medical Publishers (P) Ltd, New Delhi, India, who worked tirelessly to bring this book to fruition especially Ms Pooja Bhandari [Director–Production (Books and Journals)], Ms Sunita Katla (Executive Assistant to Group Chairman and Publishing Manager), Ms Samina Khan (Executive Assistant to Director–Educational Publishing) and Mr Rajesh Sharma (Production Coordinator) for their efforts and support in the completion of this project.

Acknowledgments

We would also like to sincerely thank Ms Seema Dogra (Cover Visualizer), Mr Deepak Saxena (Typesetter), Mr Anil Singh (Proofreader) and Mr Gopal Singh Kirola (Graphic Designer) who added hue and life to the entire book and perfected the script. Their professionalism and dedication to detail have been invaluable in the publishing process.

Lastly, we would like to thank all the readers who will embark on this journey with us. Your interest and engagement in our work make all our efforts worthwhile, and we hope that the knowledge and insights shared in these pages prove valuable to you.

Contents

1. Communication and Nurse-Patient Relationship — 1
2. Vital Signs — 10
3. Pulse Oximetry — 42
4. Hot and Cold Application — 46
5. Care of Articles — 68
6. Asepsis — 79
7. Bed Making — 88
8. Comfort Devices — 99
9. Therapeutic Positions — 106
10. Pain — 114
11. Restraints and Safety Devices — 117
12. Hospital Admission and Discharge — 124
13. Mobility and Immobility — 130
14. Bandages and Dressings — 143
15. Health Assessment — 156
16. Nursing Process — 172
17. Nasogastric Tube Insertion and Feeding — 178
18. Bed Bath — 183
19. Hair Washing — 186
20. Care of Pressure Points and Back Care — 189
21. Oral Hygiene — 199
22. Perineal Care — 203
23. Urinary Catheterization — 208
24. Assisting with Bedpan — 213
25. Insertion of Enema and Suppository — 216
26. Specimen Collection — 224
27. Oxygenation — 234

28.	Steam Inhalation	238
29.	Chest Physiotherapy	242
30.	Oral Suctioning	250
31.	Blood Transfusion	253
32.	Drug Dose Calculations	257
33.	Oral Medication Administration	262
34.	Topical Medication Administration	265
35.	Inhalational Medication Administration	268
36.	Intradermal Injection Administration	272
37.	Subcutaneous Injection Administration	275
38.	Intramuscular Injection Administration	278
39.	Instillation	281
40.	Irrigation	285
41.	Assessing the Level of Consciousness	290
42.	Care of Dead Body	296
43.	Poisoning	300
44.	Care of Newborn	314
45.	Assisting in Diagnostic Procedures	327
46.	Family Planning-Contraception	360
47.	Antenatal Care	377
48.	Postnatal Care	385
49.	Perioperative Care	389
50.	Surgical Instruments	394
	Index	*403*

CHAPTER 1

Communication and Nurse-Patient Relationship

INTRODUCTION

Communication term is derived from the Latin word 'communis', that means common. Communication refers to the reciprocal exchange or imparting of information, ideas, facts, opinions, beliefs, feelings and attitudes through speaking, writhing or any other verbal or nonverbal means between two or people.

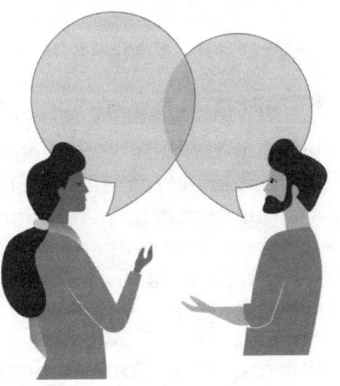

Communication is based on the concept of giving and taking information. It also involves the interpretation and understanding of the information (message).

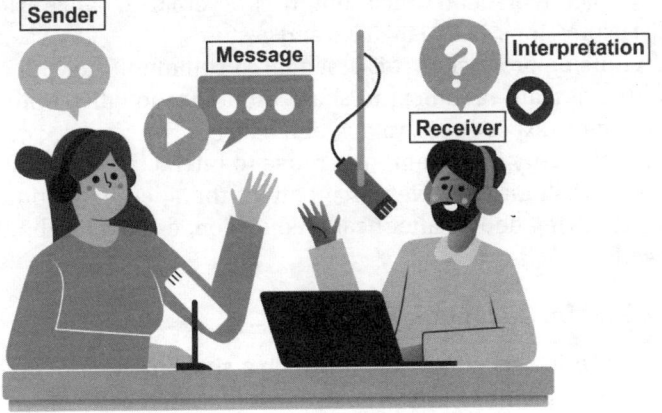

Communication and Nurse-Patient Relationship

DEFINITION

- Communication is a process by which information is exchanged between individuals through a common system of symbols and signs of behavior.

  —Webster's Dictionary

- Communication is interchange of thoughts, opinions, or information by speech, writing or signs.

  —Robert Anderson

LEVELS OF COMMUNICATION

Intrapersonal Communication

It is a powerful form of communication that occurs within self. It is also known as self-verbalization, or inner thought. Thoughts had a strong impact on perceptions, feelings, behavior, and self-concept.

Nurses' and patients use intrapersonal communication to develop self-awareness and a positive self-concept that enhances appropriate self-expression.

Interpersonal Communication

It is the one-to-one interaction between a nurse and other person that can be a patient or other healthcare team member. It is usually a face-to-face interaction which comprises of verbal exchange of ideas, facial expressions, body language and gestures.

In nursing profession, it is essential to communicate with other healthcare team members to share different thoughts, opinions, information, experiences, values, and belief.

It is also very important for a nurse to interact with her patient and establish an effective nurse patient therapeutic relationship (e.g., clarifying doubts after health education, discussing about the procedure, etc.).

Small-group Communication

It is goal-oriented interaction in which a small number of persons meet and interact (e.g., small staff meeting).

Public Communication

It is communicating with large group of people. Effective public communication creates awareness about health-related topics, health issues, and other important issues related to nursing (e.g., health education, role-play, seminars, social media post, etc.).

COMMUNICATION PROCESS

- ❖ Communication is a dynamic and circular process that involves a series of actions and reactions and takes various steps.
- ❖ It is the two-way process that involves the sender and receiver of a message.
- ❖ It is an ongoing process in which the receiver of the message becomes the sender of the response, and the original sender becomes the receiver.
- ❖ The communication process starts with the sender who encodes or formulates an idea or message to communicate to another person known as a receiver, a person who decodes the message.
- ❖ The message may be expressed verbally or nonverbally through a channel (media), and the communication process also has feedback in the form of a response, which is essential at each step.
- ❖ In between, there may be many barriers, such as noise as depicted in the **Figure 1.1**.

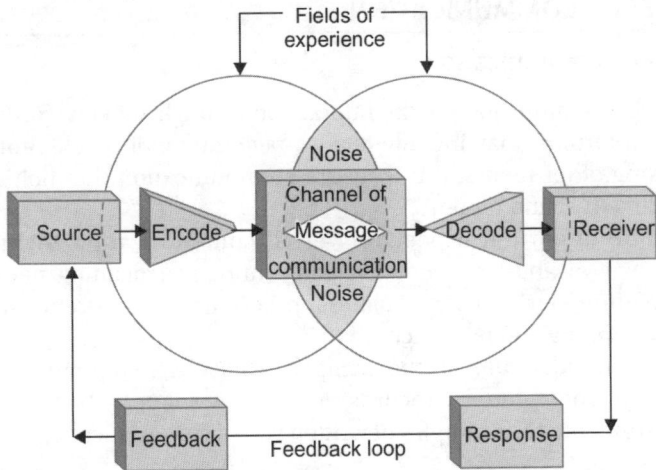

Fig. 1.1: Elements of the communication process.

Elements of Communication Process

- **Sender:** The sender is a source who initiates or encodes the communication process and takes the initiative to start a dialogue.
- **Encoding:** It is assembling the ideas, thoughts that needs to be communicated and the method of communication either verbal or nonverbal.
- **Message:** It is the thought, ideas, facts, opinions, or information. The message must be in the form that the receiver must understand it.
- **Channel:** A channel is the medium of communication; it is the way of carrying a message from the sender to the receiver. The sender must select the most appropriate channel to convey the message keeping in mind the time and urgency of the message.
- **Receiver:** A receiver is a person who receives and interprets or decodes the message. The receiver is responsible for responding and giving feedback on the information received.
- **Decoding:** Decoding is the process of understanding the message.
- **Feedback:** It is a reply from the receiver to sender. It is the backbone of effective communication. It helps to stimulate and reinforces an idea to communicate.

Noise: Noise is an interruption (barrier) that affects the communication process adversely.

TYPES OF COMMUNICATION

Verbal Communication

Verbal communication is the interaction through spoken words or written form. It may include face-to-face interaction, telephonic, or using other media. It is a secure communication that helps in building trust and rapport.

Some important aspects of verbal communication include: language, vocabulary, denotative and connotative meaning, pacing, intonation, clarity, consciousness, preciseness, comprehension, brevity, timing and relevance.

Speech and lectures are the examples of oral verbal communication whereas notes, letters, records, forms, newspapers, books, and magazines are the examples of written verbal communication.

Nonverbal Communication

It is the exchange of a message without the use of words. Nonverbal communications are essential to express emotions, attitudes, and reactions. Eye contact, gestures, movement, and postures are types of nonverbal communication. Eye contact is most useful in gaining someone's trust. Gesture allows to interest the person by showing the bigger picture of saying. Movements are used to attract people to have more interest in speech. Good posture reflects confidence, trust, and power.

Nonverbal communication may be accomplished by the following means:
- Touch
- Eye contact
- Facial expression
- Posture
- Gait
- Gesture
- Physical appearance
- Sound
- Silence

7C'S OF EFFECTIVE COMMUNICATION (FIG. 1.2)

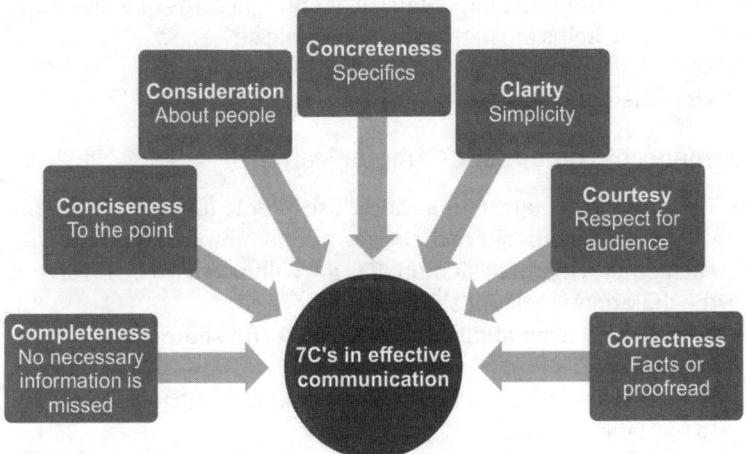

Fig. 1.2: The 7C's of effective communication.

NURSE-PATIENT RELATIONSHIP

"Nurse-patient relationship is an interaction process between two persons in which nurse fulfils her/his role by using her/his professional knowledge and skills in such a way that she is able to help the patient physically, socially and emotionally."

—Bimla Kapoor (1994)

It is a mutual learning experience for both the nurse and the patient. In this relationship, the nurse uses her competency, skills, and clinical techniques with the patient to bring about insight and behavioral change. Maintaining professional boundaries is an essential component in the provision of safe, competent, and ethical nursing care.

Goals of Nurse-patient Relationship

- The nurse helps the patient to cope with present problems
- The nurse helps the patient to understand his problem
- The nurse helps the patient to understand his active participation in an experience
- The nurse assists the patient to identify emerging problems realistically
- The nurse helps the patient to find out a new alternative for his or her problem
- The nurse helps the patient to try out new patterns of behavior
- The nurse helps the patient to communicate
- The nurse helps the patient socialize
- The nurse helps the patient to find a meaning for his illness

Elements of Therapeutic Communication

- **Rapport:** It is a harmonious and close interaction, with which the nurse and patient share their views and communicate well with each other without hesitation. It is the willingness to be involve in the therapeutic relationship.
- **Empathy:** It is an ability to understand and share the feeling of another.
- **Warmth:** It is the ability to comfort the patient and help the patient to feel being cared.
- **Genuineness:** It is the ability to be real and honest with each other.

Phases of Therapeutic Communication

❖ **Preinteraction phase:**
- It begins with the patient assignment to initiate the therapeutic relationship.
- It involves preparation for the first encounter with the patient.
- It explores the self-perception of both the nurse and patient.

Tasks of nurse	Problems
• To explore the own feelings, fantasies, and fears • To analyze own professional strength and limitations • To collect data about patient whenever possible • To plan for first meeting with the patient	• Difficulty in self-acceptance • Boredom • Anxiety • Depression • Indifference • Anger

❖ **Orientation phase:**
- This is the first interaction between the nurse and patient in which both introduce themselves.
- In this phase, trust and rapport are established.

Tasks of nurse	Problems
• Establish effective communication • Establishment of trust and rapport • Collection of baseline data • Identifying patient's strengths and limits • Define the patient's problem and plan the nursing care • Formulating nursing diagnoses • Agreement of goals • Set the priorities for the intervention	• Different perception • Different opinion • Difficulty in agreement

❖ **Working phase:**
- During this phase, therapeutic work of nurse-patient relationship is accomplished.
- Maintenance of trust and rapport that was established during the orientation phase.
- Promote the patient's insight and perception of reality.
- Continuous evaluation of the process towards the goal attainment.

Tasks of nurse	Problems
• Collection of data • Explore stressors • Facilitate behavioral change • Provide opportunities for independent functioning • Evaluate the patient's behavior	• Fear of closeness • Resistance behavior • Transference • Countertransference

- ❖ **Termination phase:**
  - ♦ This is the most tough phase, but important phase of the therapeutic relationship.
  - ♦ The goal of this phase is to terminate this therapeutic relationship.
  - ♦ Termination may be due to patient's discharged from the hospital or shift change of nurse, allocation to different department or unit etc.
  - ♦ Termination can be difficult phase for both the nurse as well as patient

Tasks of nurse	Problems
• Review progress of nursing care and therapy • Review attainment of goals • Evaluate the outcomes • Establish the reality of separation • Formulate the plans for discharge and follow-ups.	• Anger • Depression • Punitive behavior

Therapeutic Communication Techniques

- ❖ Silence
- ❖ Be specific and tentative
- ❖ Therapeutic touch
- ❖ Restating or paraphrasing
- ❖ Seeking clarification
- ❖ Giving information
- ❖ Acknowledging
- ❖ Clarifying
- ❖ Reality check
- ❖ Focusing
- ❖ Reflecting
- ❖ Summarizing
- ❖ Defensive

- Agreeing and disagreeing
- Testing
- Rejecting
- Passing judgement
- Changing topic
- Giving common advice

BARRIERS OF COMMUNICATION

- **Physical factors**—such as illness, fatigue, pain, deafness, and speech defects.
- **Emotional factors**—such as fear, suspicion, jealousy, anger, anxiety, resentment, antagonism, prejudices, lack of interest and lack of listening.
- **Intellectual factors**—such as low IQ, mental retardation, misinterpretation of words.
- **Social factors**—such as socioeconomic status, language issues, cultural issues, professional status etc.
- **Environmental factors**—such as noise, lack of privacy etc.
- **Other factors**—lack of listening, changing of subject, inappropriate use of knowledge, false reassurance etc.

CHAPTER 2

Vital Signs

INTRODUCTION

Vital signs are the signs that indicate the status of the body's vital organs **(Fig. 2.1)**. It is an objective measurement of the essential physiological functions. Assessment of vital sign is the primary step for clinical evaluation.

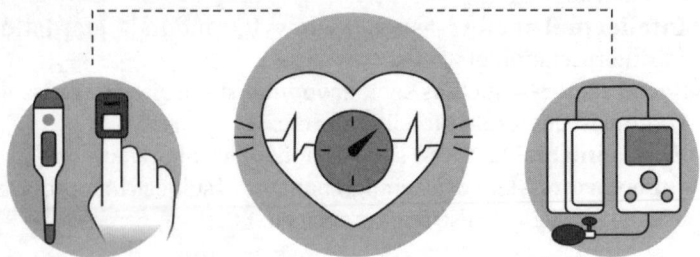

Fig. 2.1: The status of the body's vital signs.

Assessment of vital signs allows the nurse to identify nursing diagnoses, to implement planned intervention and to evaluate outcomes. When the nurse learns the physiological variables influencing vital signs and recognizes the relationship of vital sign changes to other physiological assessment findings, precise determination of the client's health problems can be made.

BODY TEMPERATURE

It is defined as the degree of heat maintained by the body. In other words, body temperature is the balance between the heat produced/thermogenesis and the heat lost/thermolysis from the body **(Fig. 2.2)**.

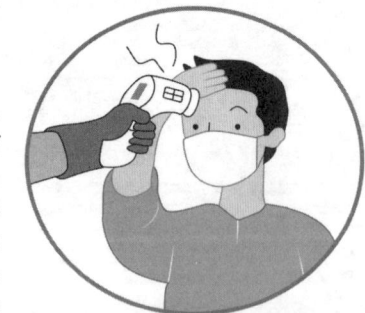

Fig. 2.2: Body temperature.

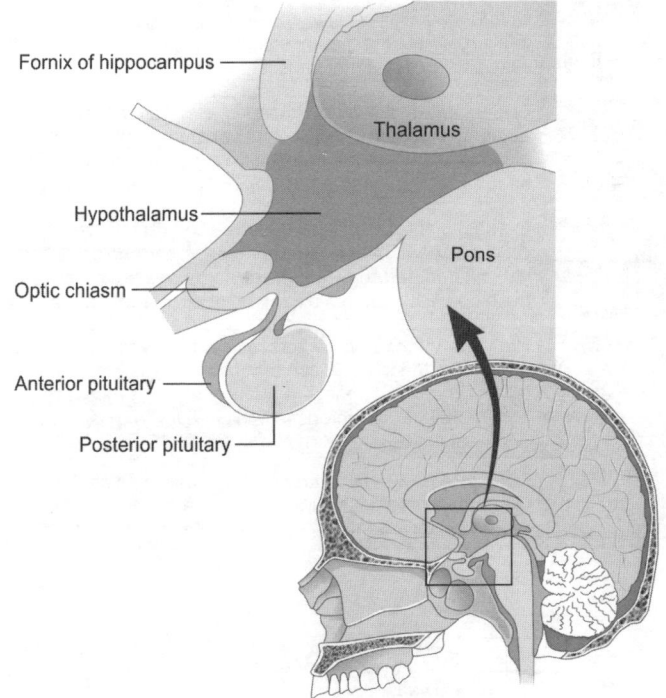

Fig. 2.3: Temperature controlling center: Hypothalamus.

Hypothalamus is the heat regulating center which is situated in the brain **(Figs. 2.3 and 2.4)**.

Types of Temperature

- **Core temperature:** It is the temperature of deep structures. It is the optimum temperature at which the internal organs and body system function. It also refers as body's internal temperature. It is constant 37°C.
- **Surface temperature:** It is the temperature of the outer surface (i.e., skin).

Ways of Heat Production

Oxidation of food	During the metabolism of proteins, carbohydrates, and fats, heat is produced as a by-product like 1 g of carbohydrate and 1 g of protein gives each 4 calories of heat and 1 g fat gives 9 calories of heat

Vital Signs

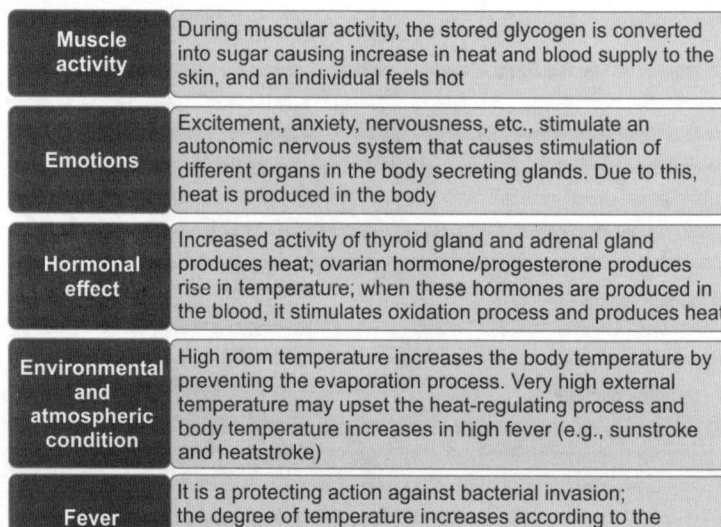

Muscle activity	During muscular activity, the stored glycogen is converted into sugar causing increase in heat and blood supply to the skin, and an individual feels hot
Emotions	Excitement, anxiety, nervousness, etc., stimulate an autonomic nervous system that causes stimulation of different organs in the body secreting glands. Due to this, heat is produced in the body
Hormonal effect	Increased activity of thyroid gland and adrenal gland produces heat; ovarian hormone/progesterone produces rise in temperature; when these hormones are produced in the blood, it stimulates oxidation process and produces heat
Environmental and atmospheric condition	High room temperature increases the body temperature by preventing the evaporation process. Very high external temperature may upset the heat-regulating process and body temperature increases in high fever (e.g., sunstroke and heatstroke)
Fever	It is a protecting action against bacterial invasion; the degree of temperature increases according to the severity of infection

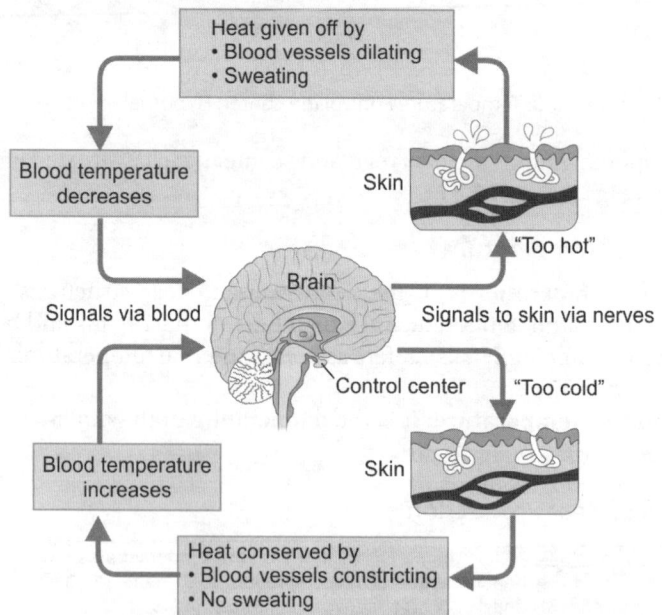

Fig. 2.4: Regulation of body temperature.

Ways of Heat Loss

The heat is lost from the body in different ways:
- **Through the skin:** Heat is controlled by the hypothalamus when the body temperature is increased the warm blood flows through the hypothalamus. It is very sensitive to heat variation in the blood and sends impulses to the skin causing vasodilatation. Due to vasodilatation, more blood comes to the skin and the heat is lost by means of conduction, convection, radiation, and evaporation.
    - *Conduction* is the transfer of heat directly through a substance from the hot part to the cold part from one molecule to the other (by direct contact). Heat is transferred by conduction from the body to any substances in contact with the body such as air, food stuffs, and water.
    - *Convection* is the method of the transfer of heat by circulating air in liquid. It depends upon the air movement and the temperature of atmosphere.
    - *Radiation* is the transfer of heat from the surface of one object to another which is not in contact with each other.
    - *Evaporation* is the process by which a substance in a liquid state is changed into vapor. The body loses a large amount of heat by evaporation of perspiration and sweat.
- **Through the lungs:** The temperature of the air which is taken to the lungs is that of the atmosphere, and it is lower than that of the body temperature. On entering the respiratory tract, it is warmed to that of the body temperature by absorbing heat from the lung tissue. As the individual breathes out, the warm air is lost through the expired air. Approximately 300 mL of water is also vaporized from the lungs daily.
- **Through the kidney:** Secrete urine which is warmed by the heat taken from the body. As the urine is excreted, the heat is also lost from the body.
- **Through the bowel:** The feces that are formed in the bowels absorb heat from the body, so as individual defecates the heat is lost from the body.

Conversion of Body Heat

The heat can be considered by the type of clothing worn, that is, cotton garments are good conductors of heat, so they are used for summer. Woolen garments and blankets are used in the winter season. Wool is a bad conductor of heat because the air is trapped in the interlocking space of the material, which thereby prevents the heat loss from the body.

Use of hot water bottle and hot drinks helps to maintain the body temperature in a client who is exposed to cold. Rubbing the skin surface increases the body temperature by friction which changes mechanical energy to thermal energy. Cold drinks and cold sponges reduce the temperature by the evaporation of moisture.

Normal Temperature Variations

The normal temperature of the body is 98°F (37°C). In a normal healthy person, the temperature varies from 97–99°F (36.1–37.2°C).

- **Age:** Temperature regulation is unstable until children reach puberty. The normal temperature in young people is higher than that of the people of old age.
- **Exercise:** Heavy exercise increases heat; rest and sleep reduce temperature.
- **Hormonal level:** Women generally experience fluctuation in temperature. Progesterone and thyroid hormone increase temperature.
- **Time of the day (circulation rhythm):** It is less in the morning and more in the evening by 0.5°C. Temperature is usually the lowest at 1–4 AM.
- **Stress:** Physical and psychological emotions cause an increase in temperature.
- **Fasting:** When a person is fasting, the body temperature decreases.

Assessment of Temperature

The body temperature can be assessed through the various types of thermometers.

Types of Thermometers

Glass Thermometer/Clinical Thermometer (Figs. 2.5A and B)

- It is available in both Fahrenheit and Celsius scales.
- It has two parts—a bulb containing mercury and a steam in which the mercury can rise on the stem in a graduated scale representing the degree of temperature.

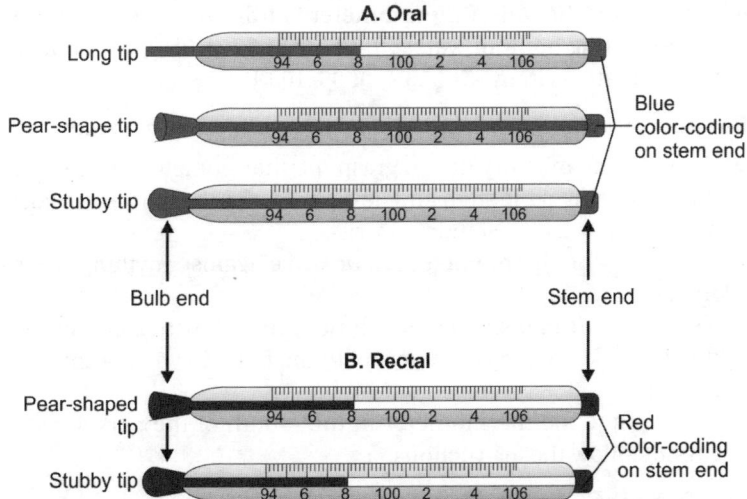

Figs. 2.5A and B: Showing oral and rectal thermometer.

- The lowest registered temperature is 35°C or 95°F and the highest is 43.3°C or 110°F, because the body temperature above or below this range is rare.
- The stem usually has a curved surface that magnifies the lines and figures on the scale and a flattened back with a sharp ridge that makes it easier to read and lessen the danger of breakage.
- The bulbs are of different sizes and shapes; the greater the surface of glass surrounding mercury, the more rapidly the thermometer registers; the oral thermometers are with long and slender bulbs, whereas the rectal ones are with short and fat bulbs.
- Mercury is a liquid metal with silvery appearance used in thermometers because it is very sensitive to temperature; expansion of mercury is uniform and easily visible; it boils in very high temperature (35.7°C) and freezes in very low temperature (39°F).
- There is a constriction above the bulb which prevents the mercury from falling into the bulb on cooling so reading can be done conveniently.

Clinical Thermometer is Different from Lotion Thermometer

- Lotion thermometer is 13.5 times heavier than water, so a small glass tube is used.
- There is no constriction.

- Grading on the lotion thermometer is from the freezing point to the boiling point of water (0–100°C or 32–212°F); the clinical thermometer is from 35–43.3°C or 95–100°F.

General Instructions to be Kept in Mind while using Thermometer
- To shake the mercury down, grasp the thermometer securely by the upper end of the stem and never hold it by the bulb and shake it down by quick movement of wrist.
- Do not let the thermometer fall or strike against anything while shaking.
- Never store it in disinfectant solution; rinse it with clean water, dry it, and keep it in containers with the bulb down on a smooth surface.
- Never place the thermometer in the mouth of the person who cannot follow the instructions.

Disinfection of Thermometers (Table 2.1)
Table 2.1: Disinfection of thermometers.

Disinfecting solution	Strength	Time
Dettol	1:40	5 min
Savlon	1:20	5 min
Lizol	1:40	3 min

Celsius and Fahrenheit Scales
Formula used to change from one scale to another:
$F = (C \times 9/5) + 32$
$C = (F - 32) \times 5/9$

Electronic Thermometer (Fig. 2.6)
- It has a battery-powered control unit and a temperature-sensitive probe.
- This type of thermometer readily provides the temperature within <60 seconds.
- Convenient, safe, accurate, and fast method and easy to read; typically, the unit beeps when the measurement is complete.

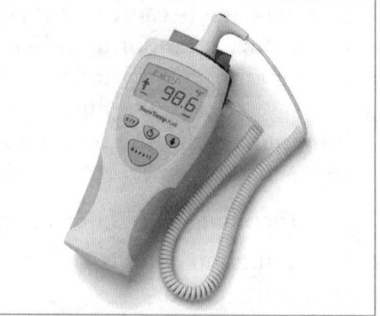

Fig. 2.6: Electronic thermometer.

Tympanic Membrane Thermometer (Fig. 2.7)
- It resembles an otoscope that can be recharged.
- Records temperature by placing a probe in the ear canal.
- It is appropriate for infants over 2 months or very young children; the recording is available in 2 seconds. It should not be used in clients who have ear drainage or scarred tympanic membrane.

Disposable Paper Thermometer (Fig. 2.8)
Single-use paper thermometers are thin strips of chemically treated paper with dots that can change color to reflect temperature in <1 mL available in Celsius and Fahrenheit scales.

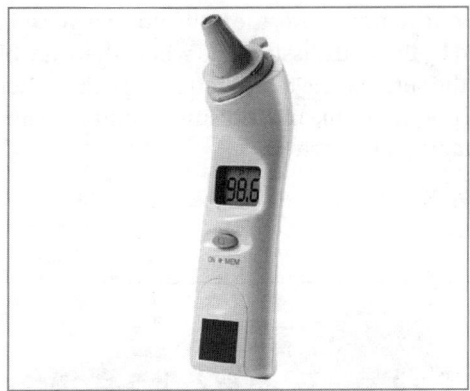

Fig. 2.7: Tympanic membrane thermometer.

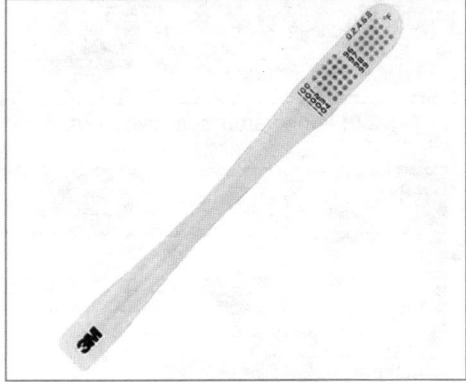

Fig. 2.8: Disposable paper thermometer.

Temperature-Sensitive Strips and Chemical Dot (Fig. 2.9)

They are usually placed on the forehead or abdomen. The skin under the strips must be dry. After the specified time, the strips change the color. The strips are removed and discarded after the color change is noted.

- **Oral digital pacifier thermometer** can be used for infants supralingually; it is ideal for children. The sheath is unbreakable.
- For the visually impaired people, **auditory thermometers** are available. The disadvantages are their high cost and need for regular maintenance.

Common Sites for Assessing Temperature

To get an accurate temperature, the bulb must be placed where it can be surrounded by the body tissues and where there are blood vessels situated near the surface; the temperature may vary when the bulb is in contact with clothing, air, and moisture. Common sites are mouth, axilla, groin, vagina, and rectum.

Temperature by Mouth

See **Fig. 2.10**.

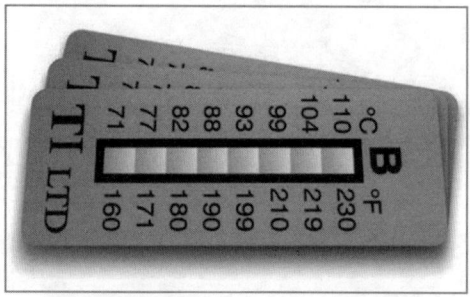

Fig. 2.9: Temperature sensitive strips.

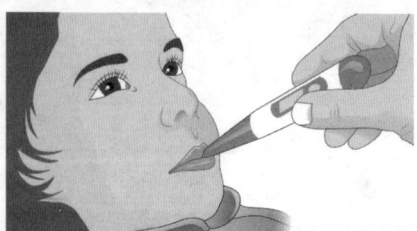

Fig. 2.10: Temperature by mouth (oral temperature).

Contraindications

- Clients who are extremely nervous, delirious, unconscious, hysterical, mentally confused, and who cannot follow instructions.
- Client having convulsions
- Mouth breather
- Injuries, surgeries, and inflammation in mouth
- Extremely weak persons not able to hold a thermometer
- Suffering from severe cough
- Children under 6 years.

Temperature by Axilla (Fig. 2.11)

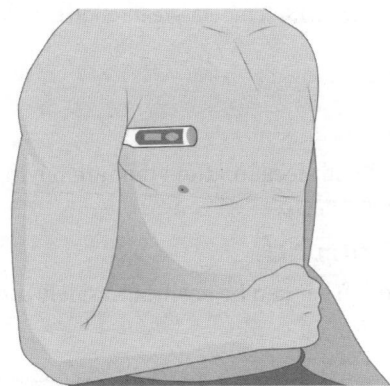

Fig. 2.11: Temperature by axilla.

Temperature by Rectum (Fig. 2.12)

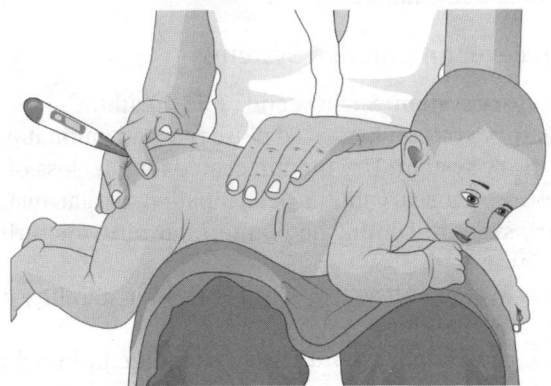

Fig. 2.12: Temperature by rectum.

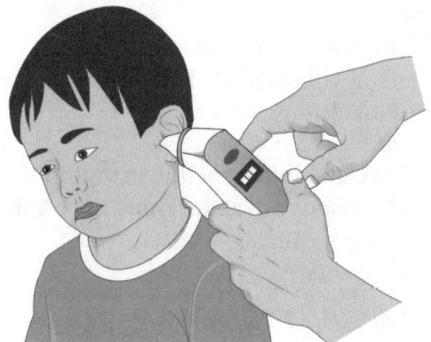

Fig. 2.13: Temperature through ear.

Contraindications
- Rectal surgeries
- Diarrhea
- Rectum packed with fecal matters that are having treatment like bowel wash, enema, etc.

Temperature by Ear (Fig. 2.13)

Temperature through ear can be easily and safely measured.

FEVER

Fever or Pyrexia is defined as a rise in body temperature above 99°F/37.2°C. The causes of fever are infections, diseases of nervous system, malignant neoplasms, blood diseases, exposure to hot environment, dehydration, etc.

Effects of Fever on Different Systems

- **Respiratory system:** Shallow and rapid breathing
- **Circulatory system:** Increased pulse rate and palpitation
- **Alimentary system:** Dry mouth, coated tongue, loss of appetite, indigestion, nausea, vomiting, constipation, or diarrhea
- **Urinary system:** Diminished output, burning micturition high colored urine
- **Nervous system:** Headache, restlessness, irritability, insomnia, convulsions, delirium
- **Muscular skeletal system:** Heavy sweating, hot flushes, goose flush, shivering, or rigors

Types of Fever (Fig. 2.14)

- **Onset or invasion:** It is the period in which the body temperature is rising, and it is a gradual process.
- **Fastigium or stadiums:** It is the period in which the body temperature reaches its maximum and remains constant at a high level.
- **Defervescence or decline:** It is the period in which the temperature is returning to normal.
- **Fevers subside:** Suddenly within few hours, means crisis and gradually means lyses.
- **True crisis:** The temperature falls suddenly by a marked improvement in the patient's condition.
- **False crisis:** Sudden fall in temperature but not accompanied by the improvement in general condition.
- **Lyses:** The temperature falls in a zigzag manner for 2–3 days or a week before reaching normal.
- **Remittent fever:** This is a fever characterized by variations of more than 2° between morning and evening but does not reach normal.
- **Intermittent or quotidian fever:** The temperature rises from normal or subnormal to high fever back at regular interval may vary from few hours to 3 days. Usually, the temperature is higher in the evening than in the morning.
- **Constant fever or continuous fever:** It is one in which the temperature varies not more than 2° between morning and evening and does not reach normal for a period.
- **Inverse fever:** Highest range of fever recorded in the morning and lowest in the evening.
- **Hectic or swinging:** The difference between high and low points is very great.
- **Relapsing fever:** One in which a brief febrile period is followed by 1 or more days of normal temperature.
- **Irregular fever:** It is entirely irregular in its course.
- **Rigor:** It is a sudden attack of shivering in which the body temperature rises rapidly to a stage of hyperpyrexia seen in malaria.
- **Low pyrexia:** Fever does not rise above 99–100°F or between 37.2 and 37.8°C.
- **Moderate pyrexia:** Body temperature rises between 100 and 103°F or between 37.8 and 39.4°C.

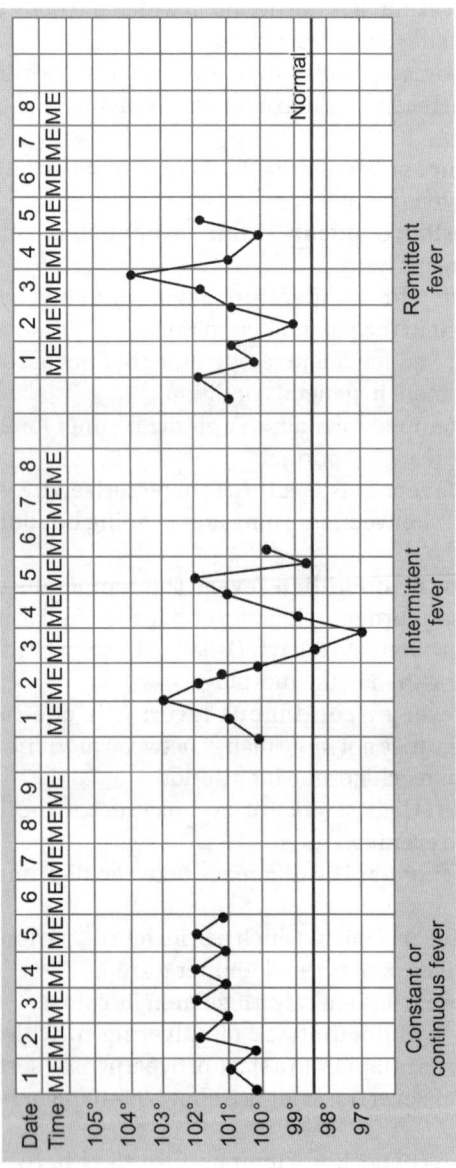

Fig. 2.14: Graphical representation of type of fever.

- **High pyrexia:** Between 103 and 105°F.
- **Hyperpyrexia:** Above 105°F.
- **Subnormal temperature:** When the temperature is below normal (i.e., vary between 95 and 98°F or between 35 and 36.7°C).
- **Hyperthermia:** When temperature is below normal or rises above 105°F or above, it is called hyperthermia.
- **Hypothermia:** Temperature below 95°F or 35°C.

NURSING CARE IN FEVER

Regulation of Body Temperature

- When a client's temperature varies, various methods of reducing the temperature can be started.
- The room should be maintained at a comfortable temperature and well-ventilated.
- Blanket and excess clothing should be removed.
- Exposure to cold by an electric fan, administration of cold drinks.
- Application of cold compress and ice bags, cold sponging, and cold packs.
- Cold bath, ice cold lavages, enema, hypothermic blankets, or mattress should prevent shivering, as it can increases the metabolic activity, produces heat, O_2 use, and increases circulation which can cause hyperventilation and respiratory alkalosis.

Meeting the Nutritional Need

- Metabolism is increased during fever. The O_2 consumption also increases by 13% for each degree Celsius therefore, a high caloric diet is suggested in fever. Since digestive process slows down, it should be easily digestible and palatable fluid food is more preferred.
- Increase the fluid intake to 3,000 mL fluid in 24 hours (if not contraindicated) to prevent dehydration. If nausea or vomiting is present, then IV fluids should be given.
- A small and frequent diet is advisable. It should be served attractively.
- A soft diet and plenty of fluids and fruits are recommended that helps to evacuate bowels regularly.

Providing Rest and Sleep

- Complete bed rest. Provide a calm and quiet environment, without bright lights and glaring places.

- Assist the patient to change position frequently.
- Clothing should be slightly loose, smooth, and nonirritating. Cotton garments are good to absorb sweating and help in evaporation.

Maintenance of Personal Hygiene

- Four hourly care of the mouth is essential to prevent cracked lips and coated tongue.
- Apply emollient to lips to prevent cracking.
- Care of skin and pressure points are essential to prevent bedsore.
- Sponge bath to be done daily.
- If high temperature persists, then cold sponging to be performed to bring down the body temperature.

Safety Factors

- Convulsion and rigor are common in fever, therefore, never leave the patient alone.
- Fever with 103°F for long time leads to delirium and convulsion.
- If high temperature persists the chance of irreversible changes are more in brain cells.
- Antipyretic drugs can be given as per the prescription.
- Sudden cooling should be done gradually as it may leads to cardiac arrhythmias; when temperature is desired to normal level, warm blankets should be provided in order to prevent from hypothermia.
- After any cold application, inspect skin for discoloration or lesions and apply cream or oil to the affected area.

Observation of Client

- Vital signs should be checked periodically.
- Any worsening that happened in the patient's condition, it should be noted and reported.

CARE IN RIGOR

It is characterized by the three stages:
1. **First or cold stage:** Client shivers uncontrollably, skin is cold, face is pitched and pale, pulse is feeble and rapid, and temperature increases to 103°F. In this stage cover with blankets, apply warmth with hot water bag, give warm drinks, and protect from falling.
2. **Hot stage:** Skin feels hot and dry, feels very thirsty, restless, and temperature rises. Remove blanket, cover with a thin blanket, give

cool drinks and cold compress to the head to relieve headache. Temperature is recorded every 10–15 minutes; pulse and respiration are carefully checked. If the temperature goes high (105°F), rapid sponging may be started. Watch for signs of sweating.
3. **Stage of sweating:** Sweating profusely, temperature falls, pulse improves, acute discomfort diminished, client may go to shock if not cared. Given quick sponge to dry up the client. Give sweet drinks to avoid fatigue, let patient sleep, and check TPR every 15 minutes.

PULSE

Pulse is an alteration expansion and recoil of an artery as the wave of blood is forced through it during the contraction of the left ventricle. Pulse can be felt by fingers at a point in which an artery crosses a bone close to the surface of the skin.

When the left ventricle contracts, it forces about 70 mL of blood into the aorta and into the arteries. The walls of the arteries being elastic, expand as an added amount of blood is forced into them. The arteries relax as the wave of blood passes, only to expand again with the next wave of blood. This expansion and recoil of arteries is the pulse and serves as an indication of frequency of heart rate.

Common Sites for Pulse Assessment (Fig. 2.15)

- ❖ **Temporal** superior and lateral to eye
- ❖ **Carotid** between trachea and sternocleidomastoid muscles
- ❖ **Apical** under 4th, 5th, and 8th intercostal space
- ❖ **Brachial** in the antecubital space
- ❖ **Radial** inner part of the elbow on the thumb side of the inner aspect of wrist
- ❖ **Femoral** alongside of inguinal ligament in the groin
- ❖ **Popliteal** best felt on knee flexion at the back of the knee
- ❖ **Posterior tibial** medial surface of ankle
- ❖ **Dorsalis pedis** on dorsum of foot draws imaginary line from middle ankle to the space between toes.

Characteristics of Pulse

Rate

Rate is the number of pulse beats per minute. The average pulse rate of a young adult is 72/min but ranges between 70 and 80/min. Common variations in heart rate may be as follows:

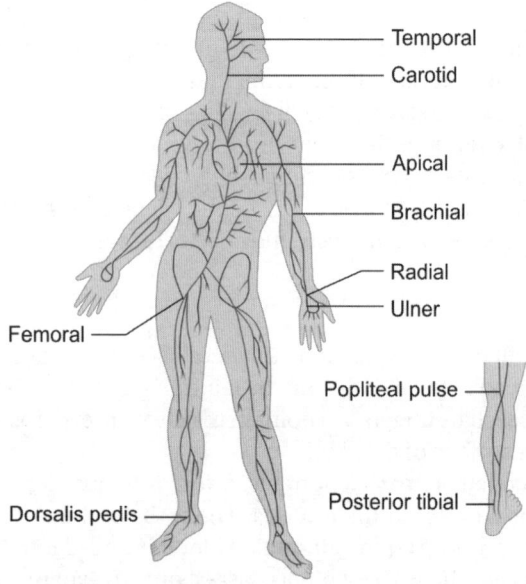

Fig. 2.15: Common sites for pulse assessment.

- **Tachycardia:** Pulse rate above 100 beats/min
- **Bradycardia:** Pulse rate below 60 beats/min.

Factors Causing Variation in Pulse Rate

- **Age:** Pulse rate decreases normally with advancement of age but in old age it decreases more, maybe, due to a weak heart or medication.
  - *Newborn:* 130–140/min
  - *Fetal heart rate:* 140–150/min
  - *Infant:* 115–130/min
  - *2nd year:* 100–115/min
  - *3rd year:* 90–100/min
  - *4–10 years:* 86–90/min
  - *10–adult:* 70–80/min
  - *Old age:* 60–70/min.
- **Sex:** A woman's heartbeat is faster than a man.
- **Exercise:** Short-term exercise increases the heart rate, but long-term exercise strengthens heart muscles causing less or normal heart rate. Rest and sleep decrease heart rate.
- **Pain:** Acute pain increases pulse rate due to sympathetic stimulation and chronic pain decreases pulse rate due to parasympathetic stimulation.

- **Anxiety** increases pulse rate.
- **Medication** like digitalis and atropine increases the heart rate.
- **Hemorrhage** loss of blood increases pulse rate.
- **Position:** Pulse rate is higher in a standing position than in a sitting position than in a lying-down position.

Rhythm

It is the pattern of pulsation and the pause between them. Normally, it is regular, and the pause uniformly occurs. If the beat is missed or is late, the individual has dysrhythmia.
- **Intermittent:** In which the beats miss at regular intervals. In this, if there is difference between apical and radial pulse, it is known as pulse deficit.
- **Extra systole:** When premature contractions are there before normal due time
- **Arterial fibrillation:** Rapid contraction of atrium causing irregular contraction of ventricles in both rhythm and force.
- **Ventricular fibrillation** is rapid twitching of ventricles; it is fatal.
- **Sinus arrhythmia** is a condition in which pulse rate is high during inspiration and slow during expiration.
- **Dicrotic pulse** is one heartbeat and two arterial pulsations giving sensation of a double beat.

Volume/Pulse Aptitude

It refers the future of artery in which reflects the strength of the left ventricular contraction.
- **Water hammer or Corrigan pulse** or collapsing pulse is a full-volume pulse rapidly collapsing due to aortic regulation.
- **Bouncing pulse:** Strong pulsation which does not disappear with moderate pressure as seen in exercise, anemia, hepatic failure, and heart block.
- **Pulsus alternans:** Rhythm is regular but with alternating strong and weak volume seen in ventricular failure, heart block, and digitalis toxicity.
- **Bigeminal pulse** is irregular rhythm in which every other beat comes early. It may be too weak to produce palpable peripheral pulse seen in myocardial infarction (MI) and digitalis toxicity.
- **Weak/wiry/thready pulse** is a small weak pulse that feels like a wire or thread on palpation of arteries signifying decreased stroke volume seen in shock, loss of fluid like diarrhea, and vomiting.

- **Paradoxical pulse:** Pulse volume becomes weak during inspiration.
- **Tension:** It is degree of compressibility; in high tension artery, it is difficult to compress and in low tension it is easy to compress.

Equality

Pulse on both sides should be assessed and compared, the characteristic of each side for equality. Inequality is due to thrombus formation or aorta dissection, etc.

Tension

It is the degree of compressibility. It is said to be high tension when the artery is difficult to compress and low tension when it is easy to compress.

Methods

- **Palpation** is done using the first, second, and third fingers of one hand. Use light pressure at first in order to locate the site afterwards forceful palpation is done to count the rate, rhythm, and quality.
- **Auscultation** of apical pulse requires a stethoscope. It should have snugly fitting earpiece and thick-walled tubing, about 12-inch long, for optimal sound transmission. The stethoscope should have a bell and a diaphragm.
- **Doppler** place transmitter of the devices over artery; sound disturbances are amplified and heard through earpiece or through speaker.

RESPIRATION

Respiration is the act of breathing. It involves two processes (i.e., inspiration and expiration followed by a pause).

Respiration may be external and internal:
- External respiration is the exchange of gases between the blood and the air in the lungs.
- Internal respiration is the exchange of gases between the blood and the tissue cells.

Characteristics of Respiration

It is observed to determine the rate, depth, rhythm, and easiness. Normal breathing is effortless, automatic, and even regular and produces no noise; it is called eupnea.

Rate

Rate is the number of full respirations per minute. Normal rate is from 16-20 minutes and the respiratory rate varies according to few factors:

- **Age:**
  - *At birth:* 30-40/min
  - *1st year:* 20-30/min
  - *2nd year:* 20-26/min
  - *Adolescence:* 20/min
  - *Adult:* 16-24/min
  - *Old age:* 10-24/min
- **Sex:** Females have slightly rapid respiration than men.
- **Emotion:** Increases metabolic rate, increases respiration.
- Changes in environmental temperature increase respiration.
- Ingestion of food and digestion: Increases respiration.
- **Disease condition:** In typhoid, respiratory disorders, and poisoning, respiration increases while in anemia, hemorrhage, brain tumors, analgesics, and sedatives, the respiration decreases.

Depth

- A normal person inspires and exhales about 500 cc of air in each respiration. If more than this, it is deep and less than this means that it is shallow respiration.
- The diaphragm moves about 1 cm down and ribs retract 1.2-1.5 cm.
- Any disease condition that reduces the vital capacity of lungs, interferes the exchange of gas by the blood, and increases the need for oxygen beyond body capacity leads to hyperpnea (deep breathing), polypnea (rapid breathing), and dyspnea (difficult breathing).
- When a person is in dyspnea, sitting position is advisable.

Rhythm

In normal respiration, rhythm is normal.

Variations Abnormal Respiration

- **Tachypnea/polypnea:** Increased breath rate over 24/min.
- **Bradypnea:** Decreased breath rate below 10/min.
- **Apnea:** Total cessation of breathing.
- **Hyperpnea:** Increases in the depth of respiration.
- **Orthopnea:** Can breathe only in upright position.

- **Stertorous respiration:** It is noisy breathing; snoring sounds are produced.
- **Stridor:** A harsh vibrating shrill sound seen in upper airway obstruction laryngitis.
- **Rale:** Abnormal rating or bubbling sound caused by mucus in air passages seen in bronchitis or pneumonia.
- **Wheeze:** The high-pitched or musical whistling sound that occurs with the partial obstruction of smaller bronchi and bronchioles as seen in asthma or emphysema.
- **Sigh:** A very deep inspiration followed by a prolonged expiration; frequent signs are signs of emotional lesion.
- **Air hunger:** A form of dyspnea in which there is deep sighing.
- **Cheyne strokes respiration:** It consists of retries of respiration that gradually become deeper and noisier until a climax is reached; when a pause occurs/apnea, then the cycle is repeated. An increase in rate and depth of respiration alters the rate with a period of apnea.
- **Dyspnea:** Difficult to labored breathing.
- **Cyanosis:** Blueness or discoloration of the skin of oxygen in the tissues.
- **Anoxia/hypoxia** is lack of oxygen in tissue.
- **Anoxemia/hypoxemia** is lack of oxygen in bloodstream.
- **Kussmaul's respiration** is abnormally deep but similar to hyperventilation seen in diabetic ketoacidosis.
- **Orthopnea** is in which a person must sit or stand to breathe comfortably.
- **Blot's respiration** is shallow breathing interrupted by an irregular period of apnea.

What to Observe When Taking Respiration
- Rate of respiration
- Regularity of rhythm
- Easiness movement of muscles
- Position of the client during breathing.

Nursing Care of Client with Breathing Difficulty
- **Psychological support:** A dyspnea client is very anxious and needs to be reassured.
- **Ventilation of the room:** Room should be well-ventilated to supply fresh air to the client.

Vital Signs

- **Ventilation of the lungs:** When the respiratory mechanism fails, it is achieved by artificial respiration.
- Positioning—Fowler's position.
- **Oxygen inhalation:** If the client is cyanosed, it indicates the lack of oxygen and it should be given.
- Clearance of air passage.
- Breathing and coughing exercise.
- Postural drainage.
- Nutrition.

GENERAL INSTRUCTIONS FOR TAKING TPR

Temperature

- Wash hands.
- Thermometer should be disinfected in a proper manner for required time. It should be changed daily.
- Before proceeding, decide the route for taking temperature.
- Before taking oral temperature, check whether the patient had a hot or a cold drink, chewing gum, etc.
- Before placing the thermometer, rinse it in cold water.
- Do not use hot water to rinse.
- Before placing it, wipe it from bulb to stem. After the procedure, wipe it from stem to bulb.
- Bring down the mercury below 35°C before and after the procedure.
- Keep it in between the tissue fold of mouth or axilla or rectum.
- Help the client to retain the thermometer in place.
- In oral temperature, instruct the patient not to bite the thermometer.
- Never leave client alone during procedure.
- Place it in site for sufficient time.
- Read it on edge level and against light.
- Never tell the client his/her temperature; he/she may get alarmed.
- Use a separate thermometer for infectious diseases.
- Never hold it by bulb.
- Do not use an oral thermometer for rectum.
- Record TPR immediately and accurately.

Pulse

- Choose an appropriate site.
- Do not apply much force on artery.

- Before taking, consider the factors that normally affect.
- Encourage the client to relax.
- Count for 1 minute; if only irregularity, count on both sides.

Respiration

- Preferably sitting or lying-down position.
- Keep in a comfortable position.
- Wait for 5–10 minutes if client is active.
- Count the inspiration only.

NURSE'S RESPONSIBILITY FOR THE PROCEDURE

Preliminary Assessment

- Identify patient.
- Check diagnosis, date, and type of surgery done.
- Ability to follow instructions.
- Any contraindications for procedure.
- Previous measurements and range of TPR.

Articles Required

- Savlon 1:40
- Plain water
- Soap solution
- Cotton swab
- Kidney tray/paper bag
- Pen
- Chart
- Watch

Steps of Procedure

Assessing Temperature with Clinical Thermometer (Table 2.2)

- Wash hands
- Explain the procedure
- Assess the site
- Remove the thermometer from antiseptic solution and rinse with cold water
- Wipe it from bulb to stem
- Read the level of mercury in good light by holding with fingers of right hand very slowly.

Vital Signs

❖ Shake the thermometer if mercury level is above 35°C by holding it between the thumb and forefinger at the tip of stem. Shake till the mercury is below 35°C.

Table 2.2: Assessing temperature with clinical thermometer.

Steps	Rationale
Remove thermometer from antiseptic solution and rinse with cold water	To remove disinfectant solution
Wipe thermometer from bulb upwards with rotating movement	To maintain asepsis
Read the level of mercury in good light by holding with fingers of right hand very slowly rotating back and forth until the silvery mercury line comes into view and read measurements	The lines are manifested and visible
Shake if mercury level is above 35°C; shake with quick movements of wrist by holding it by its stem and move away from wall or any equipment	To record temperature correctly
Ask the patient to open his mouth and place thermometer at the base of the tongue/the posterior sublingual pocket. Ask the patient to hold the lips for 2 minutes	Heat from superficial blood vessels
Count the pulse and respirations while the thermometer is still in place	
Remove the thermometer after 2 minutes and wipe it from stem to bulb with cotton swab using rotating movements	To prevent contamination
Read the level of mercury	
For axilla	
Wipe axilla with a towel and keep the thermometer in place for 5 minutes	Friction can increase temperature and moisture can decrease temperature
For rectal	
Place patient in side-lying position; screen to provide privacy. Place a lubricant cotton swab and apply about 2–5 cm from bulb	Lubricant facilitates insertion and causes less injury
Ask the client to take a deep breath and insert it by separating buttocks with the help of gauze piece about half inch into the rectum and in place for 2 minutes	Reduce friction

Contd...

Contd...

Steps	Rationale
Place patient's hands over his chest with the wrist extended and palm downward	To place fingertips above pulse point; arms placed over chest help to count the respiration without patient's knowledge
Holding watch or pulsimeter in left hand, start to count for 1 full minute	To note the pattern of breathing
Continue the palpitation for rhythm and volume, tension, and type of irregularity	To watch the rise and fall of the chest without the patient's knowledge; if he knows, he may hold his breath
Remove it, wipe it from stem to bulb with a clean cotton swab using rotating movements, and discard	To prevent cross infection
Clean with soap solution and rinse with water	To remove microorganism and soap
Read the level and shake it mercury level down and put in disinfected solution	
Aftercare	
Tidy up the unit; take the tray to utility room	Discard the soiled swabs along with paper bag; change disinfected solution as per need
Do not use hot water for thermometer cleansing, put cotton padding under bottles, and replace it with special container	Bottle should be washed with soap and water

Assessing Temperature with Digital Thermometer (Table 2.3)

Table 2.3: Assessing temperature with digital thermometer.

Steps	Rationale
Provide privacy	To ensure the dignity of the client
Adjust clothing of client to expose only axilla	Ensure proper placement of thermometer
Place the end of probe in the axilla	For accurate measurement
Ask client to hold the probe in place until beep is heard and then remove the thermometer and note the reading	For accurate measurement
Clean the thermometer from stem to bulb	To prevent contamination
Document the findings	

BLOOD PRESSURE

Blood pressure is defined as the force exerted by blood against the walls of the blood vessels as it flows through them.

Types of Pressure

- **Systolic pressure:** It is the highest degree of pressure exerted by the blood against the arterial wall during the ventricular systole as the left ventricle contracts and forces the blood from it into the aorta.
- **Diastolic pressure:** It is the lowest degree of pressure when the heart is in its resting period just before contraction of the left ventricle.
- **Pulse pressure:** It is the difference between systolic and diastolic blood pressure. It represents the volume output of the left ventricle.

The normal blood pressure of a healthy adult is 120/80 mm Hg. Hypertension is the condition when the blood pressure is abnormally high. Hypotension is the condition when the blood pressure is abnormally low.

Normal Variations in Blood Pressure

- **Age:** Blood pressure is lower in children comparatively from adults. It increases until 45-50 years of age then it decreases sharply.
- **Sex:** No specific difference between boys and girls until puberty but females have lower BP than males until menopause. After menopause females have high BP than males.
- **Body build:** Overweight person have high BP than person with normal weight.
- **Race:** Some races like Negroes have high BP than other races.
- **Climate:** BP is lower in tropical regions and higher in polar region.
- **Time of day:** BP is lowest early in the morning then reaches to peak by the evening and then it declines.
- **Exercise:** Muscle exertion increases the BP.
- **Pain:** Pain causes increase in BP.
- **Emotion:** Fear, worry, excitement, stress raises the BP.
- **Posture:** BP is lower when lying down as compared to standing or sitting.
- **Disease condition:** Diseases related to circulation, kidney, liver increases the BP and disease of heart muscle lowers the BP.
- **Bleeding:** Bleeding causes low BP as there is blood loss.

Instrument Used for Monitoring Blood Pressure

Sphygmomanometer (Figs. 2.16 to 2.19)

It is standardized instrument which is used to measure blood pressure. The word is derived from the Greek *sphygmus* (pulse) and the scientific (physical) term manometer. It is of three types—mercury, aneroid and digital.

Mercury manometers are accurate and should have no 'zero error' the mercury level should rest at zero before pressure is applied and it should fall freely as cuff pressure is released.

The cuff size should be proper and adequate for accurate reading. If it is narrow, not overlapping it will provide false reading. If cuff size is wide, then it will give low readings.

The width of cuff should be 20% more than diameter of extremity and it should long enough to encircle the extremity.

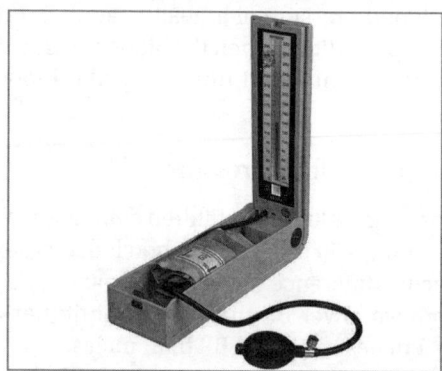

Fig. 2.16: Mercury sphygmomanometer.

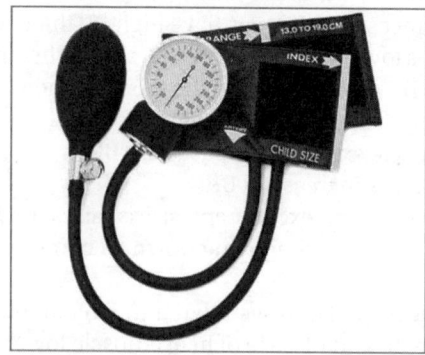

Fig. 2.17: Aneroid sphygmomanometer.

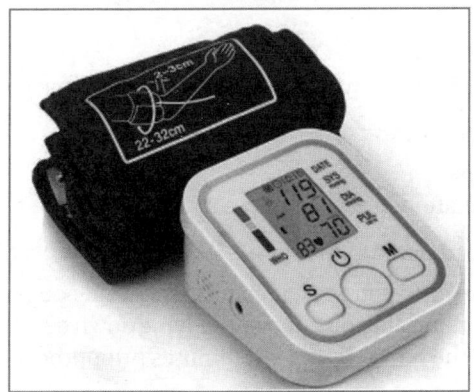

Fig. 2.18: Digital sphygmomanometer.

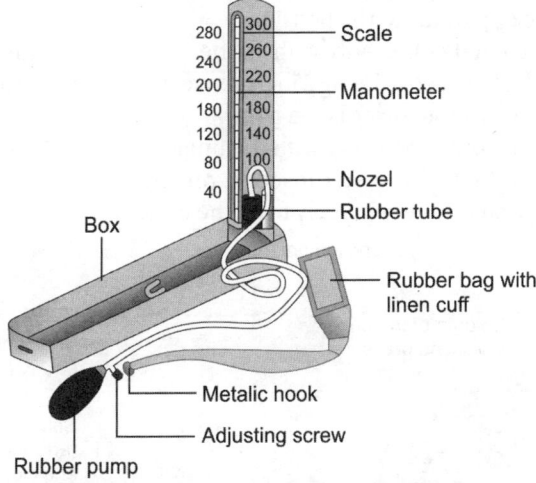

Fig. 2.19: Parts of mercury sphygmomanometer.

Assessment of Blood Pressure

Preliminary Assessment

- Identify the client
- Check diagnosis and reason for BP monitoring
- Previous measurement and range
- Assess the arm on which BP to be monitored

Don'ts of BP Measurements

- Choose the arm with IV cannulation or IV infusion

- Injured/diseased arm
- Arm with fistula
- Arm with same side where female patient had mastectomy.

Preparation of Articles

- Stethoscope
- Sphygmomanometer.

Preparation of Client

- Explain the procedure to gain confidence and cooperation.
- Provide comfortable position either lying down or sitting with arm resting on the bed at least 5–10 minutes prior procedure.

Steps of Procedure (Fig. 2.20)

- Wash hands.
- Take the apparatus to the bedside.
- Apply deflated cuff evenly with rubber bladder over the brachial artery, the lower edge being 2 inch above the antecubital fossa. The two tubes turning towards the palm.
- Palpate the brachial artery with the fingertips.
- Place the bell of the stethoscope on the brachial pulse. The stethoscope must hang freely from the ears.

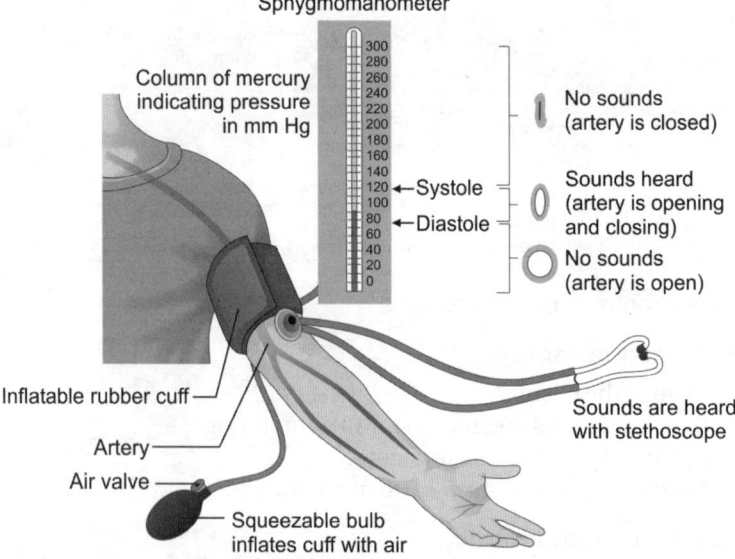

Fig. 2.20: Blood pressure measurement.

- Close the valve on the pump by turning the knob clockwise. Pump up air in the cuff until the sphygmomanometer registers about 20 mm above the point at which the radial pulsation disappears.
- Open the valve slowly by turning the knob anticlockwise. Permit the air to escape very slowly. Note the number on the manometer where the sound first begins. This is the systolic pressure.
- Continue to release the pressure slowly. The sound became louder and clearer. Note the point on the manometer where the sound ceases. This is the diastolic pressure.
- Allow the air to escape and the mercury to fall from zero. Wait for 1 minute with the cuff deflated.

After Care

- Remove the cuff rotate it and replace it
- Assist the patient to cover the arm if exposed
- Place the apparatus to its place
- Wash hands
- Documentation of reading.

Assessment of Blood Pressure: Lower Extremity

- The cuff may be wrapped around the thigh or above the ankle; thigh pressure measurement requires a larger cuff.
- Place the patient in a flat prone or supine position with cuff centered mid-thigh over the popliteal artery.
- Auscultate or palpate blood flow at the popliteal fossa.
- The systolic pressure measured at the thigh is generally 20–30 mm Hg higher than that measured in the arm.
- To measure in the ankle, place the patient in flat supine position and place a stand and arm cuff first above the dorsalis pedis artery as the cuff is deflated (**Fig. 2.21**).

Cuff Size

- The width of the cuff of the bladder should be 40% of the circumference of midpoint of the limb. The length should be 80% of the limb circumference or about twice the bladder width.
- Cuff size according to age is given below:
    - *Under 1 year:* 6 cm and 2.5-3 cm size length
    - *1–4 years:* 15 cm and 5-6 cm
    - *4-8 years:* 15-24 cm and 8-9 cm
    - *8 years and above:* 24-38 cm and 12-18 cm cuff with length.

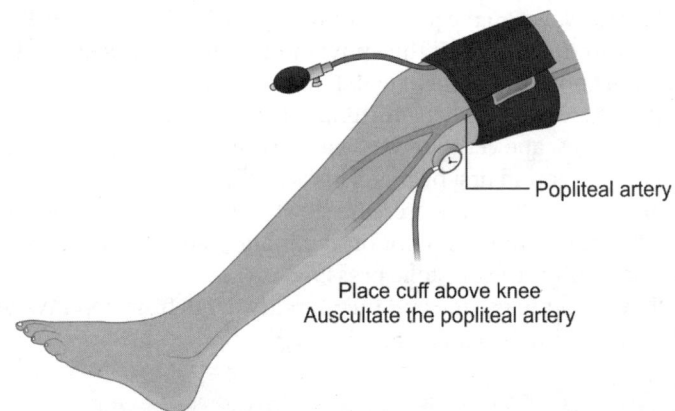

Fig. 2.21: Placement of cuff when taking BP with popliteal artery.

Sources of Error in Blood Pressure Measurement (Table 2.4)

Table 2.4: Common sources of error in BP measurement.

Cause	Effect	Intervention
Manometer		
Losses of mercury	Reading impaired	Have mercury added till "O" mark
Clogged air vent at the top	Mercury column responds sluggishly	Clean or replace air vent
Loose air vent	Mercury column bounces	Tighten cuff
Bladder		
Too narrow	High reading	Determine proper bladder and cuff size
Too wide	Low reading	Determine proper bladder and cuff size
Not centered over artery	High reading	Use proper technique cuff
Cuff		
Applied too loose	High reading	Use proper technique
Too narrow	High reading	Use large adult cuff
Too wide	Low reading	Use pediatric cuff

Contd...

Contd...

Cause	Effect	Intervention
Tubing		
Pressure leaks	Reading impaired	Check for leaks and replace
Stethoscope		
Far tips forward	Auditory impairment, low systolic, high diastolic	Use proper technique
Sensory impairment		
Hearing	Inaccurate reading	Hearing tests, correction of impairment
Sight	Inaccurate reading	Read top of meniscus of mercury column at eye level

Alternate Techniques of Measuring Systolic Pressure

❖ Palpating the pressure
  ♦ It is also known as a sensory detection method.
  ♦ It requires only the use of a sphygmomanometer for the return of the pulse by this method only systolic pressure is recorded.
❖ Doppler ultrasound: It only measures systolic pressure.
❖ Electronic indirect pressure meters.
❖ Transducer device that converts nonelectronic parameters like TPR and BP to electronic parameters.

CHAPTER 3

Pulse Oximetry

INTRODUCTION

Pulse oximeter is used in a variety of settings including critical care units, operation theatres, postanesthesia care unit, diagnosis and treatment area, general nursing unit, and home care settings. A Pulse oximeter is a handheld clip device used to measure one's oxygen saturation. Pulse oximetry is the process of using the device to measure the oxygen saturation. A probe/sensor is attached to the fingertip, forehead, earlobe, or bridge of the nose. A sensor detects changes in oxygen saturation by monitoring light signals generated by the oximeter and reflected by blood pushing through the tissue at the probe.

The normal value of SaO_2 is 95–100%; values <85% indicate that the tissues are not receiving enough oxygen and the patient needs further evaluation. The pulse oximeter sensor slips easily over a patient's finger. The oxygen saturation level appears on the monitor, and it is portable **(Figs. 3.1 to 3.3)**.

DESCRIPTION

Pulse oximetry is a noninvasive method to continuously monitor the oxygen saturation of hemoglobin (SaO_2). It is an effective tool to monitor for subtle or sudden changes in oxygen saturation.

Pulse oximetry became popular during Covid-19 pandemic. People are now well-informed about its usage and its reporting to get medical advice.

A transducer (sensor) that illuminate red and infrared light through tissues when attached to the client's body. A photo detector records the relative amount of each color absorbed by arterial blood and transmits the data to a monitor, which displays the information with each heartbeat.

It also monitors pulse rate and amplitude and can detect changes in the client's oxygenation status within 6 seconds.

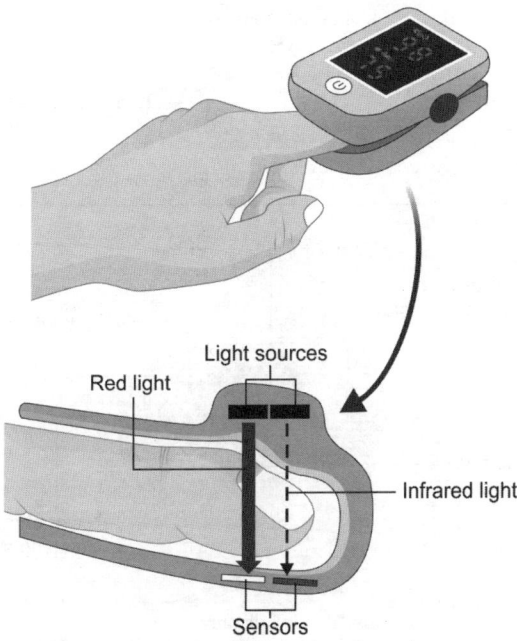

Fig. 3.1: Measuring SpO$_2$ with pulse oximeter.

PURPOSES

- It measures the SpO$_2$.
- It detects the presence of hypoxemia before visible signs develop.
- It assesses client's tolerance to tapering of oxygen therapy or activity.

STEPS OF PROCEDURE

- Explain the procedure to the patient to gain confidence and cooperation.
- Wash hands.
- Select the site to put sensor.
- Remove the nail polish if applied.
- Apply probe securely to the skin and make sure that light emitting sensor and light receiving sensor are aligned opposite to each other to ensure accurate reading.

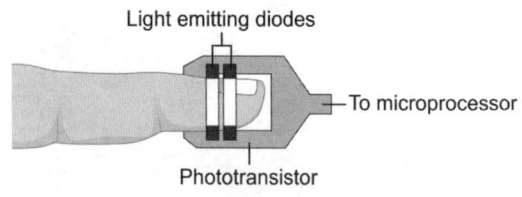

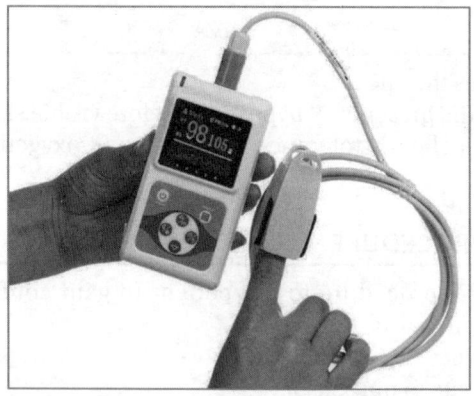

Figs. 3.2A and B: Parts of pulse oximeter.

Fig. 3.3: Measuring of oxygen saturation with pulse oximeter (probe).

- Connect the sensor probe to pulse oximeter.
- Check the saturation levels at regular intervals.
- Remove the sensor and document the reading.

Pulse Oximetry

Nursing Considerations

- If using the ear transducer, attach it to the fleshy parts of the earlobe.
- If using finger transducer, attach it to the client's index finger and keep the finger at heart level.
- Protect the transducer from exposure to strong light.
- Check the transducer site periodically to make sure the device is in place and assess the skin for abrasion and circulatory impairment.
- Rotate the transducer at least every 4 hours to avoid skin irritation.

CHAPTER 4

Hot and Cold Application

INTRODUCTION

Cold and hot are known as physical agents which are used to relieve certain conditions during illness. The procedure of application of cold and heat to body is a part of self-treatment for various kinds of ailments such as headache, muscular aches and boils because they have found it to be effective. But sometimes due to incorrect application of these agents no beneficial effect or harmful effect have been noticed. Heat application results in vasodilation, which lowers blood pressure, and cold application results in vasoconstriction, which raises blood pressure. Depending on each individual's tolerance level, the effects of applying heat or cold may vary from person to person.

DEFINITIONS

Hot application: The term "hot application" refers to the application of a hot agent that is warmer than skin, either in a moist or dry form, to the surface of the body in order to reduce muscle tone, soften exudates, relieve pain and congestion, and provide warmth.

Cold application: The term "cold application" refers to the application of a cold agent that is cooler than skin, either in a moist or dry form, is applied to the surface of the body to relieve pain, lower body temperature, anesthetize an area, stop bleeding, control bacterial growth, prevent gangrene, prevent edema, and reduce inflammation.

CLASSIFICATION OF HOT AND COLD APPLICATION (FIG. 4.1)

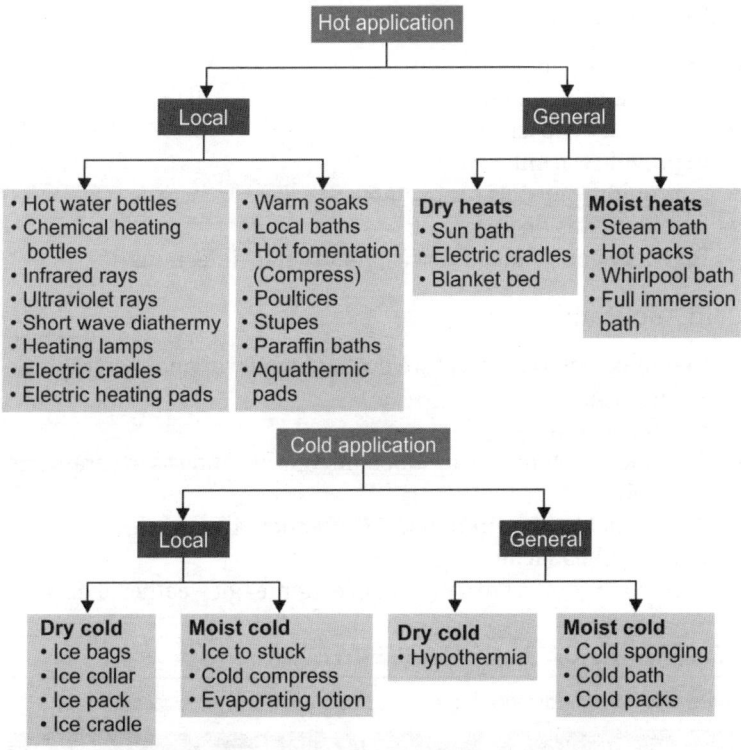

Fig. 4.1: Classification of hot and cold application.

PRINCIPLES OF HOT AND COLD APPLICATION

- ❖ Heat flows from hotter area to lesser hot area.
- ❖ Water is a good conductor of heat.
- ❖ Long-term moisture exposure cause skin vulnerable to maceration and deterioration.
- ❖ Steam increases the temperature in hot application.
- ❖ Tolerance of temperature vary from one person to another.
- ❖ Friction produce heat.
- ❖ Heat transmission can be slowed down by oil's insulating properties.

INDICATIONS

Hot Application

- To decrease pain
- To promote blood flow
- To relax any muscle tension
- To provide warmth
- To promote peristalsis movement
- To relieve tension headache
- To relieve cold, sinusitis or respiratory tract infections.

Cold Application

- To reduce body temperature during high fever and hyperpyrexia or sun stroke.
- To relieve local pain.
- To reduce swelling due to subcutaneous bleeding as in sprain and contusion.
- To control bleeding from nose or after dental extraction.
- To relieve headache.
- To provide comfort to a patient in extreme hot weather, if desired.

CONTRAINDICATIONS (TABLE 4.1)

Table 4.1: Contraindications in hot and cold application.

Hot application	Cold application
- Heart disease	- Stage of shock or collapse
- Kidney and lung disease	- Edema
- Acute inflammation	- Circulatory disorders
- Open wounds	- Infected wound
- Localized malignant tumor	- New wound
- Active hemorrhage	- Feeling of child or low temperature

HOT APPLICATION

Hot Water Bottles/Bag

Purposes

- To relieve pain of the part of the body.
- To relieve distention of abdomen.
- To relieve pain and congestion.

Hot and Cold Application

- To relieve retention of urine.
- To provide warmth to the body.

Articles Required

- Hot water
- Jug/Mug: For pouring water into bag
- Hot water bottle/bag with cover
- Bath thermometer
- Duster
- Towel

Steps of Procedure

- Identify the patient and check for any special instructions.
- Inform the patient about the procedure.
- Wash hands.
- If a private part is to be exposed make arrangement to maintain privacy by putting bed side screen.
- Fill the hot water bottle/bag with hot water at 105–115°F only.
- Use the bath thermometer to measure the temperature.
- Never fill the hot water bottle/bag completely. It should be filled half or two-third of its capacity.
- Expose all air by laying the lower half of the bag on a flat surface and forcing the water up to the neck of the bottle **(Fig. 4.2)**.
- Close the screw and check for any leakage by turning up-side down.
- Dry with towel and put the cover.
- Apply to the part of the body desired.

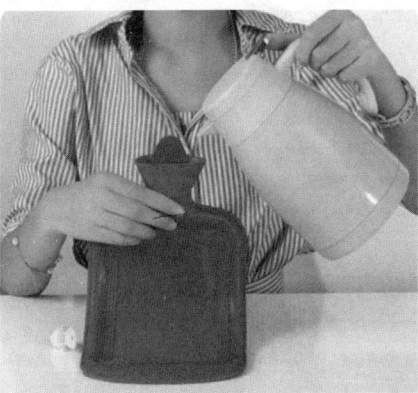

Fig. 4.2: Filling of hot water in hot water bag.

- ❖ Check the temperature at certain interval and refill with hot water intermittently.
- ❖ When the procedure is completed, wash the bottle/bag with soapy water and dry by hanging up-side down. Inflate little air into the bottle before storing.

 Note

> A hot water bottle/bag filled with warm water can be placed inside a quilt, blanket, or sleeping bag to provide overall body warmth and offer additional comfort to a needy patient, especially in extremely cold climates.
> The hot water bottle or bag warms the quilt, blanket or sleeping bag by the process of heat conduction and radiation.

Hot Compress

This is an improvised method of application of heat to a part of body where hot water bottle is not available. Though this is routinely used in houses by common people, it is not an authentic hospital nursing procedure. But still in absence of hot water bottle the procedure can be used by nurse for limited purpose of local application **(Fig. 4.3)**.

Types

- ❖ **Moist warm compress:** In this, warm water is used (e.g., Towel soaked in hot water).

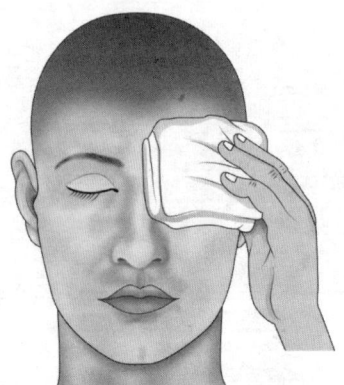

Fig. 4.3: Application of hot compress.

Hot and Cold Application

❖ **Dry warm compress:** In this, dry surface is used to transfer heat (e.g., Gauze exposed to a source of heat like heater, stove etc.).

Articles Required

- **A source of heat:** Heater, stove etc.
- Thickly fold gauze of cotton/towel.

Steps of Procedure

- Identify the patient and check for any special instructions.
- Inform the patient about the procedure.
- Wash hands.
- Make the arrangement of heat near the patient.
- Hold the folded thick gauze or compressed cotton in your right hand.
- Warm the compress bringing nearer to source of heat.
- Take care that it does not catch fire. The distance should be maintained.
- Now bring it back from source of heat and test the temperature by back side of palm of your hand to a tolerable limit.
- If it is hotter, wait a little for its cooling down.
- Now apply over the desired part of body of the patient.
- Repeat the procedure again and again to have desired effect.

General Guidelines for Application of Heat to the Body

- Make sure that the patient has no paralysis, numbness, or loss of sensation or poor circulation, which are absolute contraindications for application of heat.
- Explain procedure to obtain cooperation from patient and his attendants.
- Position the patient comfortably before starting the procedure.
- If fomentation is going to be used repeatedly cut or fold the cloth to fit the body part like the arm or foot, so that air is not allowed to circulate freely and cool the part.
- If the area that is being treated is infected, be careful to observe the necessary precautions to protect the uninfected area and dispose the soiled dressing or fomentation in hygienic way.
- Carry out the procedure quickly including covering the fomentation in order to retain the heat of the application.
- Discontinue hot application if the skin becomes red or mottled or if any rashes appear.

- Any affected area treated with heat application should be kept covered so as to retain the benefit of procedure.
- If heat is applied to a particular area for repeated time, oil or cream should be applied to keep the skin in proper condition.
- Babies or heart patients should not be given hot applications at temperature more than 115–120°F because of impaired circulation.
- Always ensure that the hot water bottle is properly wrapped before application.

Electric Heating Pads

Nowadays in certain places electric pads are used as a method of application of heat in place of hot water bottle. This is suitable for application of heat to a particular part of area of the body.

- An electric coil is enclosed in a waterproof rubber covering in electric heating pads, which also have a heat control switch to keep the temperature where it should be.
- As the current flows in constant voltage, the heat liberated by the electric pad maintains constant temperature so electric pad is a convenient method for providing evenly released heat to a part of body **(Fig. 4.4)**.
- Electric pads should not be used for comatose patient or a patient while he is in sleep. This should also never be used over moist area.
- Before handling the electric pad, it should be properly checked by a tester for any leakage or short circuit.
- Patient should be told about the electrical procedure you are going to apply on his body.

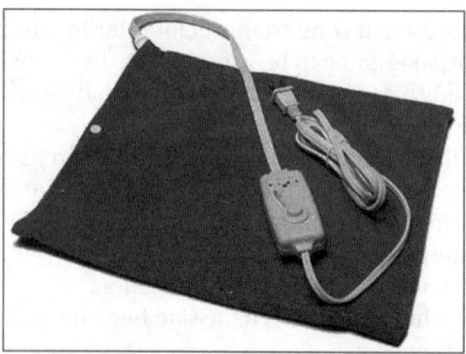

Fig. 4.4: Electrical heating pads.

Electric Cradles/Heat Cradles

- ❖ Electric cradles are used when a large portion of the body must be treated and a gown or sheets cannot be used to cover the skin.
- ❖ A special heat is mounted inside a bed cradle to provide heat.
- ❖ Electric cradles can be applied for a duration of 20-30 minutes **(Fig. 4.5)**.
- ❖ Sheet and blanket can be used to maintain the heat at a desire levels.
- ❖ Monitor the patient closely to prevent burns.

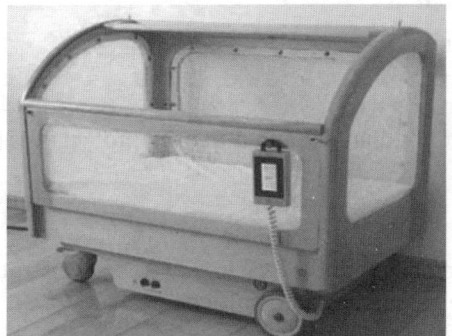

Fig. 4.5: Electric cradle.

Infrared Lamp/Infrared Rays (Fig. 4.6)

The infrared lamp is an electrical lamp which remits infrared rays. These rays are invisible rays of spectrum used for therapeutic purpose

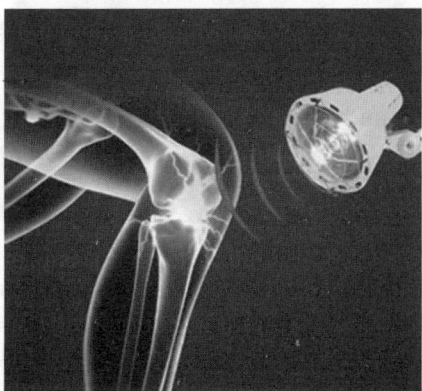

Fig. 4.6: Infrared lamp.

on patients for production of heat in tissue. The heat penetration length to tissue is about 3 mm.

Purposes

- Promote healing in bed sores.
- Relieve spasm and pain.
- It softens the connective tissue.
- Useful for drying casts.
- Use for muscle stiffness and backache.

Articles Required

- Infrared lamp
- Inch tape
- Top sheet
- Goggles for both patient and nurse: To protect eyes from infrared rays.

Steps of Procedure

- Identify the patient and check for any special instructions.
- Inform the patient about the procedure.
- Wash hands.
- Keep the patient in comfortable position.
- Keep the infrared lamp on a stool.
- Switch on the lamp.
- Expose the part to be treated.
- Keep a distance of about 18–24 inches from patient.
- The application can be continued up to 30 minutes or less.
- Caution the patient not to touch the lamp or reduce the distance.
- Lesser distance may cause burns over the skin.
- Record in detail about the procedure in chart with duration of exposure, time and date, etc.
- If used for drying casts the duration of application depends on size of cast and climatic condition.

Medical Fomentation

It may be simple when only boiled water is used for fomentation and medicated when drug is added to boiled water for fomentation. The word medicated fomentation means it is applied to unbroken skin.

Hot and Cold Application

Guidelines for Application

- The areas of application should be a larger area when applied to relieve pain and congestion in adjoining parts of internal organs.
- Whole of the back and sides of axilla are covered to relieve congestion of kidney.
- For joint stiffness or inflammation the whole of joint and some areas above and below the joint are covered.
- In case of pain in stomach area, the area of application is from xiphisternum to umbilicus and both sides of abdomen.
- For fomentation over breast, never foment the nipple. Cut a hole in the cloth to spare nipple protruding out.

Purposes

- To promote suppuration.
- To increase circulation.
- To relieve pain.
- To relieve swelling.
- To relieve congestion.

Articles Required

- Container for heating water.
- A source of heat or fire.
- A bowl or other container for moistening the cloth or dressing.
- Small cloth or dressing or flannel cloth if available.
- Large cloth or towel for wringing the small cloth.
- A large piece of mackintosh.
- A binder or bandage.
- Vaseline to prevent tender areas from burning.

Steps of Procedure

- Identify the patient.
- Explain the procedure to the patient.
- Wash hands.
- Put the patient in comfortable position.
- Uncover the body surface to be fomented.
- Put a bed side screen, if privacy is required.
- Apply Vaseline to the area.
- Place a small cloth or dressing or flannel or large cloth and roll them together.

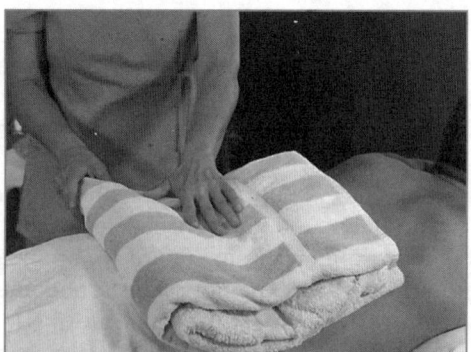

Fig. 4.7: Application of medical fomentation.

- Put the cloth in bowl or in other container and pour hot water over them while they are covered.
- Lift them out of the water and wiring them thoroughly.
- Remove the small cloth or dressing from the large cloth and shake out the steam to cool them.
- Take the temperature quickly on the back of your hand or arm.
- Apply fomentation to the affected area and if it is too warm for the patient, leave it to cool, then re-apply **(Fig. 4.7)**.
- Foment the area with either plastic or rubber in order to retain as much heat as possible.
- Bandage the area lightly to keep the fomentation in place.
- Change fomentation when it becomes cold, usually in about 20 minutes.
- Dry the area well after the fomentation has been removed and cover the area with warm cloth to prevent chilling.
- Repeat the procedure every 2, 3, or 4 hours.
- Record the procedure in chart.

Surgical Fomentation

This is a fomentation to broken part of skin like over an open wound.

Purposes

- To accelerate the process of suppuration.
- To promote better drainage.
- To reduce swelling and congestion.
- To relieve pain and muscle spasm.

Hot and Cold Application

Articles Required

- Bowl or basin.
- Solution or medicated water at 125–150°F or 51.5°C.
- Square gauze slightly bigger to the area of application.
- Two forceps.
- Mackintosh sheet.
- Towel.
- Large cloth or wringer towel.
- Bath thermometer.
- Dressing or cotton pad.

Steps of Procedure

- Wash hands.
- Collect and put all items at bed side.
- Identify the patient.
- Explain the procedure to the patient.
- Put a bed side screen for privacy.
- Put the patient in comfortable position.
- Protect the bed by spreading mackintosh.
- Place the small cloth or wringer or towel on large cloth.
- Place the cloth in a pan or container. Ensure that the ends of outer large cloths extend over the edge of the pan.
- Boil the water or solution with cloth inside.
- Remove the cloth from the pan or container making sure that the inner cloths are completely covered by outer cloth.
- Lift them up out of the water solution and wiring them out thoroughly.
- Scrub your hand thoroughly and then pick up the inner cloths by holding them by the corner.
- Shake out the steam and gently apply fomentation to the wound.
- If the heat is not tolerable, lift it up by the corner for a while then replace being careful not to touch the rest of the compress.
- Change the fomentation when it becomes cold.
- Dry the area well. Usually after 10–20-minute fomentation may be removed.
- Repeat the treatment according to the need (every 2, 3, or 4 hourly).
- Air dry the wound and reapply the sterile dressings after fomentation has been removed.
- Record the procedure in chart.

Sterile Soak

This is a type of application of moist heat over skin surface by immersing the part specially an extremity in hot water or medicated solution.

Purposes

- To apply moist heat or medicated solution to an extremity.
- To promote drainage.
- To apply medication in skin disease.
- To reduce swelling.
- To increase blood circulation to aid prevention of infection and to arrest inflammation.
- To prevent cold injury like chilblain or frostbite in extremity by process of increase in circulation.

Articles Required

- Container or basin.
- Immersion solution—plain water, boric acid, magnesium sulphate, Candy's solution 1: 5,000.
- Bath thermometer.
- Mackintosh.
- Towel.
- Sterile dressing and bandage.

Steps of Procedure

- Wash hands.
- Identify the patient and check if special instructions is required.
- Explain the procedure to the patient.
- Put the patient in comfortable position, usually a sitting position as limbs are commonly immersed.
- Boil the solution in container by putting a lid over it.
- Allow the solution/water to cool to the temperature of 110°F (43.3°C).
- If a bath thermometer or lotion thermometer is not available, the warmth of the water or solution can be approximately assessed by sprinkling over inner aspect of lower arm to test it.
- Assist the patient to immerse the part in hot water.
- Keep the affected part for 20–25 minutes.
- Add some hot water every 5–10 minutes to the container in which body part has been immersed and stir to keep the temperature

at a constant level. But first lift the affected part out of water and then add otherwise you may cause burn as you are adding more hot water.
- Dry the affected part thoroughly after the treatment has been completed.
- Apply some sweet oil or cream to the part and cover it.
- Instruct the patient to keep the part warm.
- Repeat the procedure if ordered.
- Record the procedure in chart.

Sitz Bath

This is a method of applying moist heat to a patient especially to pelvic area.

Purposes

- To relieve pelvic congestion.
- To promote drainage of rectal- or perianal abscess or furuncle.
- After surgery of anal fissure and fistula or piles.
- To relieve pelvic pain.
- To promote relaxation of bladder in case of retention of urine.
- To relieve perianal pruritus when advised.

Articles Required

- Tub with warm water (temp 99–102°F/37–39°C).
- Bath thermometer.
- Extra-arrangements for providing hot water.
- Ice bag and ice.
- Bath towel and blanket.
- Jug.

Steps of Procedure

- Wash hands.
- Identify the patient and check if special instructions is required.
- Assess the patient's condition, pain level, and the ability to ambulate to the bathroom.
- Inform the patient about the procedure.
- Maintain privacy by putting a bed side screen.
- Alternately, the patient can have sitz bath in bathroom.
- Fill the basin with warm water at a temperature of 99–102°F (37–39°C).
- Check the temperature using bath thermometer.

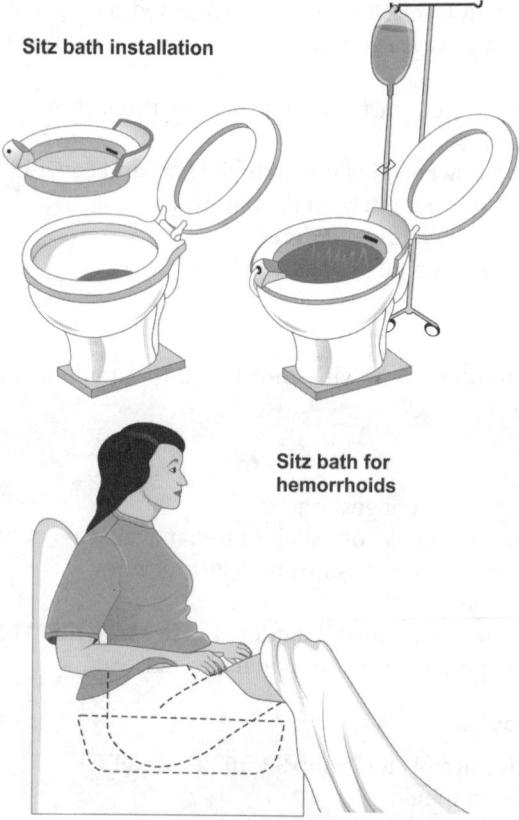

Fig. 4.8: Sitz bath.

- Keep the basin on a low stool/potty chair/toilet bowl with toilet seat up **(Fig. 4.8)**.
- Assist the patient with removal of any dressings or Peri-Pad and position and assist to sit in sitz bath basin.
- Place a towel on the patient's thigh and cover the shoulders with a sheet.
- Be with the patient till the procedure is complete.
- Instruct the patient to contact and relax the anal sphincter while taking sitz bath.
- Continue the procedure for 15–20 minutes. The duration of the bath can vary according to the patient condition.
- Assist the patient in drying and applying dressing or peripad as required.

- ❖ Assist the patient in taking comfortable position in bed and instruct to stay in bed for 20 minutes with hip elevated.
- ❖ Record the procedure.

Note

Sitz bath is done for 3–5 minutes for relief of pelvic inflammation and retention of urine and for 15–20 minutes for hemorrhoids.

COLD APPLICATION

Cold Compress

Applying a moist cold to a body part is known as a cold compress.

Purpose

- ❖ To reduce body temperature in fever.
- ❖ To relieve pain.
- ❖ To reduce inflammation.
- ❖ For treatment of sprain, bleeding from nose (epistaxis), contusion over eye by blunt injury (black eye) and abrasions.

Articles Required

- ❖ Bowl of ice-cold water (15°C/59°F).
- ❖ Cold compress: Folded lint or gauze, ice bags, gel based ice packs, cold packs.
- ❖ Mackintosh.
- ❖ Towel.

Steps of Procedure

- ❖ Identify the patient and check physician's order.
- ❖ Explain procedure to the patient.
- ❖ Wash hands.
- ❖ Put the patient in comfortable position to expose the area of application.
- ❖ Uncover the area to be treated or compressed.
- ❖ Living out the clothing thoroughly to avoid dripping of water over clothing or bedding.
- ❖ If a private part to be compressed place a bed size screen.
- ❖ Soak the compress: Thick gauze pad in cold water and apply to the area.

- ❖ If the water is very cold (i.e. ice water pour some tap water to bring temperature to a tolerable limit).
- ❖ Repeated compress at every few minutes by dipping in cold water.
- ❖ Continue applying for 15–20 minutes.
- ❖ Keep a constant watch on the color of the skin where cold is applied. Test the skin for numbness which warns for stoppage of application.
- ❖ Record the treatment in chart.

Ice Cap/Ice Bags (4.9)

Ice cap is a local dry application. In this, rubber bag is filled with small pieces of ice and salt to a specific body part. As the ice is kept in a rubber cap; the effect of cold persists without soiling or wetting the skin.

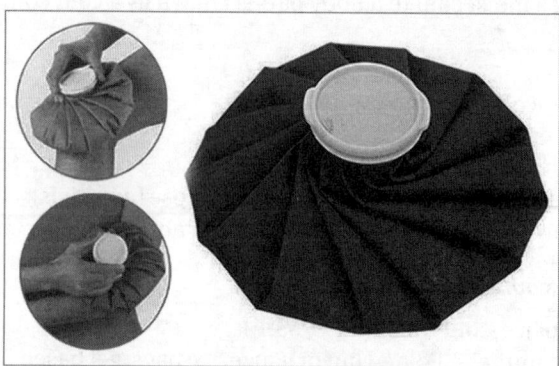

Fig. 4.9: Application of ice cap.

Purpose

- ❖ To check suppuration.
- ❖ To control bleeding.
- ❖ To reduce swelling.
- ❖ To relieve headache.
- ❖ To relieve local pain.
- ❖ To prevent cerebral congestion.

Articles Required

- ❖ Bowl with small pieces of ice.
- ❖ Ice cap or collar with cover.
- ❖ Ice pick or holder.
- ❖ Hand towel.
- ❖ Common salt.

- ❖ Duster to wipe ice cap.
- ❖ Teaspoon.
- ❖ Mackintosh.
- ❖ Kidney tray.

Steps of Procedure

- ❖ Identify the patient and check for any special instructions.
- ❖ Inform the patient about the procedure.
- ❖ Put bed side screen, if privacy is required.
- ❖ Wash hands.
- ❖ Break the ice into small pieces to go into the mouth of ice cap. Do not make very small pieces.
- ❖ Put ice in ice cap and add salt. Addition of salt prevents quick melting.
- ❖ Cap should be filled half and screw the cap.
- ❖ Dry the cap with duster or towel. Check for any leakage.
- ❖ Put a cloth over ice cap for wrapping.
- ❖ Now apply ice cap to the affected area.
- ❖ Apply about 30 minutes.
- ❖ Observe for any change of color of skin or numbness which will call for discontinuation of cold application.
- ❖ Record the procedure.

Tepid Sponging

Tepid sponging is a general application of moist cold liquid to the skin to reduce body temperature. Temperature of water for tepid sponging: 102–103°F.

Purposes

- ❖ To reduce body temperature.
- ❖ To stimulate blood circulation and respiratory movement.
- ❖ To stimulate excretion through kidney and skin.
- ❖ To decrease toxicity in case of toxemia due to some cause.
- ❖ To quite nervous and delirious patient.

Articles Required

- ❖ Wash basin.
- ❖ Bath thermometer.
- ❖ Tepid water (102–103°F)
- ❖ Large rubber mackintosh to cover whole length of bed.
- ❖ Bath towel.

- Draw sheet and bath blanket.
- Wash clothes.
- **Articles for cold compress:** Basin with ice pieces, ice cap with cover.
- Bucket for collection of waste water.
- Clinical thermometer.
- Cold drink in a feeding cup.

Steps of Procedure

- Identify the patient and check for any special instructions.
- Inform the patient about the procedure.
- Collect all materials at bed side table.
- Take patient's temperature before starting the procedure and note it.
- Fan fold top cover to the foot of bed replacing with bath blanket.
- Place rubber sheet and draw sheet under patient to cover entire mattress.
- Remove patient's clothing from body.
- Place ice cap to patient's head.
- Bath the face first and dry with towel.
- Expose upper half of the body.
- Place a cool moist cloth over axilla and groin so as to cover the large superficial vessels. This will further help in lowering the body temperature.
- Change the water when it is warm by discarding in bucket and reapply sponges and groin as needed.
- Use a downward motion. Sponge arm and neck for 3–5 minutes. The back, front and buttock should be sponged for 5–10 minute.
- Do not wipe and dry with towel. Let the water stick and evaporate by itself. Evaporation causes cooling. This is required to cool body temperature.
- Likewise sponge lower extremity for 3–5 minutes.
- While sponging one, cover other half of the body. Do not expose the whole body at a time.
- Reassess temperature and pulse every 15 minutes.
- After sponging of whole body is completed, dry the patient by putting the towel and not by rubbing it.
- Put on dress or gown to the patient.
- Remove draw sheet, mackintosh, replace top cover, remove bath blanket.
- Leave ice cap for half an hour.

- ❖ The entire sponging should take 15–20 minutes depending on temperature of body cooling and patients' tolerance or comfort.
- ❖ Record the procedure in chart.
- ❖ Intimate if any abnormality in body temperature to the attending physician.

Cold Pack (Wet Sheet Pack)

Cold pack is defined as application of moist cold using wet sheet when temperature rises to 104°F or more **(Fig. 4.10)**.

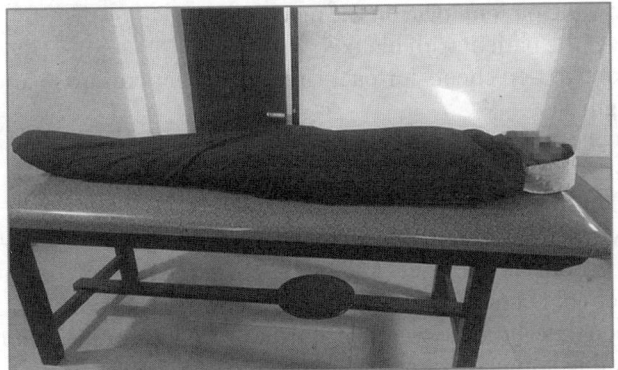

Fig. 4.10: Covering patient with wet sheet/blanket.

Purposes

- ❖ To calm an irritable and restless patient.
- ❖ To improve blood circulation and reduce pulse.
- ❖ To bring down body temperature.

Articles Required

- ❖ Tub or big basin with cold water at 65°F or 18.3°C temperature.
- ❖ Bath thermometer.
- ❖ Large wringer or two cotton sheets for pack.
- ❖ Bed side screen.
- ❖ One big mackintosh.
- ❖ Two blankets.
- ❖ Hot water bottle.
- ❖ One tray.
- ❖ Bottle of spirit.
- ❖ Bowl of extra-piece of ice.

- Ice cap.
- Feeding cup.
- Towel.
- Clinical thermometer.

Steps of Procedure

- Identify the patient and check for any special instructions.
- Explain the patient about the procedure.
- Put bed side screen.
- Put the mackintosh on the bed.
- Allow the patient to lie on the mackintosh.
- Cover the patient with blanket.
- Take two bed sheets for pack, fold one sheet crosswise and one length wise.
- Put bed sheet in tub of cold water.
- Roll patient on one side and place bed sheet folded crosswise under patient.
- Cover patient with bath blanket.
- Wiring out second sheet and place it over the front of the patient.
- Place cold compress on the head.
- When sheet becomes warm repeat the procedure for 15–20 minutes.
- Dry the patient by wiping with towel.
- Apply pack with spirit, rub and then apply powder.
- Observe for any symptom of chill or any other abnormality.
- Take temperature of the patient.
- Record the procedure in chart.

General Guidelines for Application of Cold to the Body

- Make sure that the patient who is going for the cold treatment or his attendants or relatives come to know what you are going to do so that they will assist and cooperate in your procedure.
- Have the patient assume a comfortable position.
- Maintain privacy to patient.
- If the compress is to be used repeatedly cut or fold the cloth to fit to the part like eye, ankle or wrist if locally applied.
- Apply cold compress without any covering to allow for better evaporation and better cooling.
- Cold compress must be repeated every few hours for more effectiveness or take advice of an attending doctor.

- Apply cold compress to the body or part when the part is not badly injured or where there is good blood circulation without any loss of sensation otherwise it will harm the part.
- Stop cold compress or application at area if the skin becomes blue or mottled or if numbness develops.

CHAPTER 5

Care of Articles

INTRODUCTION

Patient care equipment's and articles must be clean before and after use. Cleaning of equipment and items is an important part of health since it improves the quality of healthcare and health services. Articles must be kept clean and in good condition at all times to ensure a long and functioning life while also providing a safe and hygienic service to patients and staffs.

PURPOSES OF CLEANING

- To prevent the spread of micro-organism.
- To remove dust, dirt and bad odors.
- To maintain a clean hospital environment.
- To prolong the life of articles and equipments.
- To maintain the standard of nursing care.

ENAMEL WARE (FIG. 5.1)

Bedpans

- Before emptying the bedpan, inspect the contents.
- Remove any cotton sponges with forceps, if they are present.
- The contents of the bedpan must be emptied in the lavatory pan.
- Ensure that the side of the basin are not soiled.
- Rinse the bedpan vigorosly with water.
- Clean the bedpan with brush, soap and water.
- To disinfect the bedpan, soak it in Lysol 1:40 for 1 hour.
- Place the bed pan under the sun to deodorize and disinfect.
- Keep it dry and store them in bedpan rack.

Urinals

- Cleaning and disinfection of urinals are done in the same way as bedpans.
- Urine kept in the urinals should be discarded after a short period of time to prevent formation of any deposit inside the bedpan.

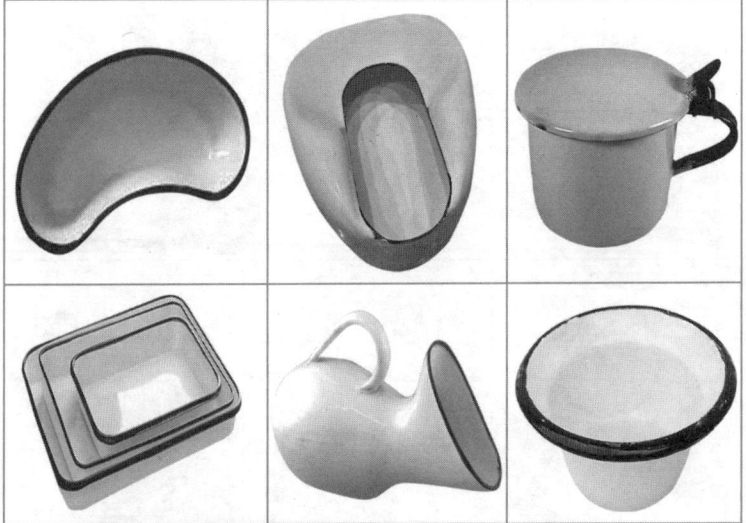

Fig. 5.1: Hospital enamel ware.

Trays and Kidney Trays

The process of cleaning and disinfection are carried out in the same manner as bedpans.

Sputum Cups

- Infectious sputum such as sputum of tuberculosis patient must be disinfected with chemicals or may be disposed by burning.
- Noninfectious sputum may be discarded into the lavatory pan.
- Ensure that the sides of the pan are not soiled.
- Cleaning and disinfection of the sputum cup is carried out in the same manner as bedpans.
- To prevent sputum from sticking to the sides of the sputum cups, a small amount of antiseptic lotion is added into the sputum cups before giving it to the patient.

RUBBER WARE (FIG. 5.2)

Mackintosh

- Spread the mackintosh on a table or flat surface.
- Wet the mackintosh with water.
- Rub the macintosh with soap and water on both surfaces using a clean cloth or towel.

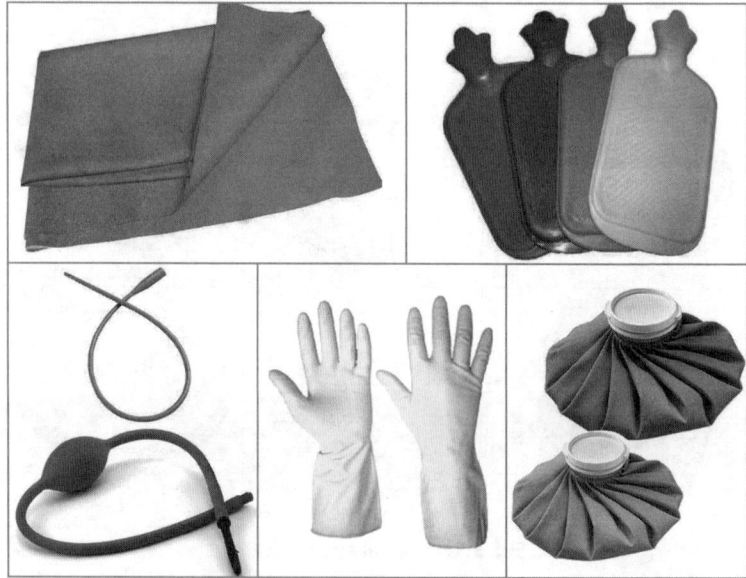

Fig. 5.2: Rubber ware use in hospital.

- Rinse the mackintosh under running water.
- Use appropriate methods to remove stains if present.
- Use Dettol or Lysol 1:40 for disinfection process.
- To dry them, hang them from a horizontal cylindrical pole in the shade. Spread them out smoothly without wrinkles.
- Sprinkle chalk powder when it is dried completely.
- When storing, ensure that the mackintosh is either flat or rolled. Do not fold the mackintosh.
- If two or more mackintosh are keep together, the surface of the mackintosh should be separated by old linen or paper. Store the mackintosh in a cool and dark place and in airtight containers.

Gloves

- Before removing the gloves from hands, wash the gloves on the hands to prevent adherence of blood and other organic materials.
- Wash the gloves with soap and cold water after removing from the hands. Wash the outside first, then invert and repeat on the inside.
- Rinse the inside and outside of the gloves with water.

- Submerge the glove filled with air in the water, if bubbles pass up through the water, it indicates that holes are present. Separate torn gloves.
- Hang the gloves to dry. When the outside is dried, then turn inside out and dry.
- Once the gloves are dried on both sides, they are powdered inside and outside and packed in pairs of the same size, right and left gloves in glove wrapper. Keep a small lump of gloves powder in a gauze mesh for powdering the hands and is kept in the cuff of the gloves.
- Autoclaving is considered the best method for sterilizing gloves.

Rubber Tubes

- Rubber tubes incudes catheters, rectal tubes, flatus tubes, Ryle's tubes, and infusion sets.
    - After using rubber tubes, wash them under running water by holding the eye upwards and allowing the water to run.
    - Lodged a small quantity of organic matter at the eye end and remove them using a swab stick.
    - Clean them with soap and warm water to remove the dirt and grease.
    - Wash them again with running water.
    - Put the tubes in boiling water and let them boil for 5 minutes.
    - Dry the rubber tubes by hanging.
    - After the rubber tubes are dried, powder and store them in airtight containers lengthwise.
    - Reboil or autoclave the rubber tubes before using.
    - Catheter that are easily destroyed by heat and moisture are disinfected using formalin tablets.
    - Hard rubber tubes that are used in medicating the body cavities are disinfected with chemicals in order to maintain the original shapes of the tips.

Air Cushion, Hot Water Bag, Ice Caps

- *Air cushion and airbeds:*
    - Do not pour water into air cushion and airbeds for cleaning.
    - Cleaning only the outside is sufficient.
    - They should not be filled with air during cleaning as it has the tendency to crack or weaken.
    - The valves of the air cushions or beds should never be immersed in water as it spoils them.

- The covers of the air cushion are disinfected and sent to laundry for washing.
- Cleaning and storing are done in the same manner as rubber goods except that they should be slightly inflated to prevent the two surfaces to come in contact with each other.

❖ **Hot water bottles, ice caps and ice collars:**
  - Empty the contents immediately after use.
  - Wash and dry in the same manner as rubber goods.
  - Hang the bags upside down to drain the water.
  - Ice bags are dried with a piece of cloth as they cannot be hung.
  - After the bags are completely dry, inflate them with air.
  - The covers are disinfected and sent to the laundry for washing.

STAINLESS STEEL AND SHARP INSTRUMENTS (FIG. 5.3)

Sharp Instruments

❖ Wash the instrument in running water after use.
❖ Immerse the sharp instrument is 0.5 chlorine for 10–20 minutes and send for sterilization.
❖ Sterilization is done by hot air sterilizer exposing them at a temperature of 160°C for 1 hour.

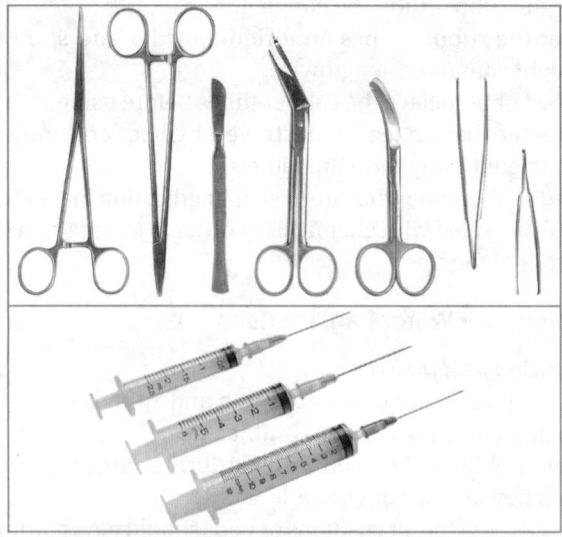

Fig. 5.3: Stainless steel and sharp instruments.

Syringe and Needles

- Syringe must be rinse immediately after use to prevent the pistons sticking to the barrels.
- If syringe is stuck, it may be placed in 25% aqueous solution of glycerin and boiled for 10 minutes or soaked in weak solution of nitric acid to separate the parts.
- If needle is stuck to the hub of the syringe, immerse it in boiling water to make the metal expand and separate them.
- The barrels and piston of the same number should be kept together for easy matching of the parts.
- Sterilization of syringe is done by hot air method of sterilization.
- After use cold water is forced through the needle with a syringe followed by detergent solution.
- Then, wash it with warm water.
- Decontaminate the syringe by flushing it with 0.5% chloride solution.
- Identify presence of hooks using a magnifying glass or drawing the point over the skin. If a hook is present, destroy the needle using needle destructor and throw it in puncture proof container.
- Sterilize the needle by boiling them for 10–20 minutes or by dry heat at a high temperature or autoclaving.

GLASSWARE (FIG. 5.4)

- Rinse the glassware immediately under cold running water to remove organic matter from the glass articles.
- Glassware used for parenteral therapy should be rinsed with freshly distilled water.
- If the distilled water leaves an unbroken film on the glass surface, it shows that the glass is clean. If any grease is present, the film will be broken and droplets will form.

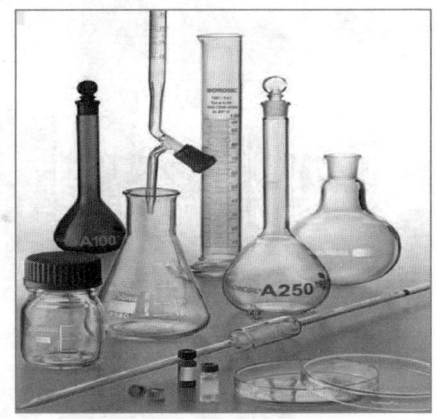

Fig. 5.4: Hospital glassware.

- Avoid exposing the glass to sudden variations of temperature to prevent breakage of glass.
- Glass containers must be arranged in an inverted manner inside the autoclave for sterilization. If kept in upright position, air trapped in them prevent steam penetration of all surfaces.
- Glass goods that are sent for boiling or autoclaving should be adequately padded to prevent breaking by rubbing with hard surfaces.

LINEN (FIG. 5.5)

Linen used in hospital includes bedsheet, blanket, curtains, cloth covers, towels, wrapper for tray and dressing set, patient's cloths, staff cloths.

General Guidelines for Care of Linen

- The linen cupboard should be kept in an orderly manner, with different items should be stocked separately and labelled.

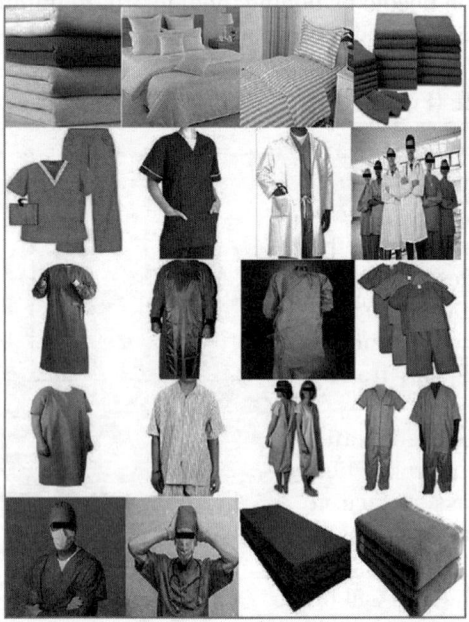

Fig. 5.5: Various types of linen use in hospital.

- The cupboard should be locked when not in use.
- Stocks of linen should be checked at regular intervals and inventory must be maintained.
- Ensure that linen should not be taken home by patients or staffs.
- Torn linen should be sent for mending.
- Everything should only be utilized for its intended usage.
- Soiled linen should not be placed on the floor.
- Damp linen if not wash immediately, should be dried to prevent it from becoming mildewed.
- Soiled linen should be rinsed with cold water first to remove the stain.
- Use appropriate stain removal to remove the stains **(Table 5.1)**.
- Linen used by patient with infectious disease should be disinfected first before they are sent to laundry.
- Use mackintosh whenever necessary to prevent soiling of linen.

Disinfection of Contaminated Linen

- Laundry box/hamper trolley must be used for collection of contaminated linen.
- Avoid putting contaminated linen on the floor.
- Dip the linen in 0.5% solution of chlorine for 10 minutes.
- Rinse the linen in cold water and send for autoclaving.
- For sterilization of linen use glutaraldehyde 0.2% for 10 hours.

Blankets

- Sheets must be used to protect the blankets over and under it.
- Blankets should never be exposed to dust.
- Occasionally brush the blanket to remove the dust.
- Clean the blanket using the dry cleaning method.
- Expose the blanket to sunlight for disinfection.
- To keep moths away from the area where blankets are stored, place naphthalene balls and cover them with dust-proof sheets.

Pillows and Mattress

- Use long mackintosh when conducting a procedure to prevent the mattress from becoming wet and stained.
- Brush the mattress at regular intervals to prevent collection of dust along the seams.
- Use washable mattress covers so that it can be changed at regular intervals.

Table 5.1: Types of stains with methods of removal.

Sl no.	Stains	Methods of removal
1.	Blood stains	• Soak immediately in cold water • Wash in warm soapy water • For old blood stain: Soak it in a mixture of hydrogen peroxide and ammonia for several hours • Wash in cold water, then with soap and warm water • For thick blood stain on mattress: Apply thick paste of starch and water and expose under the sun. Brush off the stain when it is dry and discolored
2.	Tea, coffee, cocoa	• Remove stain by pouring milk over it • Use cold or hot water with sodium carbonate • If stain still remain, use lemon juice or hydrogen peroxide
3.	Aniline dyes, gentian violet, methylene blue	• Wet cloths and bleach them in sunlight • Use chlorine water to bleach off the stain • Then, rinse thoroughly with warm water after stain disappears
4.	Candle wax	• Scrape off the wax • Place a cloth pad or blotting paper under and over the stain, press it with hot iron box
5.	Curry stains	• Immediately wash it off in cold water • Apply soap with hot water • If stains still remains bleach it in sunlight • After stain is bleached, wash them in cold water
6.	Ink stains	• Immediately wash in cold water • Use salt and lemon juice as a bleach and dry it in the sun • Apply hydrogen peroxide and dilute ammonia to remove the stains
7.	Rust marks	• Use salt and lime juice as a beach and expose in the sun • Rinse it off with cold water
8.	Iodine	• Soak the linen in rice water or apply starch paste until stain is removed completely
9.	Perspiration	• Wash it off using soap and hot water containing few drops of ammonia or bleach them in sunlight
10.	Paint or varnish	• Use turpentine, alcohol or ether to remove paint or varnish
11.	Mildew	• Soak in chlorine water and dry in sunlight • Wash it off with cold water • Acetic acid can also be used to remove mildew stain

- Use canvas between the mattress and the bedstead to prevent rusting of the mattress from the wires or springs.
- After patient is discharged the mattress should be thoroughly brushed and examined for stains and tears.
- The mattress is disinfected by exposing it to sunlight.
- Turn the mattress daily for airing, ensue that the mattress is not bend at acute angles.
- Mackintosh should be used to protect the pillows from becoming wet with blood, bodily discharges or by other fluids.
- Pillow covers can also be used to protect pillows and should be change at regular intervals.

FURNITURE (FIG. 5.6)

Furniture in the hospital may be made of wood or iron, it includes bedstead, tables, charts, lockers, stools, cupboards etc.
- Wooden furniture must be dust with damp duster daily.
- Clean the furniture with soap and water if necessary and keep them dry.
- Remove stain by scraping and polishing.
- Iron furniture is clean with a dry duster to prevent from rusting.
- If the iron becomes rusted, it is painted.
- Articles inside the cupboard should be arranged according to their size, shape and use.
- The shelves of the cupboard should be lined with paper to give a neat appearance and to prevent it from getting dirty.
- Articles must be kept inside the cupboard only when it is dry. Do not store wet or damp articles inside the cupboard.

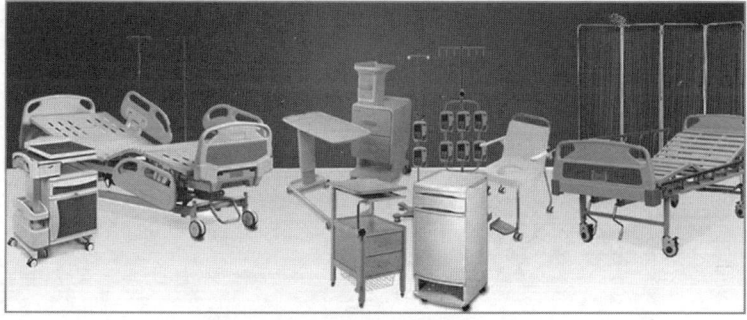

Fig. 5.6: Furniture's used in hospital.

- Use naphthalene balls to protect the articles from moths.
- Always keep the door closed.

Kitchen and Pantry

- Dishes and utensils must be cleaned, dried and kept in proper places after use.
- Ensure that the kitchen sink are not blocked.
- Use sodium carbonate solution/soap with hot water to remove the stains.
- Food store in the kitchen should be covered in a tight container.
- Kitchen/pantry garbage should be discarded properly.
- Defrosting and cleaning of the refrigerator should be done at regular intervals.
- Wash and dry any metal utensils immediately after use to prevent cross infection.

WARD INVENTORY

- Articles in the hospital required a daily count in order to maintain and trace equipment's.
- Articles such as flashlights, scissors, thermometer, BP apparatus etc. disappear easily, maintain inventory makes it easier to trace the missing items.
- Different on the types of articles, they are counted daily, weekly and monthly. Actual count of articles in the ward is known as physical inventory.
- Article must be checked and send for repairs if necessary.
- Articles that cannot be repaired are replace with a new one.

CHAPTER 6

Asepsis

INTRODUCTION

Asepsis is an accepted method to prevent contamination of wounds and other susceptible sites by organisms causing infection. Patient's protection from preventable infection is nurse's duty. Hence, an aseptic technique should be implemented during any invasive procedure.

DEFINITION

Asepsis is defined as the absence from infection or prevention of contact with micro-organisms.

HANDWASHING TECHNIQUE

Indications of Handwashing (Fig. 6.1)

- Before contact with patient.
- Before performing invasive procedure.
- After contact with patient.
- Before and after handling, dressing or touching open wounds.
- After handling contaminated equipment and organic material.

Medical Handwashing (Fig. 6.2)

Medical handwashing is the process that involves mechanical and chemical action that involves washing the hands with soap and water facilitating the removal of micro-organism, dirt and oils.

Articles Required

- Warm running water
- Antimicrobial agent/soap
- Paper towels/hand drier

Steps of Procedure

- Remove wristwatch, rings, bracelets and any jewelry items before handwashing.

Asepsis

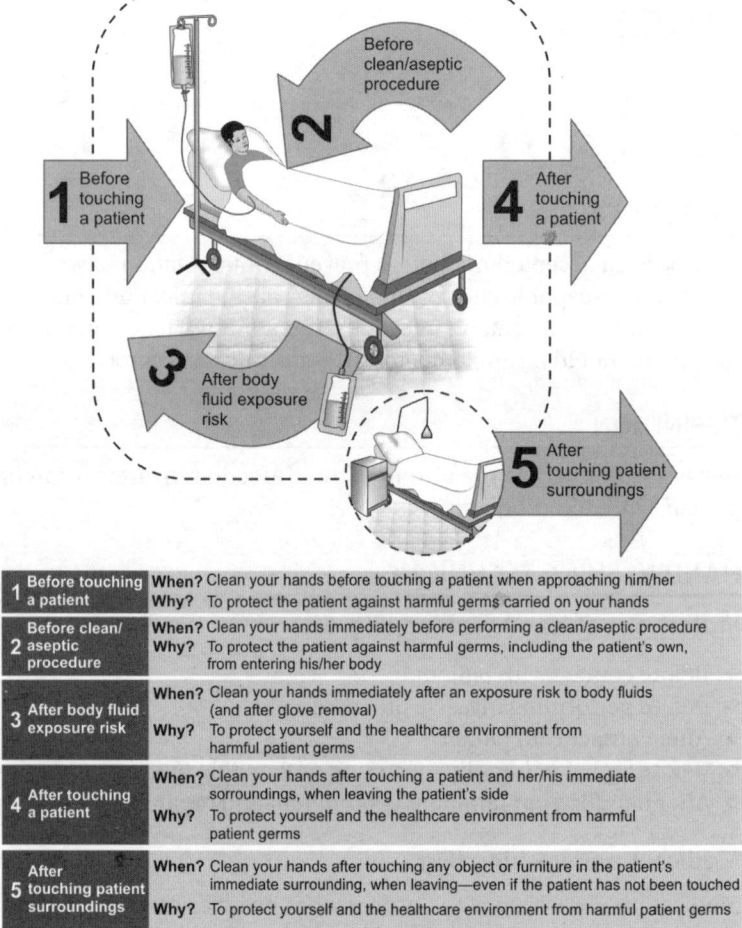

Fig. 6.1: Five moments of handwashing.

- Inspect the surface of hands for cuts, lesions.
- Stand in front of the sink, keeping a gap between the sink and uniform/clothes.
- Turn on faucet with a clean paper towel.
- Adjust water to acceptable temperature.
- Put soap on hands.
- Lather all areas of hands and wrists.
- Rub palms against one another.

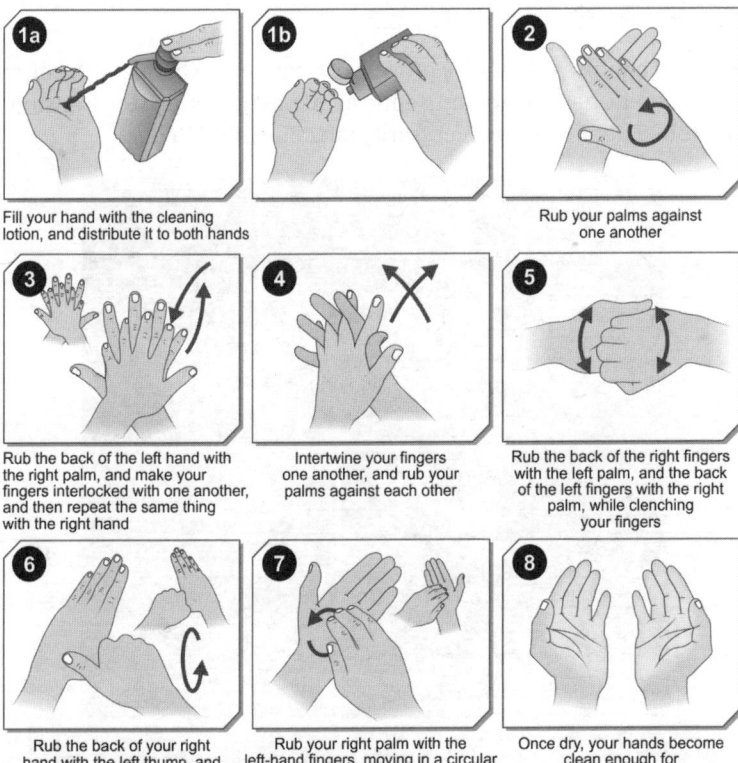

Fig. 6.2: Steps of medical handwashing.

- Rub the back of the left hand with the right palm and fingers interlocked with another. Repeat the same with the right hand.
- Interwined fingers with one another and rub palms against each other.
- While clenching fingers, rub the back of right fingers with left palm, and back of left fingers with right palm.
- Rub back of the right hand with left thumb, and back of left hand with right thumb in a circular motion.
- Rub right palm with left fingers in circular motion, and vice versa.
- Rinse thoroughly, running water down from wrists to fingertips.
- Pat dry with paper towel.
- Turn off faucet with paper towel and discard towel immediately.
- Handwashing must be performed for 40–60 seconds.

Surgical Handwashing (Fig. 6.3)

Surgical handwashing is the process of treatment of hands with either an antiseptic handrub or antiseptic handwash to reduce the transient microbial flora without necessarily affecting the skin flora.

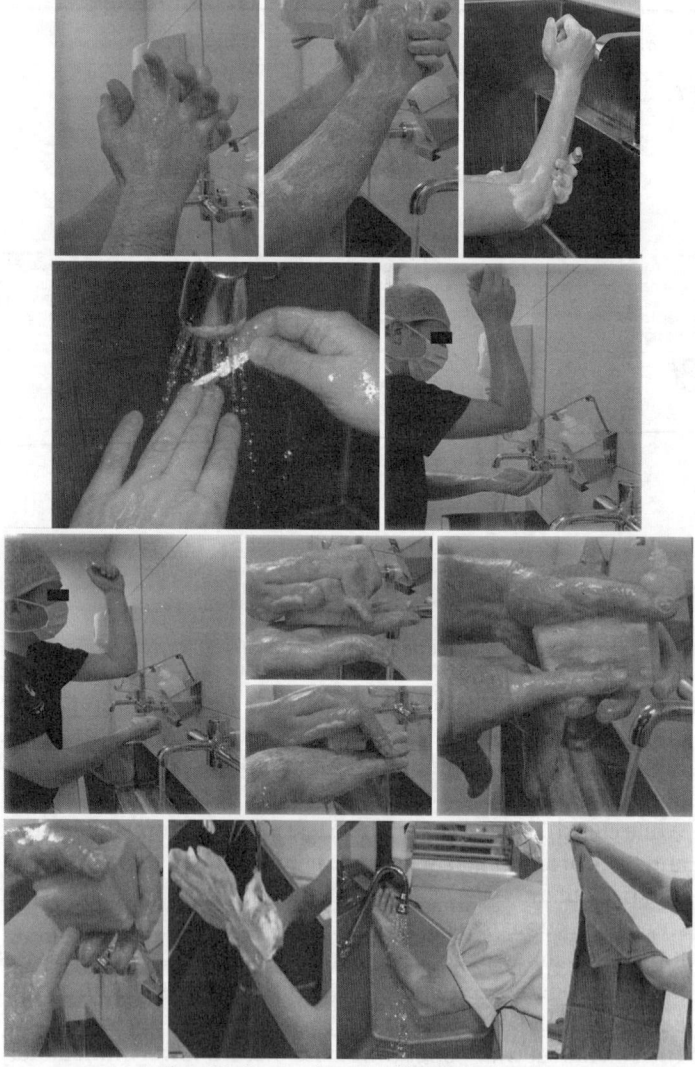

Fig. 6.3: Steps of surgical handwashing.

Articles Required

- Warm running water
- Soap
- Antimicrobial agent/solution
- Surgical hand scrub/brush
- Nail file
- Towels

Steps of Procedure

- Remove wristwatch, rings, bracelets and any jewelry items before handwashing.
- Nails must be cut short and trimmed, remove nail paint if present.
- Inspect the surface of hands for cuts, lesions.
- Ensure that sleeves must be folded 2–3 inches above the elbows.
- Stand in front of the sink, keeping a gap between the sink and uniform.
- Turn on faucet and check if water is warm and regulate the flow.
- Wet hands and arms with running water till 5 cm above elbow, lather with antiseptic agent/soap over it.
- Keep hands above the elbows.
- Thoroughly wash the hands till elbow, each side of each finger, between fingers, and clean nails using nail file.
- Dispense the needed amount of antiseptic solution into both hands and brush.
- Scrub the palm, back of the palm, each side of the thumb and fingers with 10 strokes each.
- Keep hands above the elbow, scrub each side of the arms from wrist to elbow in up and down motion for 1 minute.
- Ensure that scrubbing is done for at least 15 strokes.
- Flex the arms and rinse by letting the water run down from fingertips to elbows.
- Turn off the faucet with elbow, foot or knee control with hands elevated (depending on the type of faucet). Do not touch the faucet by hands.
- Keep hands above the waist, grasp the sterile towel with one hand and dry the other hand from the fingertips towards the forearm till the elbows in a rotating motion. Repeat the same with the other hand.
- Place the towel in soiled linen hamper/laundry basket.

STERILE MASK, GOWN AND GLOVES

Sterile mask, gown and gloves are worn after performing surgical handwashing, it is used in the operating and delivery room.

Articles Required

- Sterile Cheatle Forceps in a container of disinfectant solution.
- Sterile drums containing sterile reusable gowns or disposable gowns.
- Sterile mask.
- Sterile gloves.
- Sterile gown.

Steps of Procedure

Donning of Mask (Fig. 6.4)

- Take the sterile mask by holding the top two strings.
- Place the top edge of the mask above the bridge of the nose.
- Pull both the upper strings above the ears towards the back of the head and make a tie.
- Pull the two lower strings under the chin towards the back of the head and make a tie.
- Ensure that the mask fits properly by gently pinching upper portion of the mask around bridge of nose.

Doffing of Mask

- Wash hands.
- Remove the lower strings of the mask first, then the upper strings.

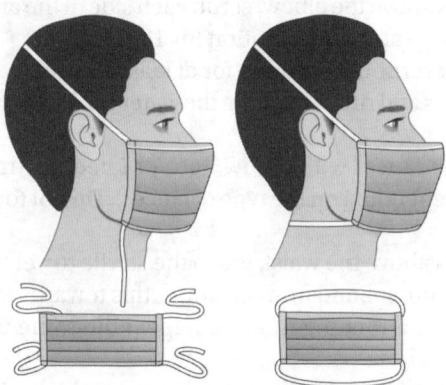

Fig. 6.4: Sterile masking.

Asepsis

- Hold the mask from the strings and discard it in the appropriate bin.

Donning of Gown (Fig. 6.5A)
- Take the folded gown by grasping the gown at the neck.
- Ensure that the gown is unfolded freely by keeping the gown away from the body.
- Hold the gown from inside at the shoulder level and put both the hands alternately into the armholes.
- While putting arms through the arm hole, extend the arms and hold hands upward at the level of the shoulder.
- The circulating nurse provide assistance from the back by pulling the gown from inside.
- The circulating nurse then fasten the gown at the back of the neck and the waist, open edges are folded or held together.

Doffing of Gown (Fig. 6.5B)
- Untie the gown's strings at the back.

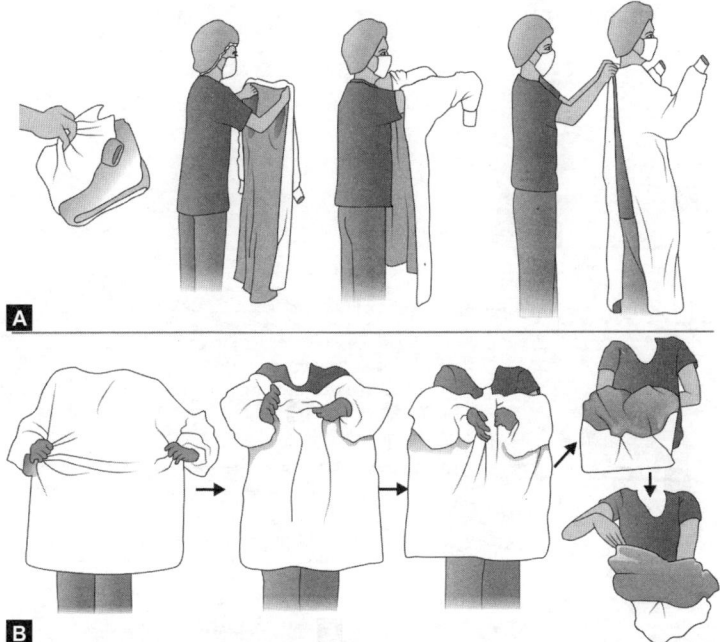

Figs. 6.5A and B: (A) Donning of gown; (B) Doffing of gown.

- ❖ Grab the gown at the waist or hip in a clump and pull down away from the sides of the body.
- ❖ Once the gown is off from the shoulders, pull the arm of the gown sleeves alternately.
- ❖ When the gown is bunched at the wrist, fold/roll the exposed side of the gown inward.
- ❖ Dispose gown in appropriate bin.

Donning of Sterile Gloves (Figs. 6.6A to E)

- ❖ Open the sterile gloves package in a dry, flat, clean area/surface.
- ❖ Remove the outer package by separating and peeling apart the sides.
- ❖ Grasp the inner surface of the sterile gloves and laid it in a dry, flat, clean surface at the waist level.
- ❖ Open the package, top flap away from the body, bottom flap towards the body, side flap without contaminating the inner surface of the wrapper.
- ❖ Identify the right and left gloves.
- ❖ Glove the dominant hand first. Grasp the edge of the cuff of the glove of the dominant hand using thumb and index finger of non-dominant hand.

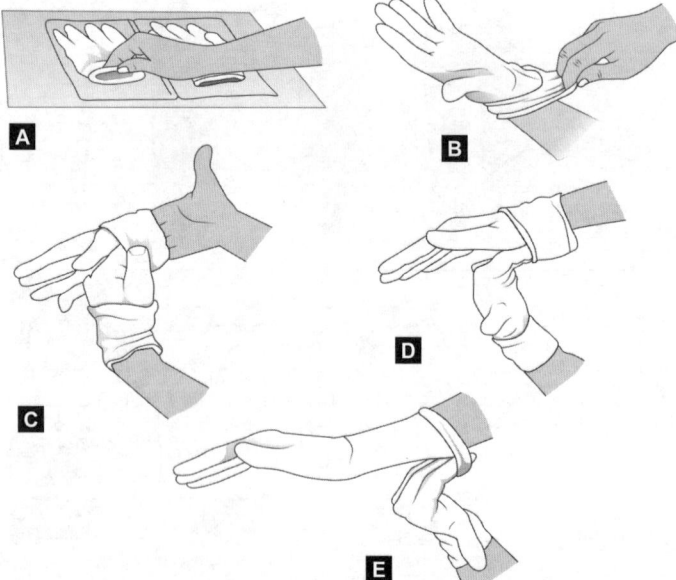

Figs. 6.6A to E: Donning of sterile gloves.

Asepsis

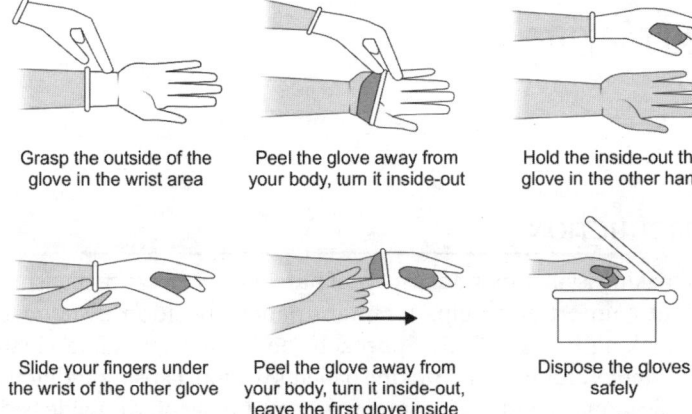

Fig. 6.7: Doffing of sterile gloves.

- Lift out the glove and carefully pull the glove over the hand, ensuring that the surface is not touch.
- Slip in the fingers of the gloved dominant hand under the cuff of the other glove. Keep thumb of gloved dominant hand abducted back to avoid touching of exposed non-gloved hand.
- Slip the glove onto your non-dominant hand making sure that the fingers slip into the proper spaces.
- Interlock the fingers of the gloved hands to ensure that the glove is fit onto each fingers.
- Ensure that the gloved hands must be positioned above the waist level.

Doffing of Sterile Gloves (Fig. 6.7)

- Grasp the outside of one cuff with the other gloved hand.
- Ensure that the skin remains untouched.
- Pull the glove off, turning it inside out and gather it in the palm of the gloved hand.
- Dispose the gloves in appropriate bin.
- Tuck the index finger of your bare hand inside the remaining glove cuff and peel the glove off inside out and over the previously removed glove.
- Dispose gloves in appropriate bin.
- Perform hand washing.

CHAPTER 7

Bed Making

INTRODUCTION

Bed making is an important aspect of nursing care because it ensures patient comfort and helps maintain patient position as needed. Bed making is a scientific approach; beds must be made clean, comfortable, and adaptable for the patients without causing additional complications. In order to promote care, the nurse must provide beds based on the patient's condition and it must be patient-centered.

DEFINITION

The process of setting up various types of beds in accordance with patients' needs is known as bed-making.

GENERAL RULES FOR BED MAKING

Bed making is a fundamental of nursing work. The systematic procedures followed in bed-making are as follows:
- The uniform of nursing staff should not touch the bed while making a bed.
- Soiled linens should not be thrown on floor.
- First lift the mattress while loosening the bed-linen or removing the sheets. The sheets should not be pulled forcefully.
- The bed linens should be folded from top to bottom or side to side. This applies to fold the mattress also while making an un-occupied bed.
- As self-precaution while tucking bedding under mattress, the palm of the hand should face downwards to prevent injury of nails.
- The open end of the pillow should not face to the entrance of ward. The beds should be in one line for better look.

TYPES OF BED MAKING

- Open/Unoccupied bed.
- Occupied bed.

- Postoperative bed.
- Cardiac bed.
- Amputation bed.

OPEN OR UNOCCUPIED BED (FIG. 7.1)

The technique of preparing a bed that is comfortable and suitable for the hospitalized patient. In open bed, the bed is yet to be occupied by the admitted patient.

Purposes

- To promote rest.
- To provide comfort.
- To prevent the spread of microorganisms.
- To maintain a clean and neat environment.
- To prevent complications.
- To prevent skin irritation.

Articles Required

- Spring or metaled-sheet bed.
- Mattress.
- Pillow.
- One mackintosh (Rubber draw sheet).
- Two large sheets.
- One draw sheet.
- Pillowcase.
- One blanket (Optional).

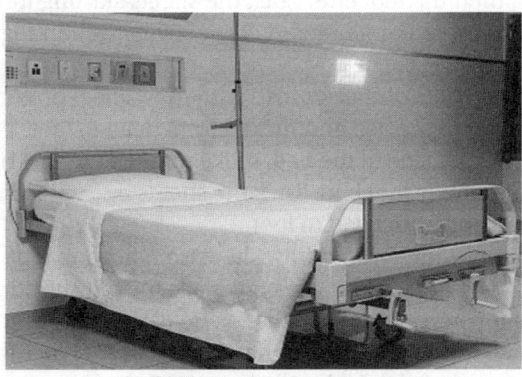

Fig. 7.1: Open bed.

- Bed spread or bed cover.
- Mattress cover.
- Chair or stool to keep the clean linen.
- Duster/cloth: Dry and damp.
- Kidney tray.
- Laundry bag for soiled linen.

Steps of Procedure

- The bed should be put where it is required.
- Assess whether there is need for change of linen and collect fresh linen as needed.
- Wash hands.
- Keep all clean linens on the stool or chair. The items should not be brought one by one from the store or storing place.
- Place kidney tray on the bedside locker.
- Clean the top of the mattress with a dry duster from head end to foot end and collect the dirt in kidney tray.
- Fold the mattress from top to bottom and clean the under surface of the mattress with a dry duster.
- Clean the cot with a damp duster.
- Then, fold the mattress from bottom to top and clean the under surface of the mattress and body of the cot from middle to foot end as described above.
- Keep the mattress flat and put on the mattress cover.
- Place the bottom sheet in the middle and is spread over now with the wide hem at the top or head end.
- Once the bottom sheet is spread, make mitered corners of the head end and then the foot end. Tuck the sheets starting from head to foot. Steps for making mitered corners are given in **Figures 7.2A to D**.
- The rubber sheet or mackintosh with draw sheet on top is spread at the center of the bed and tucked from head to foot.
- Go to the other side of the bed, make mitered corners of the head end and then the foot end. Tuck the sheets by pulling it with both hands starting from head to foot.
- Tuck the mackintosh and draw sheet from head to foot.
- Move to the initial side of the bed, place the top sheet in four-fold with the top end at level with head end of the mattress.
- Spread the top sheet evenly. On top of the sheet place the blanket at the center of the bed with its top 15–20 cm approximately

Bed Making

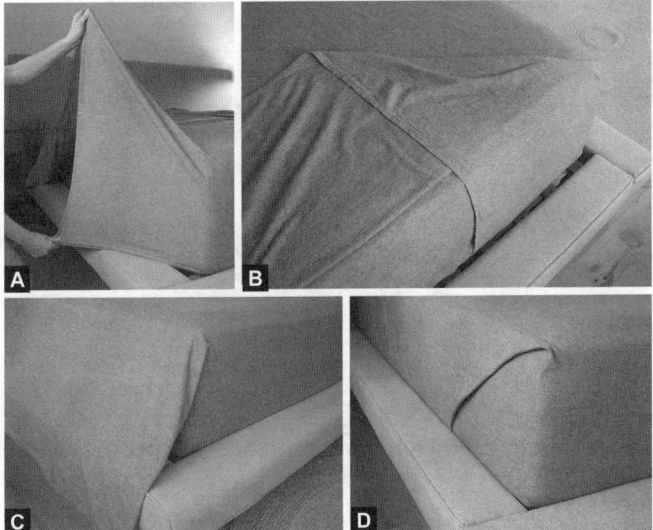

Figs. 7.2A to D: Steps for making mitered corner.

from top of the mattress. The top sheet is folded back over the blanket.
- Tuck the top sheet and blanket together at the foot end and make a modified/half mitered corner at the foot end to allow the sides to hang free.
- Change pillow if required. Put on pillow clean pillow covers and place the pillow in such a way that the free end of the pillow is facing away from the entrance of room or door.
- Place dirty linen in the laundry room.
- Replace all articles and wash hands.

OCCUPIED BED (FIG. 7.3)

Occupied bed is making a bed which is already occupied by the patient. For an occupied bed, the care is taken to make a comfortable bed without much disturbance to the patient. So, the procedure is entirely different than making an un-occupied bed.

Purposes
- To change dirty bed sheets, blankets, pillows and pillowcases for bed ridden patients.

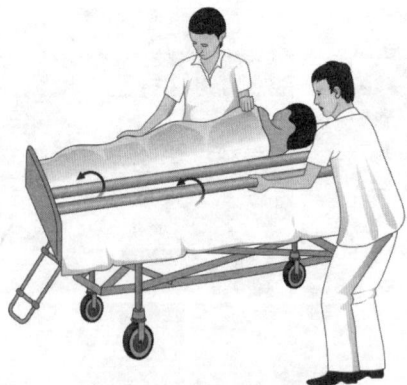

Fig. 7.3: Occupied bed.

- Reduce skin irritation and formation of bed sores for bed ridden patients.
- To provide comfort to the patients.
- To maintain a wrinkle free, neat and clean bed.

Articles Required

- Chair/stool.
- Chair to keep the clean linen.
- Clean bed linen.
- Laundry bag for soiled linen.
- Dusters-2.
- Basin with disinfectant.
- Kidney tray.

Steps of Procedure

- Assess the patient's condition and see if there are any special instructions especially movement restriction.
- The patient or the bed attendant should be told that fresh linen is to be put in and used ones are to be removed. This knowledge of bed making or notice to the patient will lessen his annoyance or disturbance.
- The stool is placed at the foot end of the bed.
- The linens are kept ready on the chair. Keep kidney tray on the bedside locker.
- A bedside screen may be placed for better privacy and less annoyance to the patient.

Bed Making

- Remove any personal items of the patient and handover it to patient or attendant.
- If there is no restriction, ask/assist patient to get out of bed and sit comfortably on a chair placed near the bed.

If patient movement is restricted/In case of bed ridden patient

- If the patient is in Fowler's position the head is lowered first before changing the linens.
- The top bedding is first loosened.
- Then the bedspread is slowly removed.
- The patient's head is lifted and all pillows are removed except one, taking help by one more assistant.
- Pull the mattress up. Never allow the patient to put himself up. You can take the help of another staff. Loosen the bottom bedding and remove the top sheet by pulling it down from under cover.
- Move the pillow to one side. Turn patient on side away from you. Roll or fanfold the draw sheet against the patient's back.
- Brush or clean the mackintosh sheet and fold it back loosely over the patient.
- Now roll the bottom sheet as far as under the patient's back as possible.
- At times the bottom sheet can be replaced with the top sheet.
- The clean sheet is spread straight length wise with fold at center of bed. 30 to 40 cm is left at the head to tuck under mattress.
- Tuck in at the top making a square corner. Also tuck at the sides and bottom.
- Bring back the mackintosh lying over the patient. Pull tighten and tuck well.
- Place the clean draw sheet widthwise fold at the center of the bed. Push it as far under the patient as possible. Tuck in both the fold and the upper layer of the draw sheet under the patient as far as possible. Tuck in the free end tightly under mattress.
- Now lifting the top bedding, turn the patient on his side towards you.
- Then go to the other side of the bed, pull out soiled linen which has been folded under patient.
- Keep soiled linen in the laundry bag.
- Now pull the clean bottom sheet under the patient, then fold draw sheet and mackintosh over the patient.
- Pull and tighten the bottom sheet under the patient, then fold draw sheet and mackintosh over the patient.

- Pull and tighten the rubber sheet and tuck well.
- Pull and tighten the draw sheet and tuck well.
- Place clean top sheet over the patient with large hem at the head with wrong side of the hem up. Then tuck in sheet making a square corner at the foot end of the bed.
- Place bed spread on the top of the bed. Unfold and make a half square corner at the foot end of the bed.
- Turn the top of the bed spread under the blanket.
- Turn the top sheet back over the blanket and bed spread.
- Now go back to the other side, fold and tuck in top of bedding as on the first side.
- Hold pillow under your arm and change the pillow cover. Now put it under patient's head by lifting and supporting the head if the patient is unable to do so.

POSTOPERATIVE BED (FIG. 7.4)

Postoperative bed is a special type of bed meant for patient who undergone surgical procedure, they can either be in anesthetized form or otherwise.

Purposes

- To protect the patient from immediate complication of anesthesia or choking.
- To make the patient more comfortable.

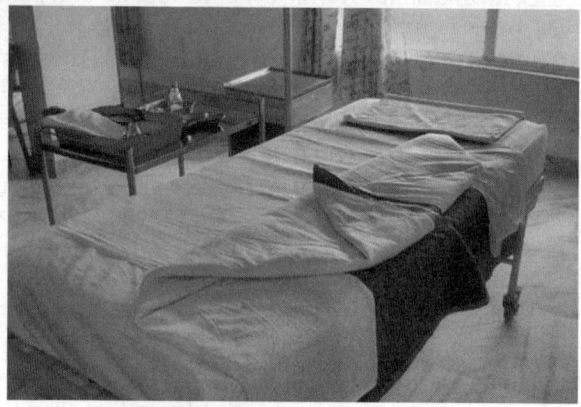

Fig. 7.4: Postoperative bed.

Bed Making

- To provide proper position of the patient postsurgery.
- To protect the mattress and other linens from blood, vomitus, and other discharge.
- For easy and quick transfer of patient from trolley to bed.

Articles Required

- Take same articles used in open bed.
- Rubber sheet or mackintosh sheet.
- Small hand towel.
- One sponge holder.
- One basin for vomitus.
- Two mouth gag.
- Airway.
- Tongue depressor.
- Temperature tray.
- BP apparatus.
- Transfusion set.
- Hot water bags or bottle.
- Suction apparatus.
- Articles required for oxygen administration.
- Kidney tray.

Steps of Procedure

- A simple bed is made as per normal procedure of bed making.
- The bottom corner of top bedding should not be mitered and must be left untucked.
- The upper bedding is fan folded to one side opposite the stretcher.
- In cold season the hot water bottle is placed in middle of the bed and covered with fan folded top bedding.
- The small mackintosh sheet covered with towel is kept at open side at top end of the bed.
- The basin for collection of vomitus is placed at bed side stand.
- The transfusion stand is kept ready at bed side.
- Articles required for oxygen administration, mouth gag, tongue depressor, temperature tray, BP instrument, pulse meter can be kept ready at bed side stand.
- In special case where required, the suction apparatus is also kept ready at bed side.
- Wash hands.

CARDIAC BED (FIG. 7.5)

Cardiac bed is a special type of bed designed for heart patients that aids the patients in assuming sitting position.

Purposes

- To prevent dyspnea or breathlessness.
- To provide comfort to the patient.
- To reduce the workload of heart.
- To prevent complications or acceleration of symptoms.

Articles Required

- The same materials used in open bed making.
- Cardiac table.
- Back rest where Fowler's bed is not available.
- Extra pillow for back.
- Air ring and footrest board.
- Basin with disinfectant solution (1:20 Savlon).

Steps of Procedure

- Arrange all articles near the bed and fold the linen on the stool in the order of use.
- Prepare the bed same as open bed.
- Instruct the patient to sit comfortably in bed.
- The back rest is placed at the back of the patient and for extra comfort one or two pillows are placed on it.

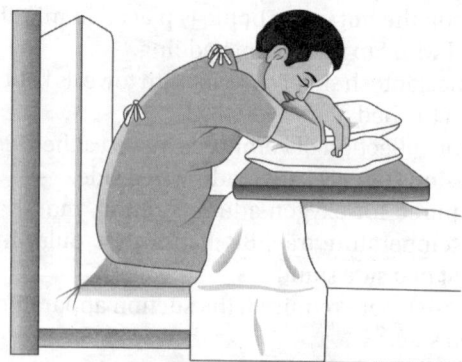

Fig. 7.5: Cardiac bed.

- ❖ The cardiac table is placed in front of the patient with one pillow.
- ❖ Place pillows under the knees and arms.

AMPUTATION BED/STUMP BED (FIG. 7.6)

A special type of bed meant for amputated patient specially the amputation of lower limb.

Purposes

- ❖ To provide easy availability of the stump.
- ❖ To facilitate proper dressing of the stump.

Articles Required

- ❖ The same materials used in open bed making.
- ❖ A set of top bedding.
- ❖ Blankets and bed covers.
- ❖ Bed cradle.
- ❖ Tourniquet.
- ❖ Pillow and plastic cover.
- ❖ Sandbag.

Steps of Procedure

- ❖ Prepare the bed same as open bed.
- ❖ Both the blankets are spread next to the patient's body.
- ❖ The bottom half of the bed is prepared.

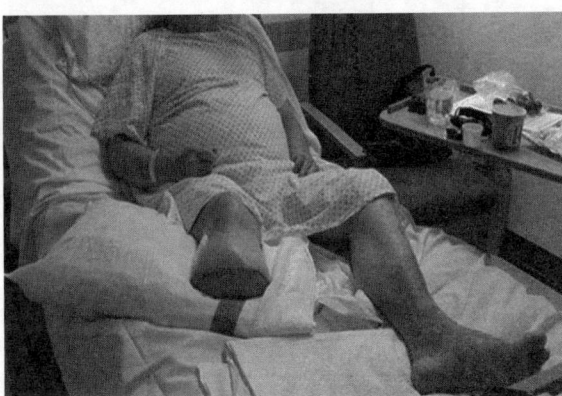

Fig. 7.6: Amputation bed.

- The bed sheet is folded at the center of the bed at bottom, tucked in and corners are made.
- The other sheet should be folded in half with the right hand side up. About 6 inches of sheet at top is folded back over top bedding. The two halves should overlap about 3 inches at the meeting places of two sheets.
- The blanket is placed at 9-10 inches from top of mattress and the top sheet is folded down over it.
- The bedspread is also folded in the same manner as blankets.

CHAPTER 8

Comfort Devices

INTRODUCTION

Since patient comfort is a crucial component of nursing care, comfort devices play a significant role in encouraging comfort and relief among patients. Comfort devices are tools that appear in a variety of forms and sizes. The primary function of using a comfort device is to relieve discomfort and maintain correct posture.

DEFINITION

Comfort devices are equipment or tools that are design to alleviate pain, reduce stress, and improve the overall well-being of patients. These devices helps patient feel more comfortable, relaxed, and at ease.

PURPOSES

- ❖ To provide comfort and relaxation.
- ❖ To immobilize a body part.
- ❖ To relieve pressure on parts of body.
- ❖ To prevent from falls and accidents.
- ❖ To stimulate blood circulation.

TYPES

- ❖ Pillows
- ❖ Back rest
- ❖ Bed cradle
- ❖ Cardiac table
- ❖ Air/water mattress
- ❖ Trapeze bar
- ❖ Footboard
- ❖ Trochanter roll
- ❖ Sandbags
- ❖ Hand wrist splint

Pillows (Fig. 8.1)

Pillows are a type of comfort device that is used to support body parts, relieve pain, and keep the patient in position.

Uses

- It gives support to the head and neck, arms, legs, and parts of back.
- It relieves pain on abdominal muscles.
- Used in maintaining positions for the patients.
- It helps in prevention of fatigue.

Back Rest (Fig. 8.2)

Back rest is an adjustable mechanical device that is used for giving support for back of the patient in Fowler's position.

Uses

- To support the back in Fowler's position.
- To relief dyspnea.
- Useful for positioning cardiac patients.

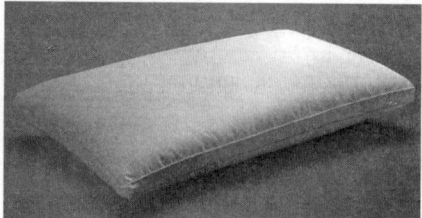

Fig. 8.1: Pillow.

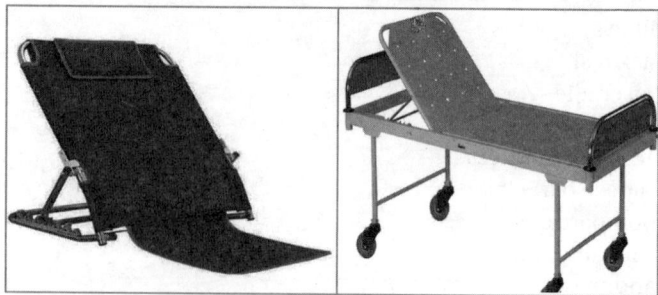

Fig. 8.2: Back rest.

Bed Cradle (Fig. 8.3)

A bed cradle is a device that supports the weight of the upper bed clothing, preventing it from coming into touch with the patient's body.

Uses

- Used in burns patients to prevent the skin from coming in contact with the patient's body.
- To observe patients with lower limb amputation.
- Used when the applied plaster cast is yet to be dry.

Cardiac Table (Fig. 8.4)

Cardiac table is a device that is intended as an over-bed table and is put in front of the patient while they are in the Fowler's position.

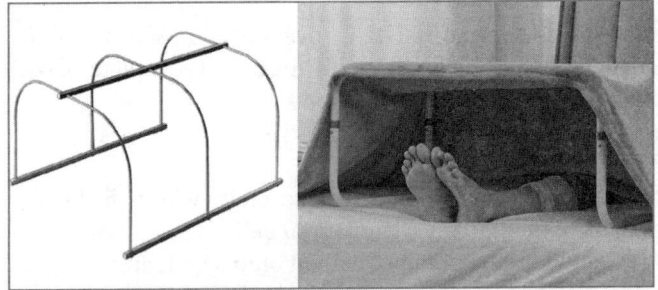

Fig. 8.3: Bed cradle.

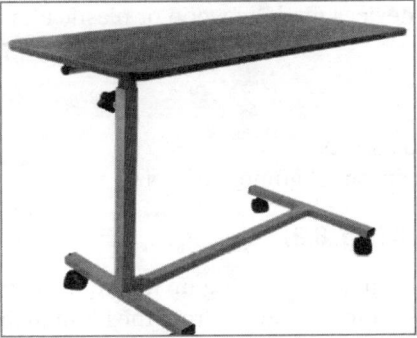

Fig. 8.4: Cardiac table.

Uses

- Used for cardiac patients to lean forward on a pillow placed over the bed.
- Used for positioning a patient during thoracentesis procedure.
- It can be used by patient as a table to take food in bed.

Air/Water Mattress (Figs. 8.5A and B)

Air/water mattress is a special type of mattress filled with air or water. In this, the pressure exerted by the body is equally distributed in all directions.

Uses

- To prevent pressure sore in bed ridden patients.
- It relieves muscle tension and reduce backache.

Trapeze Bar (Fig. 8.6)

A trapeze bar is a device that hangs over the bed frame and allows the patient to move around easily within the bed. It is a means of self-help for patients.

Uses

- It helps the patient in carrying out exercise within the bed.
- It enable patient to raise trunk from bed.
- It is useful for movement of patient onto a bedpan.
- It is useful for patient to move from bed to wheelchair.

Footboard (Fig. 8.7)

Footboard are devices made of wood or plastic attached to the foot end of the bed.

Uses

- It prevents foot drop.
- To maintain proper alignment of feet.

Trochanter Roll (Fig. 8.8)

Trochanter roll is made by rolling up a bath towel or blankets. It is place under the buttocks and roll from the ilium to the midthigh.

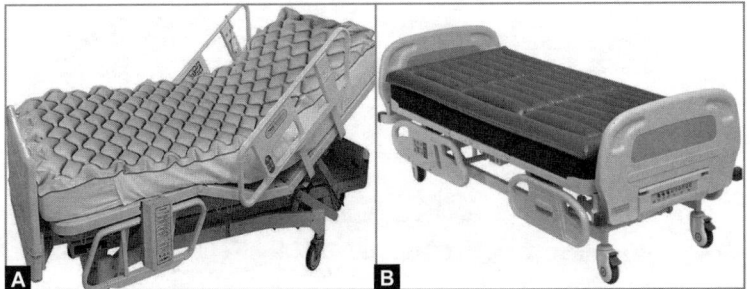

Figs. 8.5A and B: (A) Air mattress; (B) Water mattress.

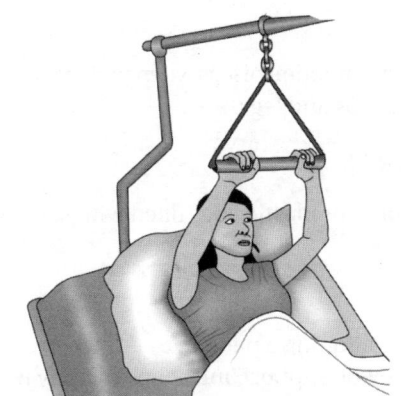

Fig. 8.6: Trapeze bar.

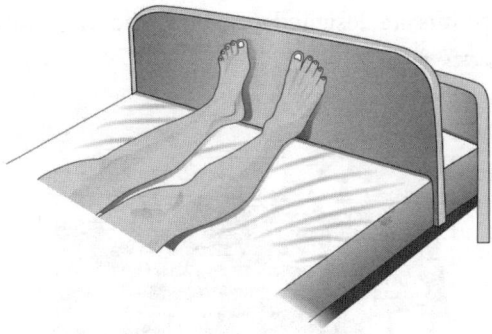

Fig. 8.7: Footboard.

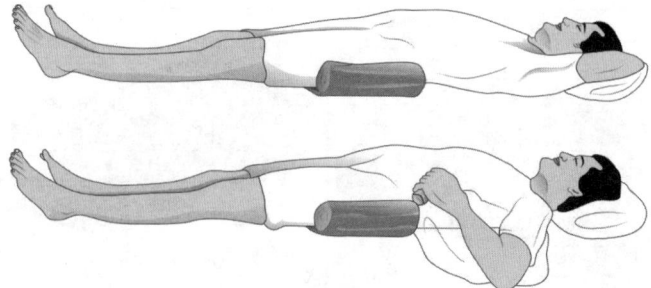

Fig. 8.8: Trochanter roll.

Uses

- It prevent external rotation of legs when patient is in supine position.
- It supports the hips and legs.

Sandbags (Fig. 8.9)

Sandbags are rubber or plastic bags filled with sand. It is available in various sizes.

Uses

- It is used for positioning a patient.
- It is used to provide support and shape to body parts.
- It is used to immobilize a body part.

Hand Wrist Splints (Fig. 8.10)

Hand wrist splints are designed to stabilize the wrist and it looks like a fingerless gloves.

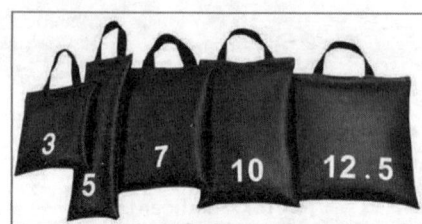

Fig. 8.9: Sandbags.

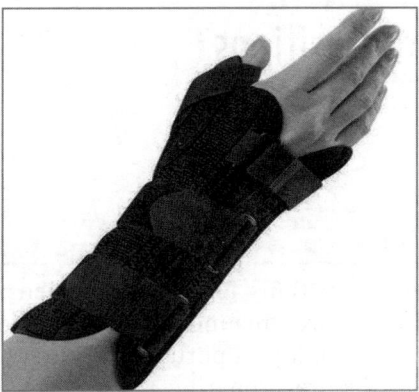

Fig. 8.10: Hand wrist splints.

Uses

- To support the weak joints of the wrist and their surrounding structures.
- It is used for minimize the pressure in condition such as carpal tunnel syndrome.
- It is used to immobilize the wrist and fingers.

CHAPTER 9

Therapeutic Positions

INTRODUCTION

There are various positions for patients which are important for providing better care, treatment or examination of patients. The positions are equally important for nurses, doctors and patients as well. Before preparing a patient for operation or examination or in postoperative cases, a nurse should know correctly the positions as these will be ordered from time to time by doctors.

DEFINITION

It is defined as placing a patient according to the required posture and alignment as needed therapeutically.

PURPOSES

- To provide comfort and relaxation.
- To prevent deformities associated with musculoskeletal system.
- To restore normal body functions.
- To prevent complications cause by immobility.
- To stimulate blood circulation.

TYPES

- Fowler's position
- Supine/dorsal recumbent/back lying position
- Prone position
- Sim's position
- Lateral or side lying position
- Lithotomy position
- Cardiac position
- Knee-chest position
- Trendelenburg's position

Fowler's Position (Fig. 9.1A)

Fowler's position is a standard patient position. It is also known as sitting position.

Purposes

- For relief in breathlessness.
- For good drainage from abdomen, and pelvic cavity postoperatively.
- For better blood circulation to prevent thrombosis.
- For good relaxation of muscles of abdomen, back and thighs.

Steps of Procedure

- Explain to the patient regarding the position and its purposes.
- Place the patient in sitting position by elevating the head end of the bed. The head end of bed should be elevated as follows:
  - Standard Fowler's position/Fowler's position. Elevated at 45°–60°.
  - Low Fowler's position: Elevated at 15°–30°.
  - Semi-Fowler's position: Elevated at 30°–45° **(Fig. 9.1B)**.
  - High Fowler's position: Elevated at 80°–90°.

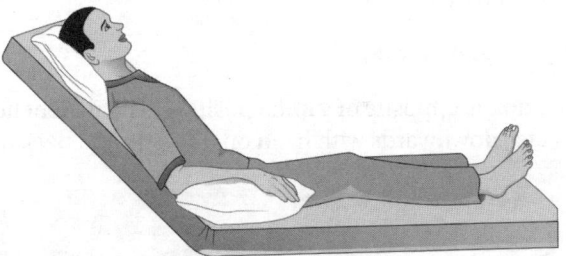

Fig. 9.1A: Fowler's position.

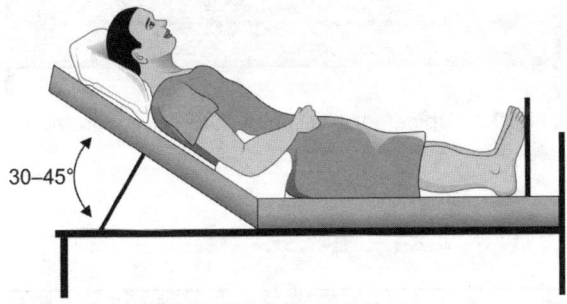

Fig. 9.1B: Semi-Fowler's position.

- Use a small pillow to rest the head against the mattress.
- Place foot board at the bottom of patient feet, if required.
- Place pillows wherever necessary.

Supine/Dorsal Recumbent/Back Lying Position (Fig. 9.2)

The patient lies flat on bed with one pillow at the head end.

Purposes

- For patient with abdominal or back pain.
- For examination of the anterior parts of body.

Steps of Procedure

- Explain the position to the patient.
- Place the patient flat on back with legs extended.
- Place patient hands at the side or over the abdomen.
- In case of patient with low blood pressure, use pillow at the leg end and no pillow at the head end.
- Place pillow under the head, neck and shoulder.
- Place foot board if required.

Prone Position (Fig. 9.3)

Prone position is opposite of supine position. The patient lies flat on bed with face downwards with head on one side and back upwards.

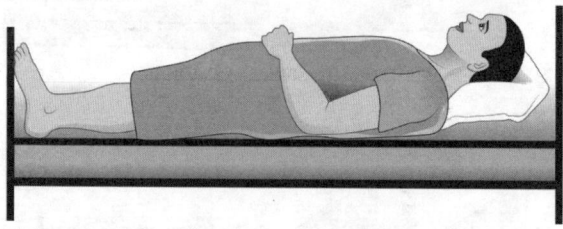

Fig. 9.2: Supine/dorsal recumbent/back lying position.

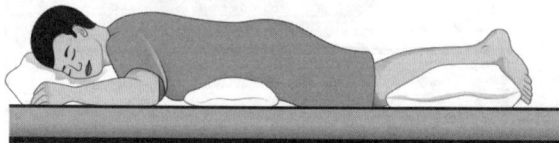

Fig. 9.3: Prone position.

Purposes

- For postoperative cases such as tonsillectomy.
- For patients with back injury and lower limb amputation.
- For prevention of bed sore.
- For patients with burn over the back.
- For relieving of abdominal distension.
- For postural drainage.

Steps of Procedure

- Provide explanation to the patient regarding the position.
- Place flat on bed with face downwards and back upwards.
- Turn the patient face on one side and support with a small pillow.
- Place the hands of the patient folded over pillow.
- Place pillow under the abdomen and legs.

Sim's Position (Fig. 9.4)

Sim's position is also called as semiprone position.

Purposes

- For examination of rectum or vagina.
- For administration of enema.
- For position in sigmoidoscopy and proctoscopy.
- For relaxation in antenatal exercise.

Steps of Procedure

- Explain the position to the patient.
- At first, place patient in supine position.
- Turn patient in left lateral position slightly prone with buttocks drawn slightly backward the edge of the bed.

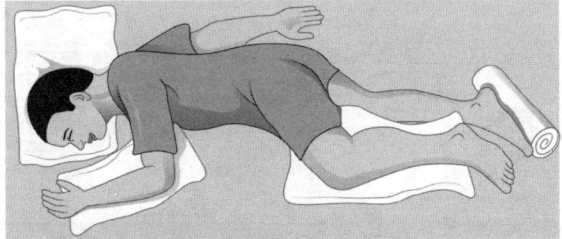

Fig. 9.4: Sim's position.

- ❖ Place the right arm in front of the patient while left arm rests behind the patient.
- ❖ Place the right knee well flexed against the abdomen.
- ❖ Place the left leg straight on the bed.
- ❖ Place a small pillow under the head, upper arm, upper leg and abdomen for better comfort.

Lateral or Side Lying Position (Fig. 9.5)

The patient lies either on the left lateral or right lateral side of the body.

Purposes

- ❖ For giving back care in bed ridden patients.
- ❖ For colonic irrigation.
- ❖ For rectal examinations.
- ❖ For immediate postoperative patients to prevent aspiration.

Steps of Procedure

- ❖ Explain the position to the patient.
- ❖ Place the patient to side of the bed.
- ❖ Turn patient on his left or right side with legs flexed.
- ❖ Place the patient thighs and knees with buttocks towards the edge of the bed.
- ❖ Position the patient so that the upper leg is flexed more than the lower leg.
- ❖ Place one pillow for resting of upper leg behind the lower leg.
- ❖ Position both arms in flexed position. Upper most arm is supported by pillow on level with shoulder.

Lithotomy Position (Fig. 9.6)

The patient lies in supine position with the legs flexed at 90°.

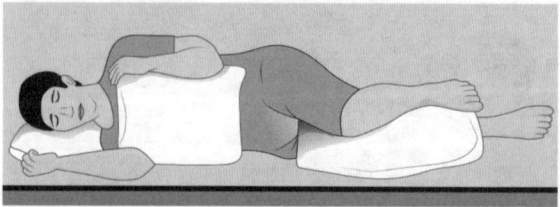

Fig. 9.5: Lateral or side lying position.

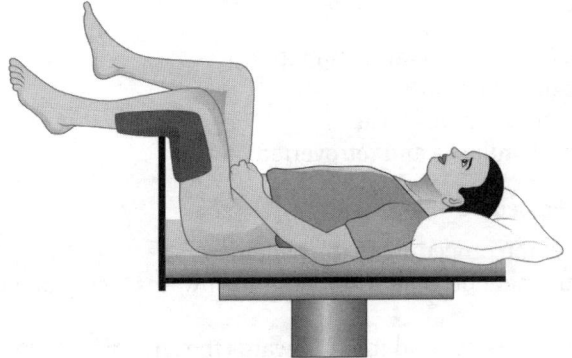

Fig. 9.6: Lithotomy position.

Purposes

- For pelvic and vaginal examination.
- For vaginal delivery.
- For vaginal and rectal surgeries.

Steps of Procedure

- Explain the position and procedure to the patient.
- Place the patient in supine position.
- Instruct the patient to flexed both the legs, knees and hips at 90°. The legs must be supported on stirrups.
- Place pillow under the head.

Knee-chest Position (Fig. 9.7)

Knee-chest position is also called as genupectoral position. The patient rest on the knee and chest with the head turned to one side.

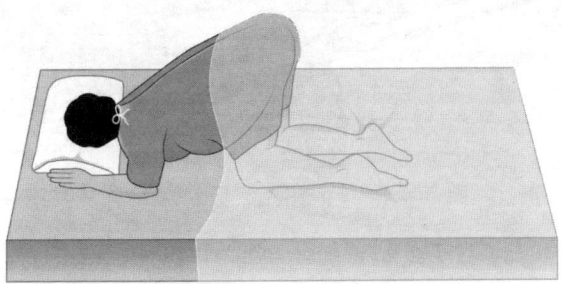

Fig. 9.7: Knee-chest position.

Purposes

- For vaginal and rectal examination.
- For sigmoidoscopy.
- For postpartum exercise.
- For cord prolapse and retroverted uterus.

Steps of Procedure

- Explain the procedure to the patient.
- Instruct patient to lie with chest downwards facing down on the bed.
- Flexed the knees and thighs towards the chest with buttocks high up in air.
- Turn the patient head to one side with one cheek on a pillow.
- Flexed the hands at elbow and rests on either side to give support to keep body in stable position.
- Place a pillow under the chest.
- The weight should rest on the chest and knees which are flexed so that the thighs are at right angles to the legs.

Trendelenburg Position (Fig. 9.8)

Trendelenburg position is also called as raised pelvic position and is applied on the operating table. This position is credited Friedrich Trendelenburg who was a prominent *German surgeon* in the late 19th and early 20th century.

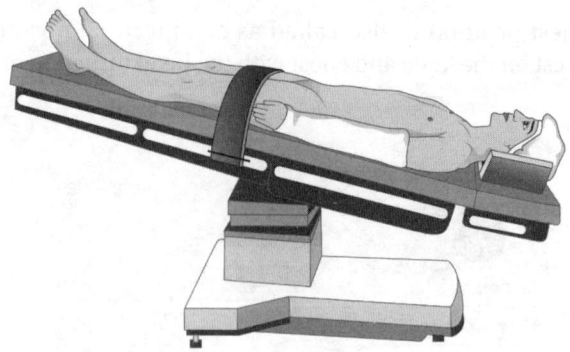

Fig. 9.8: Trendelenburg position.

Purposes

- For shock and hemorrhage.
- For surgery of pelvic organs to displace intestines into upper abdomen.
- For postural drainage.
- For patients with deep vein thrombosis.

Steps of Procedure

- Explain the procedure to the patient.
- Place the patient in supine position.
- Lower the patient head while the body lie on inclined plane with hips higher than the head.
- The patient knees are flexed over adjustable lower section of the table which can be adjusted according to desired height.
- Applied a good padding over shoulder to keep the patient from sliding towards lower end of the table.
- Avoid giving pressure on the knees and shoulder.

CHAPTER 10

Pain

INTRODUCTION

Pain assessment and management is the most fundamental part of the nurse's responsibility (considered as the 5th vital sign). Pain is a subjective experience for the patient and can be characterized in many ways: burning or tingling, sharp or dull, or generalized aching. Pain management is an important component of comprehensive patient care. Therefore, nurses must be proficient in assessing and managing pain in order to provide the best care possible to the patient.

DEFINITIONS

- Pain is an unpleasant sensation and emotional experience that links to tissue damage.
  —*International Association for the Study of Pain (IASP)*
- Pain is a subjective, unpleasant, sensory, and emotional experience associated with actual or potential tissue damage.

TYPES

- **Acute pain:** Short duration, healing process in 30 days.
- **Chronic pain:** It persist for the more than 3-6 month.
- **Physiological pain:** It leads to potential tissue damage.
- **Somatic pain:** It involves superficial tissues (skin, bone, muscle, joints)
- **Visceral pain:** It involves organs (heart, stomach and liver)
- **Neuropathic pain:** Changes in the nerve cells.

ASSESSMENT

- Pain is a subjective feeling. Assess the pain with respect to onset, the aggravating and relieving factors, quality, its radiation, severity and whether the patient has taken any earlier treatment. Pain can be assessed as per the acronym 'OPQRSTUV'.

- O: Onset
- P: Provoking and palliating
- Q: Quality
- R: Region or radiation
- S: Severity
- T: Treatment
- U: Understand how it impacts

❖ Assess the characteristics of the pain.
  - Severity of pain.
  - Quality, location, duration, and rhythmicity of pain.
  - Pain tolerance
❖ Assess whether the pain is acute or chronic.
❖ Observe for the following behavioral responses.
  - Physiologic manifestations (changes in pulse, blood pressure, respiratory rate, etc.)
  - Verbal statements
  - Vocal responses
  - Facial expressions
  - Body movements
  - Alteration in response to the environment
  - Physical contact with others
  - Adaptation of physiological and behavioral responses
  - Effect of pain on ability to communicate and carry out usual activities of daily living.

PAIN ASSESSMENT TOOLS

❖ **Numeric pain rating scale:** It is the simplest and most commonly used numeric scale in which the individual rates the pain from 0 (no pain) to 10 (worst pain) **(Fig. 10.1)**.

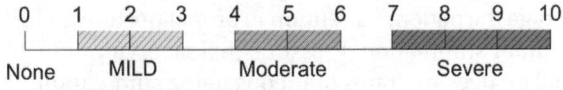

Fig. 10.1: 0–10 numeric pain rating scale.

❖ **Visual analogue scale/graphic rating scale:** It consists of straight line at extremes end point, one with no pain and other with severe pain. In this scale patient is asked to point the pain on the line between the end points **(Fig. 10.2)**.

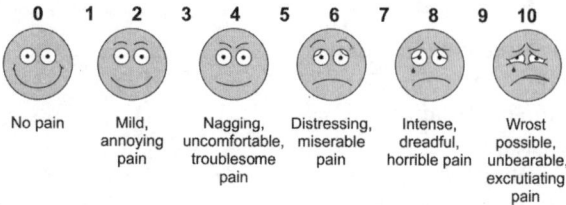

Fig. 10.2: Visual analogue scale/graphic rating scale.

MANAGEMENT

Management of pain depends upon the underlying condition. For the severe episodic spasmodic pain antispasmodics can be given. Analgesics can be given to tide over the situation depending upon the severity and response to the given drugs as per the prescription of physician.

Pharmacological Measures (as per the Doctor's Prescription)

- Anticholinergics (hyoscine butylbromide—buscopan) for colicky pains (ureteric, intestinal, biliary).
- Nonsteroidal anti-inflammatory drugs (NSAIDs) such as diclofenac or ibuprofen are used.
- Pentazocine or morphine can be administered to manage emergency severe pain.
- Tamsulosin or other alpha-blockers can be used for ureteric colic.

Non-pharmacological Measures

- Immobilize or rest affected area.
- Relieve pressure areas with turning or pressure reduction devices such as air-fluidized support systems.
- Provide therapeutic positioning.
- Encourage the patient's attention to proper posture and alignment.
- Use counter stimulation: Pressure, massage, vibration, heat/cold, external analgesics, transcutaneous nerve stimulation.
- Provide a supportive environment.
- Provide diversional therapy or music therapy.
- Discuss strategies to reduce enhancement of pain.
- Provide touch, especially for infants or for disoriented or unresponsive patients.

CHAPTER 11

Restraints and Safety Devices

INTRODUCTION

An environment that is safe and healthy is one that is lacking injuries, with a focus on preventing poisoning, fires, burns, falls, and electrical injuries. The nurse must be aware of potential safety problems and must know how to report and respond when safety is threatened.

The responsibility for providing and maintaining a safe environment involves the patient, visitors, and members of the healthcare team. Both protection and education are primary nursing responsibilities.

DEFINITION

A "restraint" is defined as any physical or chemical means or device that restricts client's freedom to and ability to move about and cannot be easily removed or eliminated by the client. It is the intentional restriction of a person's voluntary movement or behavior.

A "safety device", also referred to as a protective device, is defined as a device that is customarily used for a particular treatment. An intravenous arm board that is used to stabilize an intravenous line is an example of a safety device which is not considered a restraint.

PURPOSES

- To carry out the physical examination.
- To provide the safety to individual.
- To complete the diagnostic and therapeutic procedures.
- To protect the immediate safety of the patient or others.
- To prevent patients from falling.
- To prevent a confused patient form removing any life support equipment.
- To reduce the risk of injury to others.

GENERAL PRINCIPLES FOR USE OF RESTRAINTS

- It should be selected to reduce client's movement only as much as necessary.
- Nurse should carefully explain type of restraint and reason for its use.
- It should not interfere with treatment.
- Bony prominences should be padded before applying it.
- It should be secured away from client's reach.
- It should be attached to bed frame not to side rails.
- Frequent circulations checks should be performed when extremity is used.
- Explain the need for application and type of restraints.
- Consider the emotional impact of application on family and friends.
- Restraints shouldn't be applied without doctor's order.
- Consent should be obtained before application of restraints.
- Restrains should be used with greatest care.
- Circulation must not be occluded.
- Untie the restraint at least every 4 hours.
- Skin folds should be clean and dry prior to application of restraint.
- Ensure that there are no wrinkles in restraints.

TYPES OF RESTRAINTS

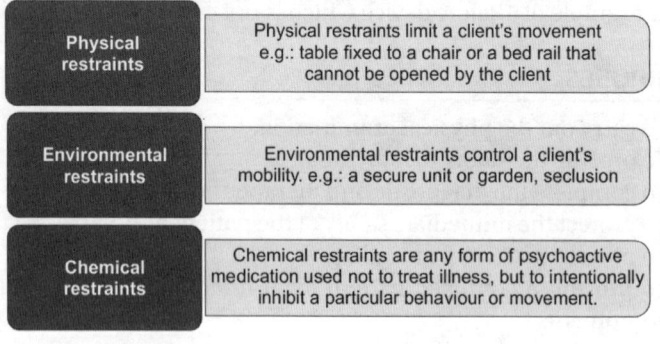

Types of Physical Restraints

Mummy restraint 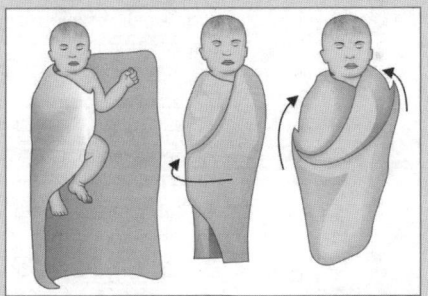	• Short type of restraints which is used in infants to immobilize the arms and legs for a short period of time. • It involves securing a sheet or blanket around the child's body in such a way that his arms are held to his sides and his leg space movements are restricted
Elbow restraint 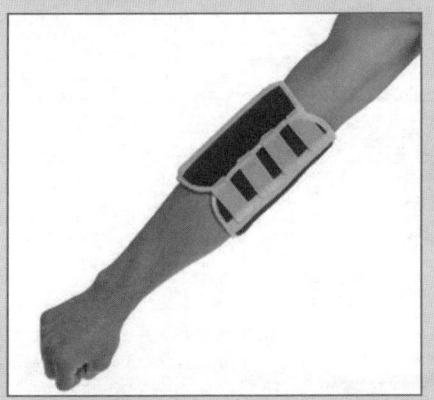	• It is used to prevent flexion of the elbow in an extended position so that individual cannot reach the face. • It is commonly used for NG tube feeding, vein infusion, etc.
Jacket restraint 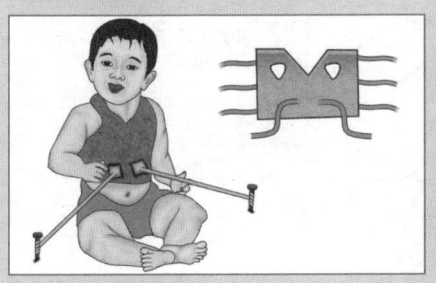	• It is used to help the child to remain flat in a supine position or to prevent the child from falling from crib, highchair, wheelchair. • The jacket is put on with the strings and the opening in the back and tied securely.

Restraints and Safety Devices

Clove-Hitch restraint 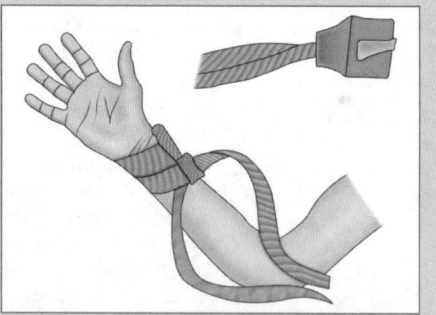	• It is used to immobilize the arm or leg. It is prepared from a piece of gauze or soft cloth or crepe bandage. • The wrist or ankle is placed in the loops of the device. The ends of the device are pulled to make it firm and tied to the cot frame. It should be tight enough to prevent slipping off the hand or foot.
Mitten or finger restraint 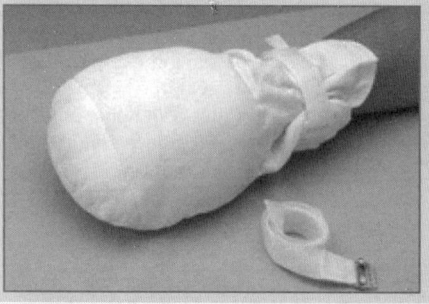	• Mitts are used for infants to prevent self-injury by hands in case of burns, facial injury or operations, eczema of the face or body. • Mitten can be made wrapping the child's hands in gauze or with a little bag putting over the baby's hand and tie it on at the wrist.
Safety belts 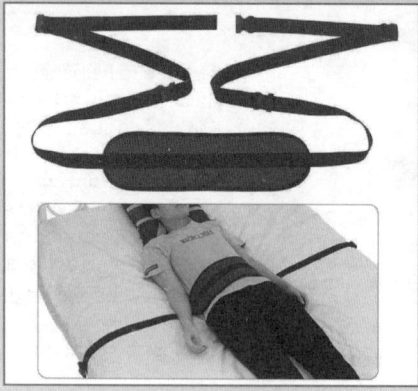	It is made of electrically nonconductive materials. These are frequently used on stretchers and operation tables to prevent the client from falling.

Other Safety Devices

Side rails 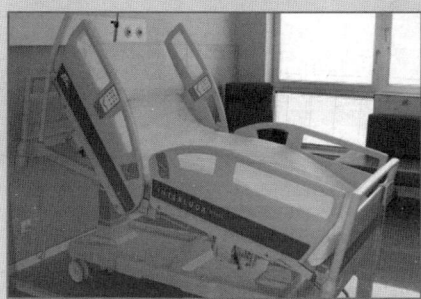	• Side rails are attached to both sides of the bed to prevent the client from getting out or falling out of the bed. • It must be kept raised on beds of all clients who have altered level of consciousness.
Trapeze 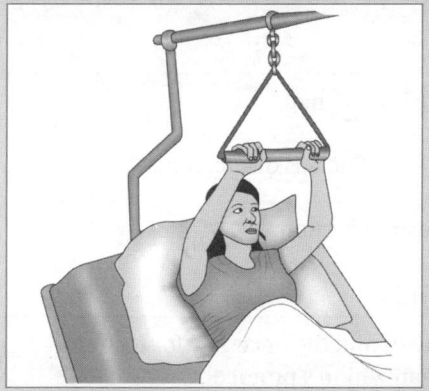	• A trapeze, a horizontal bar hanging on chains, is often attached to a large overhead frame, which itself attaches to the bed. • The trapeze is used by the client to pull up to a sitting position or to lift the shoulders and hips off the bed.
Grab bars 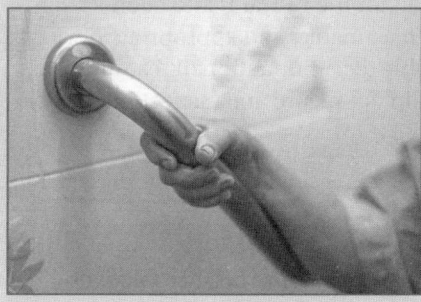	Grab bars or wall bars are the safety devices that are designed to enable a person to maintain balance, lessen fatigue while standing, comfortably redistribute their weight while maneuvering, and, most importantly, give them something to grab onto in case of a slip or fall.

Non-skit slippers

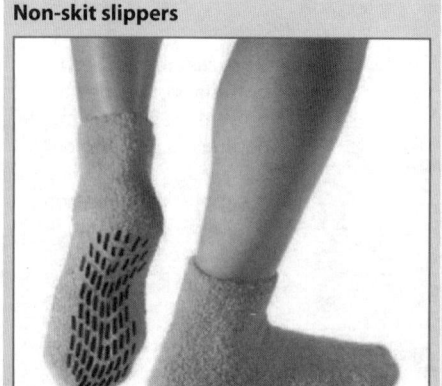

They are the specialized slippers that prevent fall and slipping.

HAZARDS OF RESTRAINTS

- Patients feel that he or she is punished.
- Foot drop or wrist drop.
- Damage to other parts of body such as dislocation.
- Development of pressure sores.
- Tissue damage due to constant friction.

NURSING RESPONSIBILITIES

- Evaluate the client's behavior and the necessity for restraint.
- Obtain consent as per organization's protocol.
- Must communicates with the client and family members.
- Explain the client the reason for the restraint and cooperation.
- Apply the least restrictive, reasonable, and appropriate devices.
- Consider the earliest possible discontinuation of restraint.
- Document the use of restraint for record and inspection purposes.

NURSING PROCEDURE

- Check for the physician order.
- Identify the client.
- Explain the procedure to the patients and his/her relatives.
- Allow the patient to ask question and encourage his/him to participate in the procedure as much as possible.
- Ensure patients privacy.

- ❖ Wash and dry hands.
- ❖ Arrange the articles near the patient's bed side.
- ❖ Make sure that the restraints are correct size for the patients build and weight.
- ❖ Obtain adequate assistance to manually restrain the patient.

Role of Nurse in Restraints

- Monitor a patient in restraint every 15 minutes for:
  - Signs of injury
  - Circulation and range of motion
  - Comfort
  - Readiness for discontinuation of restraint
- Documentation in every 2 hours for:
  - Release the patient, turn, and position.
  - Institute a trial of restraint release.
  - Hydration and nutrition need.
  - Elimination needs.
  - Comfort and repositioning needs.

CHAPTER 12

Hospital Admission and Discharge

INTRODUCTION

Patient admission, hospital stay, and discharge are the planned nursing activities as per the organization policy. Patients requiring long-term care and repeated hospitalization, these activities must be coordinated so that the nursing care is continuous. The specific medical treatment prescribed by the doctor, and the nursing regime followed by the nurse, are administered by the nurse to meet patient needs. The nurse monitors patient responses throughout the stay **(Flowchart 12.1)**.

ADMISSION

DEFINITION

Admission of a patient is the hospital stay for observation, investigation, diagnosis, treatment, and care. It is for therapeutic/diagnostic purposes.

PURPOSES

- To welcome patient.
- To establish a positive relationship with patient, nurse-patient relationship.

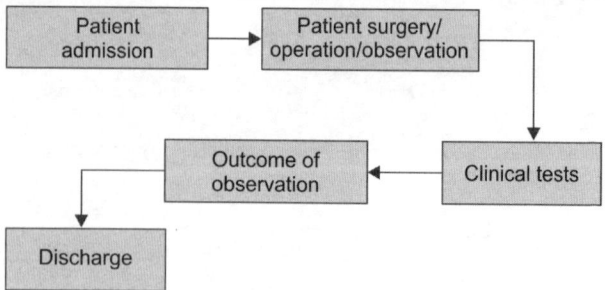

Flowchart 12.1: Patient's journey from admission to discharge.

Hospital Admission and Discharge

- To establish guidelines regarding admission of patients.
- To make the patient feel comfortable and at ease.
- To acquire vital information regarding the patient.
- To assess the patient from which the nursing care plan can be initiated and implemented.
- To assist patient in adjusting to the hospital environment.
- To obtain information that will serve as a basis of care.
- To offer immediate management and care in acute disease conditions.

ADMISSION PROCESS (FLOWCHART 12.2)

An entering to the healthcare agency for nursing care and medical or surgical treatment to meet patients' healthcare needs. During the admission process, nurses provide a holistic care and establish the basis for how patients will respond to and evaluate the remainder of their stay.

ARTICLE REQUIRED

- Prepared bed
- Thermometer tray

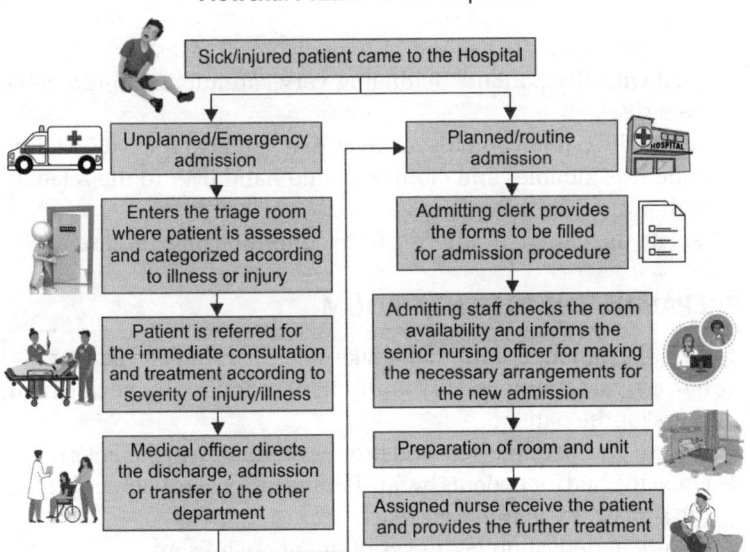

Flowchart 12.2: Admission process.

- ❖ BP apparatus
- ❖ Weighing machine (scale)
- ❖ Admission advisory form (from admitting department)
- ❖ Documents such as:
  - ◆ Doctor's order sheet
  - ◆ TPR sheet
  - ◆ Nursing assessment form
  - ◆ Nurses' record
  - ◆ Progress record/notes
  - ◆ Laboratory master sheet
  - ◆ Additional sheets as indicated, such as diabetic urine chart, intake output chart, and specific flow sheets, admission consent form.
- ❖ Kidney tray or emesis basin
- ❖ Tissue paper
- ❖ Bedpan and/or urinal
- ❖ Bath towels and wash cloth

GENERAL INSTRUCTIONS

- ❖ The nurse should address the patient by their name and proper title.
- ❖ Make proper observations of the patient's condition, record, and report.
- ❖ Observe policies in dealing with medicolegal cases.
- ❖ Deal with the patients belonging very carefully communicable diseases.
- ❖ Orient the patient and his relatives to hospital and ward policies.
- ❖ Patient's valuables and clothes should hand over to the relatives with proper recording.
- ❖ Isolate the patient if suffering from communicable diseases.

PREPARING THE PATIENT'S ROOM

- ❖ Before a patient is admitted, make sure the room is ready for his/her arrival with necessary equipment, admission checklist and dress for the patient.
- ❖ Ensure the adequate light and proper ventilation in patient's room.
- ❖ Open the bed for patients by fan-folding the covers back and attach the signal cord within easy reach.
- ❖ Ensure patient supplies and equipment are present.

PROCEDURE

- Greet the patient and introduce yourself.
- Receive the patient cordially and seat comfortable.
- Introduce him to another person in the ward.
- Complete the admission record.
- Collect history and carry out simple physical examination.
- Carry out the prescribed treatment and keep a record.
- Help the patient to maintain personal hygiene and change into hospital clothes.
- Orient the patient to the ward—toilet, bathroom, drinking water supply, nurse's station, and treatment room.
- Handover the patients valuable to his relatives.
- Issue visitor pass.
- Encourage patient to take hospital diet especially when therapeutic diet is ordered.
- Obtain local address or telephone number, relatives lodge room and document in admission record.
- Ensure the call light is within patient's reach, bed is in lowered positioned and raised side rails.

DISCHARGE

DEFINITION

Discharge planning is a centralized, coordinated, multidisciplinary process. Discharge of patient from the hospital means, reliving a person from hospital setting, who admitted as an inpatient in that hospital. It is the termination of care from a hospital (**Flowchart 12.3**).

REASONS FOR DISCHARGE

- Cured
- Transfer to other hospital
- Discharged on request.
- Discharged against medical advice.
- Death.

PRELIMINARY ASSESSMENT

- Physician's written order for discharge.

Flowchart 12.3: Discharge process.

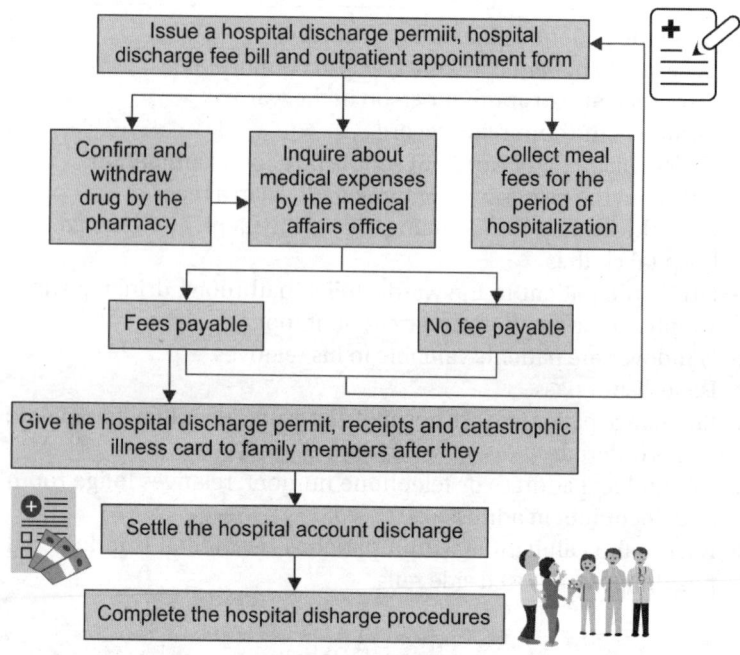

- Inform patient and relative about discharge.
- Document relevant discharge information.

DEPARTMENTS TO BE INFORMED

- Drug return to pharmacy department
- Diet cancellation
- Oxygen/ventilator charges summary
- Billing section

ARTICLES REQUIRED

- Wheelchair or stretcher.
- Patient relevant documents: Discharge booklet, prescription order

PROCEDURE

- Verify physician's written order for discharge.
- Inform the patient and relatives about discharge.

- Document relevant discharge information.
- Ensure that all costs, including those for specific investigations, special items or gadgets, physician or surgeon fees, and any narcotics used, are included (if any).
- Obtain discharge prescription after retaining the medicines to be continued for that day and after discharge. Send all other continued for that day and after discharge. Send all other medicines for refunding (include ward replacement).
- Send a chart with the necessary information to the billing section.
- One bill is prepared, and the ward has received the chart back; make sure the bill is paid. Verify the discharge bill's signature is that of the cashier.
- Assist the patient in obtaining the discharge summary, medical certificate, and drugs.
- Ensure that patient is instructed regarding medication follow up, outpatient visit, etc.
- Accompany the patient up to transport near exit gate.

CHAPTER 13

Mobility and Immobility

INTRODUCTION

Body alignment is a key factor for a nurse. She needs to serve the patient in various ways, such as lifting, transferring, moving, and shifting. She needs to use proper balance and technique to maintain body alignment. She also needs to ensure stability with base support, avoid straining the lower back, face the patient and prevent injury, and do it with minimal effort.

NORMAL MOBILITY

Normal movements are possible with musculoskeletal system, central and peripheral nervous system. The musculoskeletal system provides structural framework to the body and involved in body movement. The nervous system coordinates the complex act of movement.

The cerebellum, cerebral cortex and basal ganglia are responsible for control of motor functions such as the mechanism of alignment, posture, and balance for coordinated movement.

BODY MECHANICS

Body mechanics is defined as using alignment, posture, and balance in a coordinated effort to perform activities such as lifting, bending, and moving.

Good body mechanics means practicing good posture throughout the day. Use good body mechanics all the time.

Proper body mechanics is essential for nurses and other healthcare professionals to prevent injury to themselves and their patients.

Some tips to maintain proper body mechanics:
- **Keep a wide base of support:** Keep the feet shoulder-width apart to maintain a stable base of support.
- **Bend at the knees:** When lifting or bending, bend at the knees rather than at the waist to reduce stress on your back.

- **Use your legs:** Use the leg muscles to lift, push, or pull rather than the back muscles.
- **Keep the back straight:** Keep the back straight and avoid twisting the spine.
- **Don't lift alone:** Always ask for help when lifting or transferring patients who are too heavy or require more than one person.

When assisting patients in moving, turning, or logrolling, nurses should use proper body mechanics to prevent injury to themselves and their patients. They should position themselves close to the patient, bend their knees, and avoid twisting their spine. They should also communicate with the patient and provide clear instructions during the process.

Principles of Body Mechanics

The principles of body mechanics are all about maintaining proper posture and using the correct movements during physical activity to prevent injury and promote efficient use of energy. Some of the key principles of body mechanics are:

- Proper balancing of all body parts helps to conserve energy.
- Stability of the body is maintained by having a greater base of support.
- Keep your spine in a neutral position.
- Bend at the hips and knees, not at the waist.
- Use your legs to lift, not your back.
- Keep objects close to your body when carrying them.
- Avoid twisting your spine while lifting or carrying objects.
- Use your larger, stronger muscles to do the heavy lifting.
- Take frequent breaks and change positions often.
- Use proper ergonomics in the office or work environment to minimize strain on your body.

IMPACT OF IMMOBILITY AND INACTIVITY

Refer **Table 13.1**.

EXERCISE

It is an activity that requires alignment, posture, balance and coordinated movement. It is beneficial for psychological and physiological body functioning.

Table 13.1: Impact of immobility and inactivity on organ systems.

Organ system	Effect
Musculoskeletal	
Muscles	Reduced strength, endurance, flexibility, and bulk
Joints	Reduced flexibility, joint contractures
Bone	Osteopenia and osteoporosis
Cardiovascular	• Reduced stroke volume, cardiac output, and exercise capacity • Reduced orthostatic tolerance and venous return • Deep vein thrombosis
Respiratory	• Atelectasis • Pneumonia
Integumentary	Pressure ulcers
Psychological	• Reduced self-image and stress tolerance • Anxiety • Depression

Classification of Exercise

Refer **Flowchart 13.1**.

Aerobic Exercise

Aerobic exercise is any physical activity that increases the heart rate and breathing rate for an extended period of time. This type of exercise primarily relies on oxygen to produce energy.

Examples: Brisk walking, running, cycling, or swimming.

Flowchart 13.1: Classification of exercise.

```
                    ┌─ Based on source ─┬─ Aerobic
                    │  of energy        └─ Anaerobic
        Exercise ───┤
                    │                   ┌─ Isotonic
                    └─ Based on muscle ─┼─ Isometric
                       tension          └─ Isokinetic
```

Anaerobic Exercise

Anaerobic exercise is defined as any physical activity that involves short bursts of intense activity that are not sustained over an extended period of time. This type of exercise primarily relies on energy sources in the body other than oxygen.

Examples: High-intensity interval training (HIIT), weightlifting, or sprinting.

Isotonic Exercise

Isotonic exercises involve movements that cause the muscle contraction and muscle tension, such as lifting weights or doing push-ups. These exercises help to improve muscular strength and endurance, as well as joint flexibility.

Examples: Squats, lunges, bicep curls, push-ups, and pull-ups.

Isometric Exercise

Isometric exercises involve holding a static position, such as a plank or wall sit, without any movement. These exercises help to improve muscular strength and endurance, as well as joint stability.

Examples: Planks, wall sits, and bridges.

Isokinetic Exercise

Isokinetic exercises involve movements that are performed at a constant speed, usually with the help of specialized equipment. These exercises help to improve muscular strength and endurance and are often used in physical therapy to help people recover from injuries.

Examples: Using a rowing machine, stationary bike, or leg extension machine that controls the speed of movement.

Range of Motion Exercises

Range of motion (ROM) exercises are designed to help improve the flexibility and mobility of joints and muscles. They are often used to help people recover from injuries or surgeries, or to manage conditions that affect joint mobility.

Methods of Doing ROM Exercises

- Flexion (bending or folding movements), extension (straightening movements) **(Fig. 13.1)**.

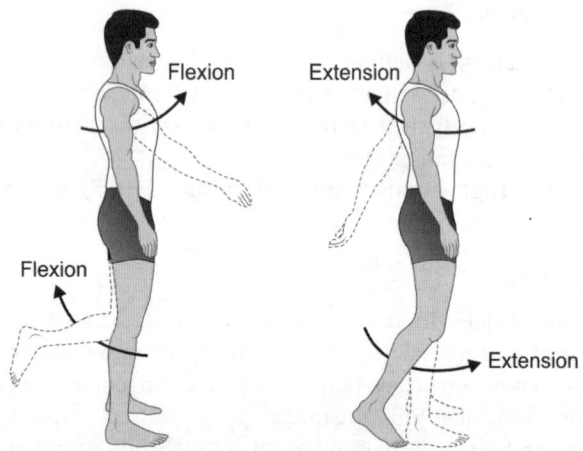

Fig. 13.1: Flexion and extension.

- Hyperextension (straightening beyond than normal) **(Fig. 13.2)**.

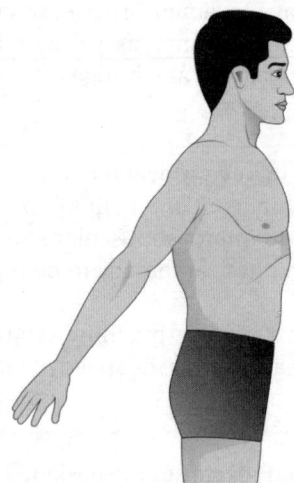

Fig. 13.2: Hyperextension.

- Abduction (moving bone away from middle part of the body) and adduction (moves the part towards the middle of the body) **(Fig. 13.3)**.

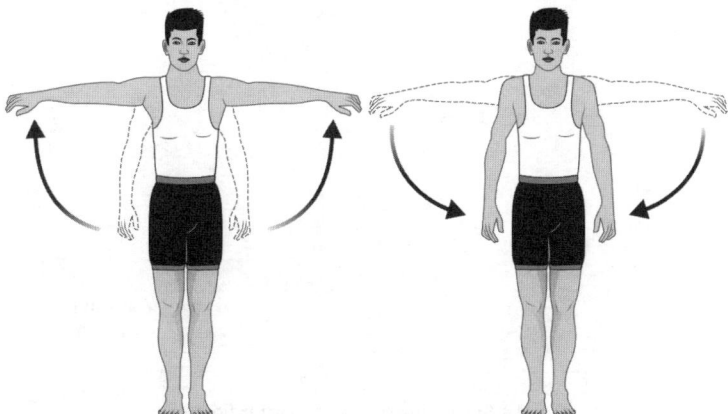

Fig. 13.3: Abduction and adduction.

- Inward rotation and outward rotation (moving of a bone upon its own axis) **(Fig. 13.4)**.

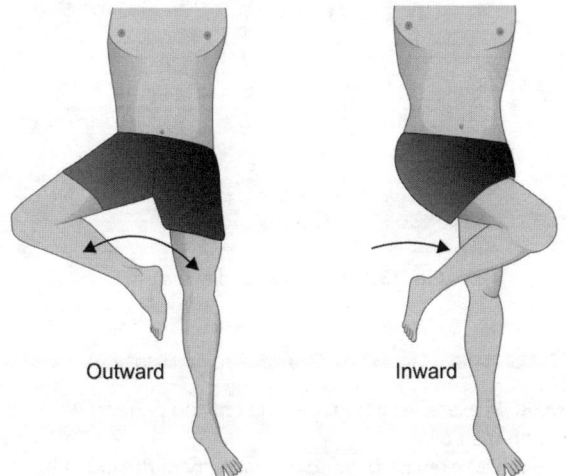

Outward   Inward

Fig. 13.4: Inward and outward rotation.

- Movements of the feet and toes are also important. The ankle joint permits dorsal flexion and planter flexion **(Fig. 13.5)**.

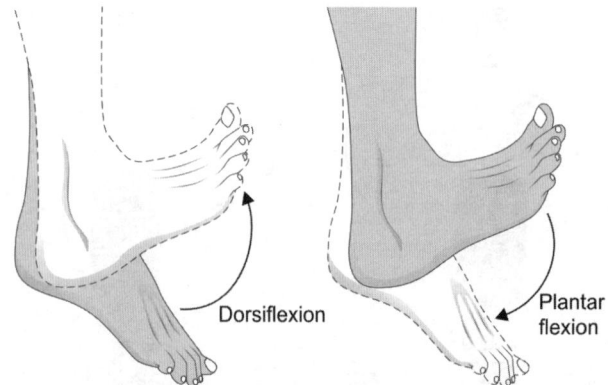

Fig. 13.5: Dorsiflexion and plantar flexion.

- Inversion (turns the sole of the foot inward) and eversion (turns it outward) of feet also needs to be done **(Fig. 13.6)**.

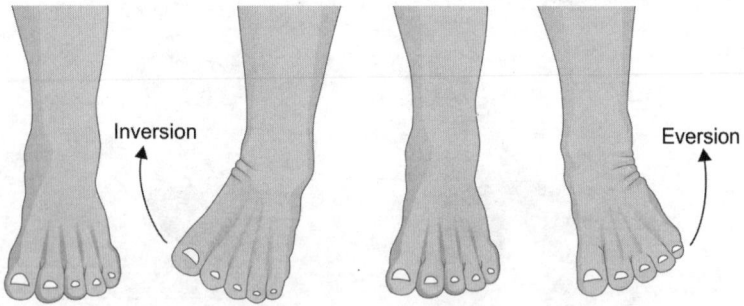

Fig. 13.6: Inversion and eversion.

Note

- Passive ROM exercise should be done only on patients who are unable to do it on their own.
- Never do ROM exercise beyond the capacity of the individual that is to the point of discomfort.
- Move body parts smoothly, slowly, and rhythmically.
- Expect heart rate and respiratory rate to increase during exercise, which should return to resting levels within 3 minutes, if not, exercises are strenuous for patient.

Mobility and Immobility

Preliminary Assessment
- Check the doctors order for any specific instructions such as position, movements, etc.
- Assess the general condition and diagnosis of the patient.
- Assess the self-care ability of the patient.

Preparation of the Patient
- Explain the sequence of the procedure.
- Provide privacy.
- Adjust the height of the bed if possible.
- Place the patient in comfortable position.

Steps of Procedure
- Wash hands thoroughly.
- Support the extremity or the part to be moved above and below joint.
- Do not hold the joint.
- Perform all movements smoothly and slowly.
- If pain or strong resistance is present, do not force movement.
- Perform each movement three times during exercise periods per day.
- Exercise period may be incorporated to an activity such as bed bath.
- Start providing passive ROM exercise from the head downward.
- **Neck (Fig. 13.7):**
  - Move head through flexion, extension, lateral flexion, rotation, and hyperextension of the neck.
  - Movement of head is contraindicated in spinal surgery, spinal trauma, and other central nervous system trauma and for patients having central venous line.

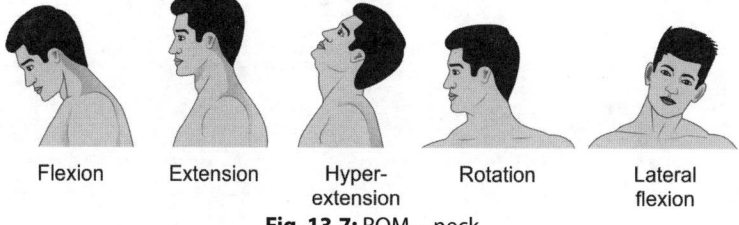

Flexion   Extension   Hyper-extension   Rotation   Lateral flexion

Fig. 13.7: ROM—neck.

- **Shoulder (Fig. 13.8):** Flexion, extension, hyperextension, abduction, adduction, and circumduction, external rotation, and internal rotation. Shoulder should be supported proximally and distally.

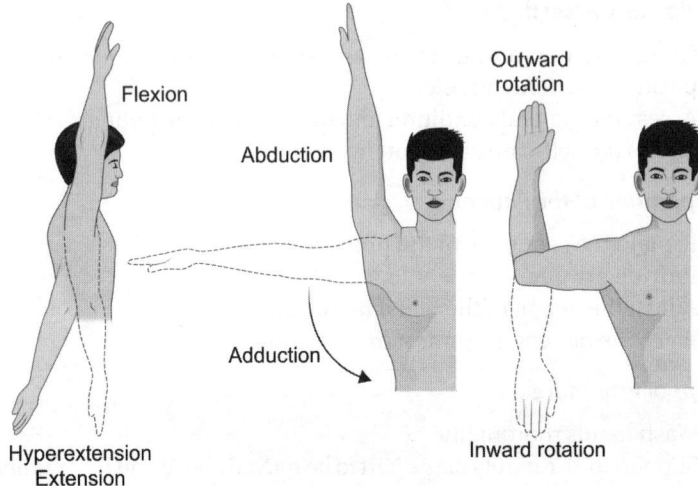

Fig. 13.8: ROM—shoulder.

- **Trunk (Fig. 13.9):** Flexion, extension, hyperextension lateral flexion, and rotation of the trunk.

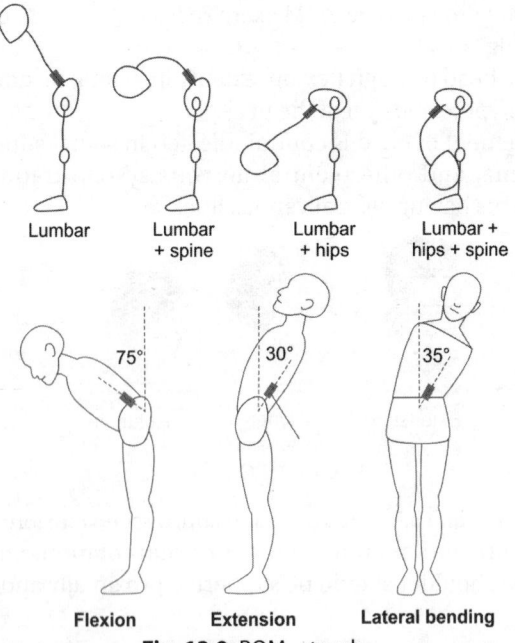

Fig. 13.9: ROM—trunk.

- ❖ **Elbow:** Flexion, extension, pronation, and supination. Support elbow joint both proximally and distally **(Fig. 13.10).**

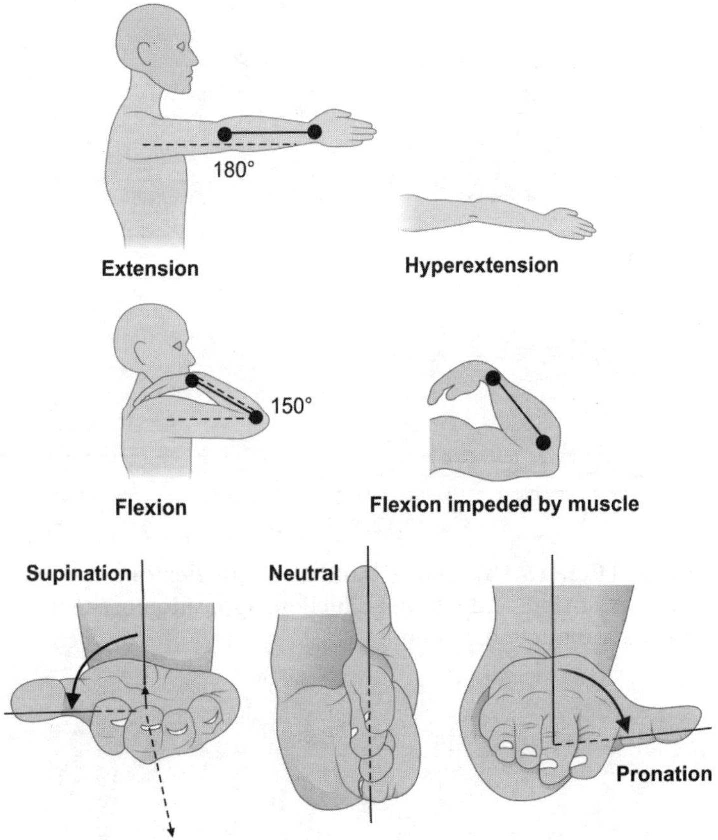

Fig. 13.10: ROM—elbow.

- ❖ **Forearm (Fig. 13.11):** Pronation and supination. Position wrist in functional position.

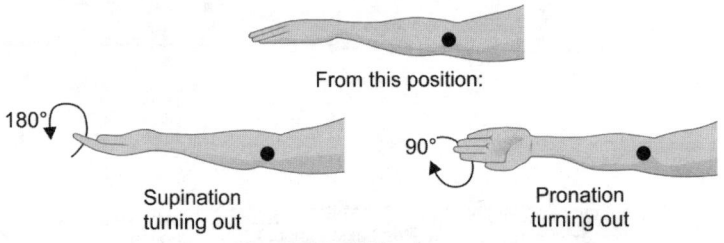

Fig. 13.11: ROM—forearm.

- **Wrist (Fig. 13.12):** Flexion, extension, hyperextension, and lateral flexion (radial and ulnar). Position wrist in functional position.

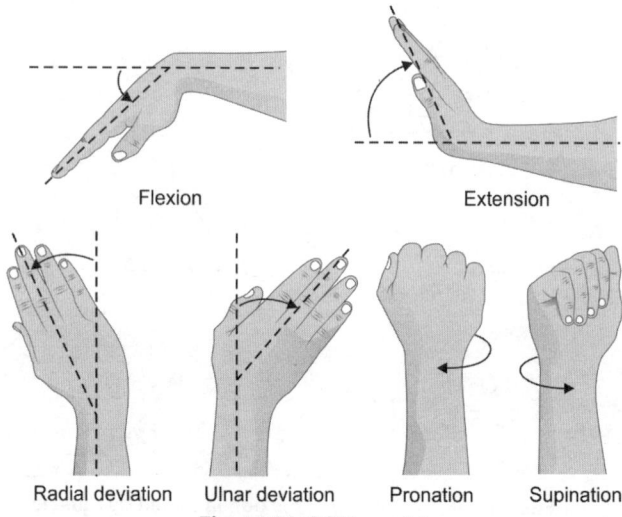

Fig. 13.12: ROM—wrist.

- **Hand (Fig. 13.13):** Move hand through flexion, extension, hyperextension, abduction, adduction, apposition of the thumb, and circumduction of thumb.

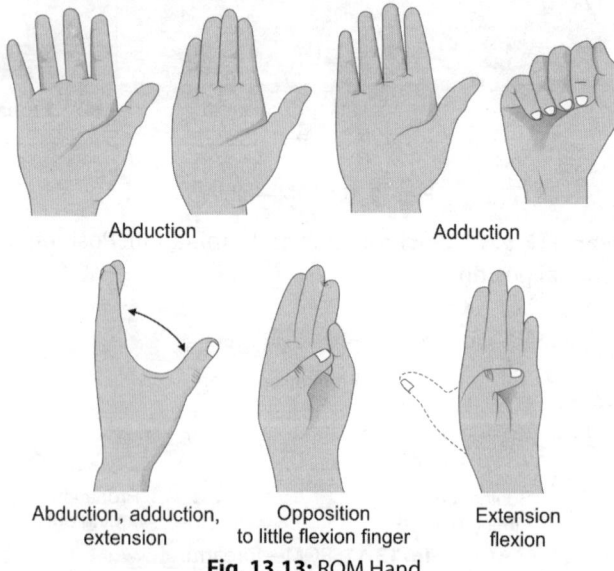

Fig. 13.13: ROM Hand

❖ **Hip (Figs. 13.14A to E):** Move hip through flexion, extension, abduction, adduction, internal and external rotations, and circumduction with support of the above and below joints.

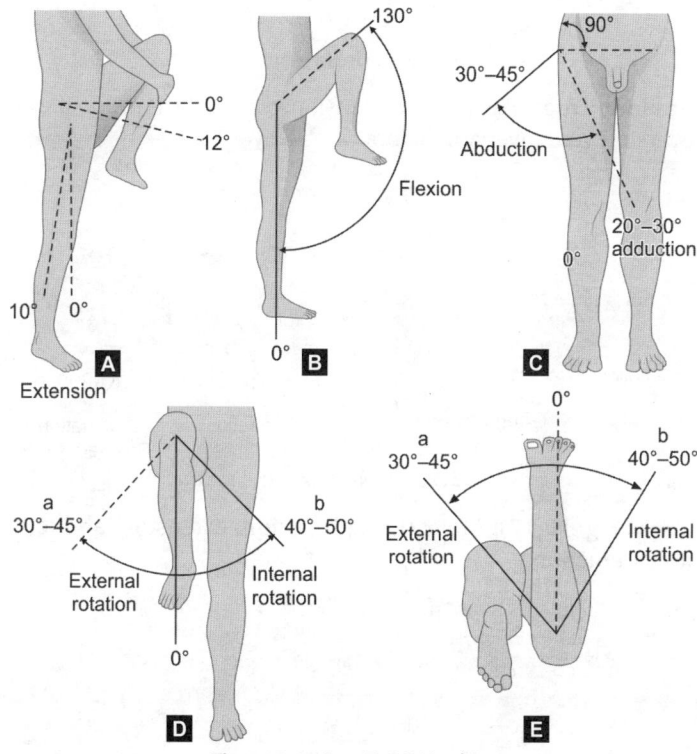

Figs. 13.14A to E: ROM—hip.

❖ **Knee (Fig. 13.15):** Move knee through flexion and extension.

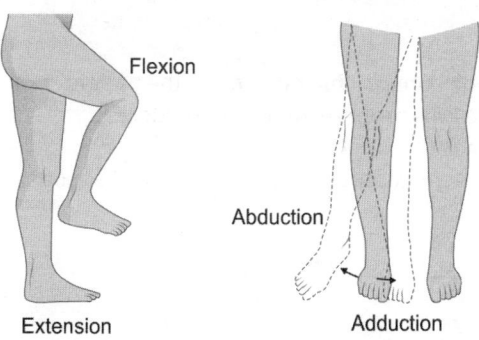

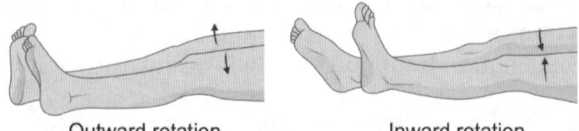

Fig. 13.15: ROM—knee.

- **Ankle and foot (Fig. 13.16):** Extension, plantar flexion, dorsiflexion, eversion, and inversion of foot.

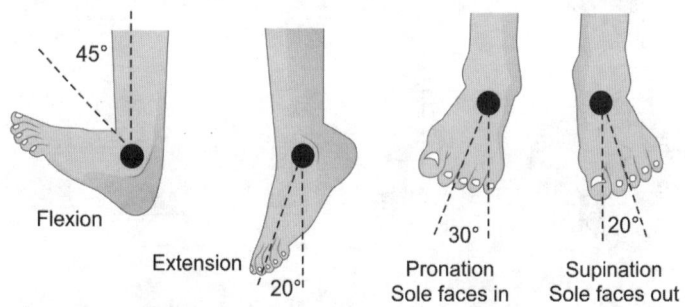

Fig. 13.16: ROM—ankle and foot.

- **Toes (Fig. 13.17):** Move through flexion, extension, abduction, and adduction.

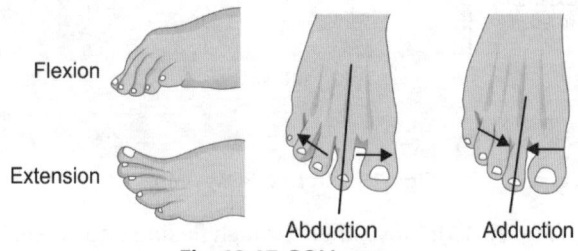

Fig. 13.17: ROM—toes.

After Care

- Provide the comfortable position to the patient.
- Place side rails properly to promote safety.
- Wash hands thoroughly.
- Record the procedure in the nurse's record sheet.

CHAPTER 14

Bandages and Dressings

INTRODUCTION

Bandages and dressings are used to provide support and to limit the movement of a bodily part. In some instances, a dressing is applied directly to the wound and a bandage is used to keep it in place. A dressing is used to contain bleeding by covering a skin break.

BANDAGES

Bandages are soft, absorbent gauze or other material that is applied to a limb or other part of the body.

Purposes

Bandage may be used for the following purposes:
- To reduce movement of a joint.
- To retain a splint in position.
- To serve as an improvised tourniquet.
- To keep dressings, poultice or splints in position.
- To give support to a limb or tissues.
- To reduce or prevent swelling.
- To correct deformity.
- To control bleeding.
- To limit movement.

Bandages can be improvised by using any soft clean pieces of cotton cloth such as a handkerchief, a towel or pieces of sheeting. Bandages may be either triangular or long strips. The bandage can be used in three forms:
1. In the triangular form.
2. In the broad-fold form.
3. In the narrow-fold form.

Principles of Bandaging
- It entirely covers the dressing and yet is not cumbersome to the patient.

- It should be firm enough to keep the dressing in place, yet not so tight that it causes discomfort, or impedes circulation (except in case of a bandage applied to stop bleeding).
- It is neat in appearance.

Patterns Used in Bandaging

1. **Circular turns:** Circular turns is used to bandage the proximal aspect of a finger or a wrist **(Fig. 14.1)**. Steps includes:
   - Apply the bandage's end to the area of the body that needs bandaging.
   - Encircle the body part several times or as close as possible, with each turn directly covering the previous turn.
   - Over a healthy area, fasten the bandage's end with tape, metal clips, or a safety pin.

   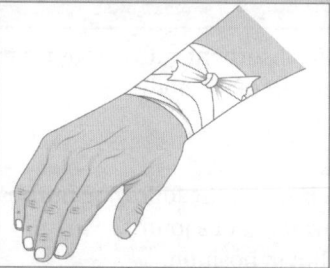

   Fig. 14.1: Circular bandage.

2. **Simple spiral/spiral turn:** Body parts with relatively uniform circumferences, like the upper arm or upper leg, are bandaged using spiral turns **(Fig. 14.2)**. Steps include:
   - To secure the bandage, make two circular turns.
   - Continue making spiral turns at a 30° angle, overlapping each turn by two-thirds of the bandage's width.
   - Wrap the bandage twice in a circle to finish

   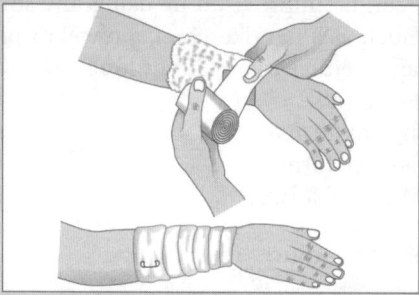

   Fig. 14.2: Simple spiral bandage.

3. **Reversed spiral:** Reverse spiral is used on limbs where, owing to varying thickness, a simple spiral bandage would not lie smoothly. It is applied on cylindrical body parts. Steps include **(Fig. 14.3)**:
   - Make two circular turns and bring the bandage upwards at about 30° angle.
   - On the upper edge of the bandage, place the thumb of the free hand.
   - Unroll the bandage around about 15 cm (6 inches) then turn the hand so that the bandage falls over itself.
   - Continue wrapping the bandage around the limb, overlapping each previous turn by two-thirds the width of the bandage, and making each bandage turn at the same position on the limb so that the bandage turns are aligned.
   - Secure the bandage with two circular turns.

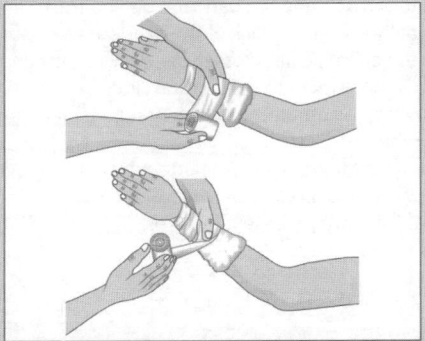

Fig. 14.3: Reversed spiral bandage.

4. **Figure-of-eight:** Figure-of-eight **(Fig. 14.4)** may be used on limbs instead of the reversed spiral, and for the hand and foot. Following steps shows knee bandage using figure-of-eight.
   - Flex the knee and place the bandage's outer side against the inner side of the knee (medial).
   - Make two straight/circular turns around the kneecap.

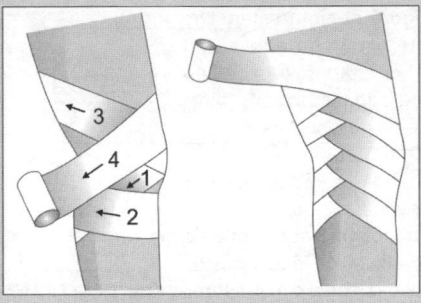

Fig. 14.4: Figure-of-eight.

- Turn below and above to cover one-third of the previous turn.
- Turn below and above the joint until the entire knee is covered.
- Finish with two circular turns around the thigh to secure the bandage.
- Use adhesive tape or a safety pin to secure the end.

5. **Spica:** The spica is a figure-of-eight in which one turn is significantly larger than the other. It is used for joints that are at right angles to the body, such as the shoulder, groin, and thumb as shown in **Figures 14.5A and B**. Steps include (Spica of thumb):
   - Place patient's hand in neutral position such that the thumb is slightly flexed at the base.
   - Hold one end of the bandage between the thumb and index finger.
   - Bring the bandage around the wrist, making one or two turns to secure the starting point.
   - From the wrist, bring the bandage behind the thumb and then diagonally across the back of the hand to the opposite side.
   - Once the bandage has crossed the back of the hand, bring it around the wrist once more to the starting side.
   - After wrapping around the wrist, bring the bandage behind the thumb once more.
   - Continue the figure-of-eight pattern by crossing over the back of the hand, wrapping around the wrist, and passing behind the thumb. Repeat this pattern for several turns.
   - Secure the bandage

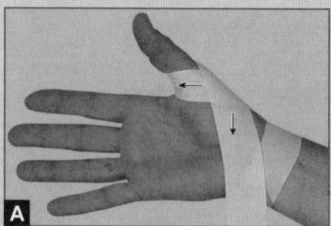 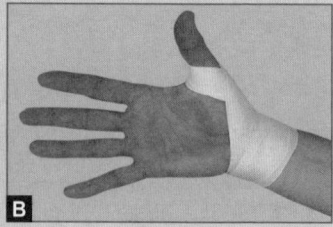

Figs. 14.5A and B: Spica of thumb.

6. **Divergent spica:** It is a variation of the figure-of-eight where the turns alternately go above and below a fixed starting turn ending above and is applied to bend joints like the elbow or heel as given in **Figure 14.6**. Steps include:
   - The bandage should be 2.5 inches wide.
   - Start bandaging at the middle of the elbow or joints and fix with two or three circular turns then, reverse the elbow.

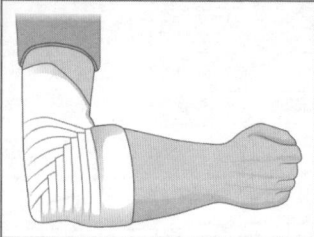

Fig. 14.6: Divergent spica of elbow.

- Once the forearm is fixed, place the middle of the bandage over the point of the elbow.
- Take the bandage from within forwards and outwards and over lower part of preceding turn.
- Then turn to the inner side again and outwards and over upper part of the first turn and so on.
- Finally, close the elbow with figure-of-eight.

7. **Recurrent bandage:** Recurrent bandage is used to cover blunt body parts, tips of fingers or a stump (amputated limb) and are fixed by using circular or spiral turns as shown in **Figures 14.7A to E**.
   - On the blunt body part, the bandage is repeatedly applied from one side across the top to the opposite side.
   - Not only the wound, but the entire length of the blunt body part should be covered in order to effectively fix the recurrent turns.
   - Successive turns are made to cover the preceding turn fully or partially

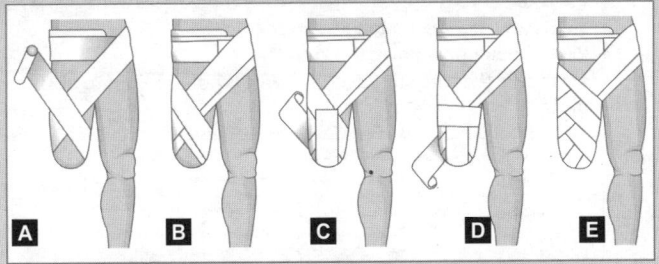

Figs. 14.7A to E: Recurrent bandage of stump.

8. **Capeline (head) bandage (Figs. 14.8A to E):** Capeline (head) bandage is used to cover whole scalp using double headed roller bandage.
   - Apply the dressing and keep it in place with a ring pad.
   - Stand in front of the patient and apply the triangular bandage to the head, so that the point hangs down at the back of the neck, and the base comes onto the forehead. Fold in the base if necessary.
   - Carry the ends around the head to cross below the back of the head and take back to the front to tie off at the front. Fold the point upon the head and pin.

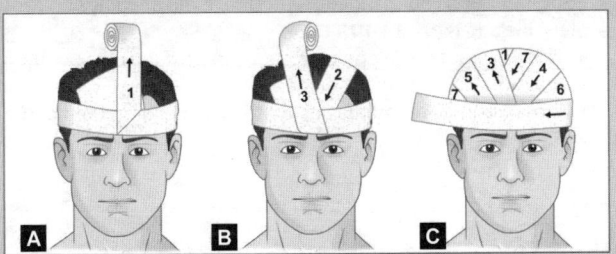

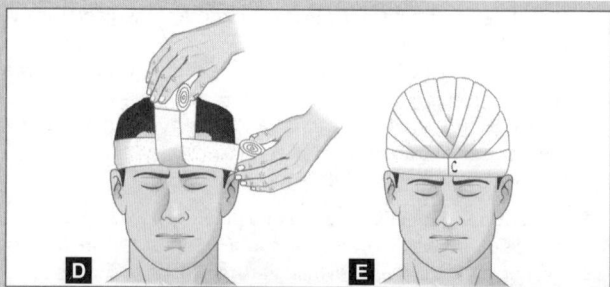

Figs. 14.8A to E: Capeline bandages of head.

9. **Hand bandage:** Hand bandage is used for retaining hand dressings. Steps include **(Figs. 14.9A to D)**:
   - Place the hand on the open bandage with fingers toward the point.
   - Bring the point down over the hand above the wrist.
   - Cross the ends round the wrist (two or three times as necessary).
   - Tie the ends of the bandage over the wrist.
   - Pin the point down over the knot.
   - Make sure that the knot over the wrist is not too tight to obstruct the pulse.

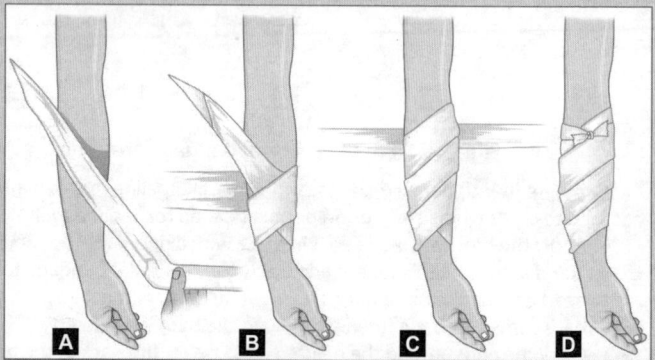

Figs. 14.9A to D: Triangular hand bandage.

10. **Foot bandage:** Foot bandage is used to retain dressings on the foot. Steps include **(Figs. 14.10A to E)**:
    - Place the foot on an open bandage, toes towards the point.
    - Bring the point up to the ankle.
    - Cross the ends round the ankle and tie the ends in front of the ankle.
    - Pin the point down over the knot

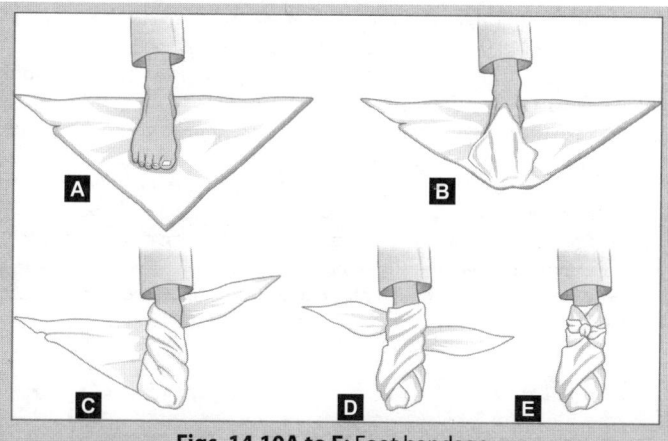

Figs. 14.10A to E: Foot bandage.

11. **Joint bandaging (Fig. 14.11):** The method of using the open triangular bandage is essentially the same for every joint. It is used to retain dressings, where a roller bandage would be bulky and uncomfortable.
    - Apply the triangular bandage to the part, pointing uppermost, and adjust the size by folding up the base as necessary.
    - Take the ends in each hand and carry them round behind the part. Cross them, thus changing hands at the back.
    - Bring the ends round to the front and tie them.
    - Pin down the point of the bandage.

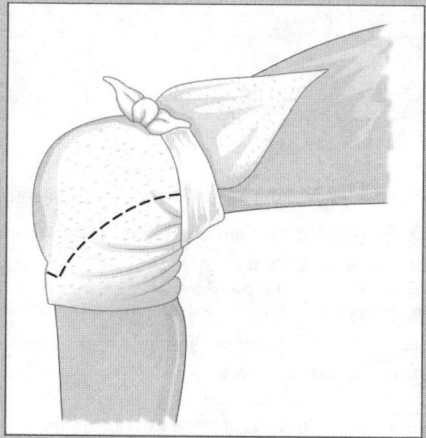

Fig. 14.11: Joint bandaging.

12. **Shoulder bandages:** Shoulder bandages is used for compression and support of shoulder. Steps include (**Figs. 14.12A to F**):
    - Wrap 3–4 inch bandage around the upper portion of the arm in spiral turns.
    - Take the bandage and make 2–3 reverse spiral turns round the upper arm till it reach the shoulder.
    - Take the bandage over the shoulder, across the back and under the opposite arm.
    - Continue the bandage across the chest and arm round under the armpit and over the shoulder.
    - When the entire shoulder is wrapped, pin it over the injured shoulder.

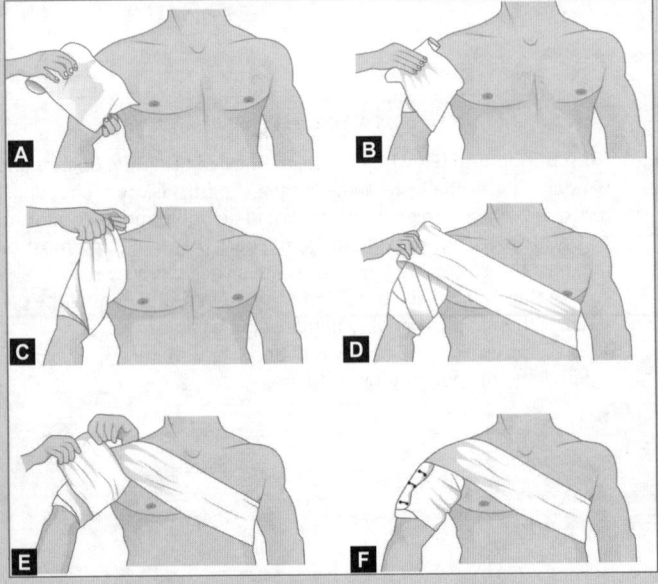

Figs. 14.12A to F: Shoulder bandages.

13. **Hip bandage (Fig. 14.13):** Hip bandage is applied for compression and stabilization of the hip joint.
    - Place the outside of the bandage about 6 inches below the groin on the inner side of the leg.
    - Take the bandage around the limb and make 3 or 4 ascending reverse spiral turns round the thigh.
    - Pass the tape from medial to lateral over the front of the groin, up around the hip and back, and over the prominence and hip bone on the opposite side.
    - Bring the bandage down, over the abdomen, to the exterior side of the thigh, and continue the figure-of-eight around the body and thigh until the hip is covered.

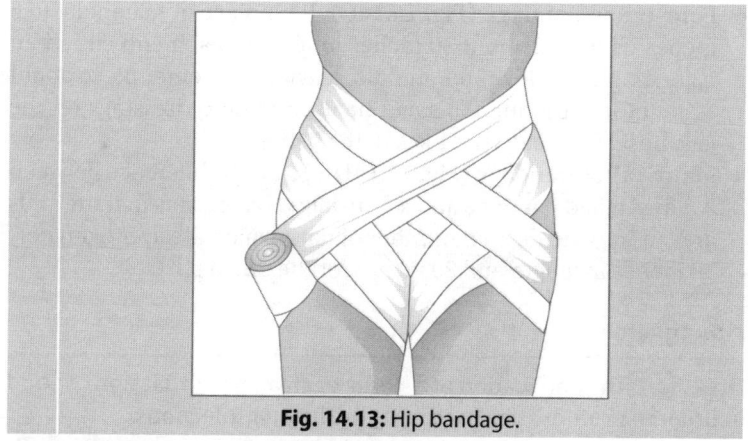

Fig. 14.13: Hip bandage.

Special Bandage: Tailed Bandages

Tailed bandages are used when roller bandages are not applicable. The tailed bandage includes:

- **T- bandage (Fig. 14.14A):** It is shaped like a "T" and is made up of a vertical strip of material sewn or pinned to the center of a horizontal strip. This can be used to bandage the scalp, ear, eye, or perineum.
- **Double T- bandage (Fig. 14.14B):** To do this, sew two vertical strips of fabric, spaced about 4 inches apart, to the centre of a horizontal strip. It can hold dressings for the perineum, back, or chest.

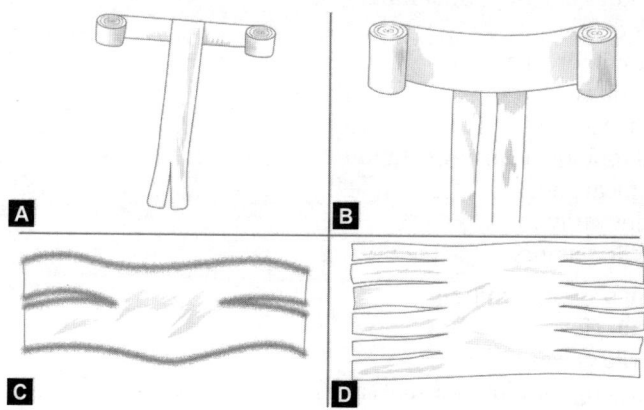

Figs. 14.14A to D: (A) T-bandage; (B) Double T-bandage; (C) Four-tailed bandage; (D) Many-tailed bandage.

- **Four-tailed bandage (Fig. 14.14C):** It's a piece of material 4 to 6 inches wide and about 30 inches long, with each end cut about 12 or 14 inches down the middle, leaving the center piece about 12 or 14 inches long. This can be used to hold dressings on the jaw, nose, forehead, and back of the head.
- **Many-tailed bandage (Fig. 14.14D):** The only difference between a many-tailed bandage and a four-tailed bandage is that the ends are cut into the desired number of tails, which are approximately 16 inches in length and 20 inches for the uncut part.

DRESSING

Dressing is the application of a sterile or clean pad to a lesion/wound in order to promote healing and avoid further infections.

Purposes

- To control bleeding and absorb wound drainage.
- To protect the wound from contamination with microorganisms.
- To promote wound granulation and healing.
- To reduce chances of scarring.
- To maintain adequate exchange of gases.

Wound Dressing

Articles Required

Sterile dressing tray containing:
- Artery forceps
- Thumb forceps
- Cotton swabs
- Gauze pieces
- Gallipot for cleansing solution
- Surgical pads
- Kidney tray
- Sterile scissors

A clean tray containing:
- Clean gloves
- Sterile gloves
- Cleaning solution (normal saline)
- Ordered medications
- Adhesive plaster

- Bandage scissors
- Plastic bag
- Waterproof pad or Mackintosh
- Culture tubes (optional)

Steps of Procedure

- Identify the patient.
- Explain the procedure to the patient and needs for change of dressings.
- Arrange all articles near the bedside.
- Check for any specific instruction from the physician's order.
- Instruct patient to lie in position that provide easy access to the wound area, position of patient may vary depending on the location of the wound.
- Place an open plastic bag near the bed.
- Gently loosen the dressing bandages; if the tape is soiled, use gloves.
- Put on clean disposable gloves and carefully remove soiled dressings from a more clean to a less clean area.
- Discard the dressings in a disposable bags.
- Assess the wound for color, odor, moisture, swelling, drainage.
- Remove gloves inside out and discard them in the proper container.
- Open the sterile tray using sterile technique.
- Pour sterile solution into the sterile cup and soaked cotton balls.
- Don sterile gloves.
- Using artery forceps take the soaked cotton and clean from top to bottom or from center to outward (surgical wound).
- In case of contaminated wound, clean from periphery to center in circular motion.
- Discard cotton swab after each wipe.
- In case of wound drainage clean around it, moving from center to outward in a circular motion **(Fig. 14.15)**.
- Drop the medication/ointment on a sterile a dry sterile gauze and apply it over the wound.
- Place a layer of sterile dressing over wound **(Fig. 14.16A)**.
- Use sterile scissors to slit a guaze in the center, then place on side under and around the drain (in case of wound drainage).
- Apply a second layer of gauze to the area of the wound, with a surgical pad acting as the top covering.
- Remove gloves and secure the dressing using adhesive tape **(Fig. 14.16B)**.

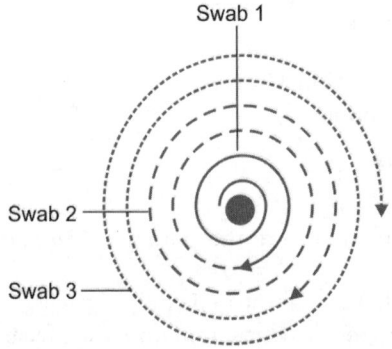

Fig. 14.15: Center to outward cleaning of wound.

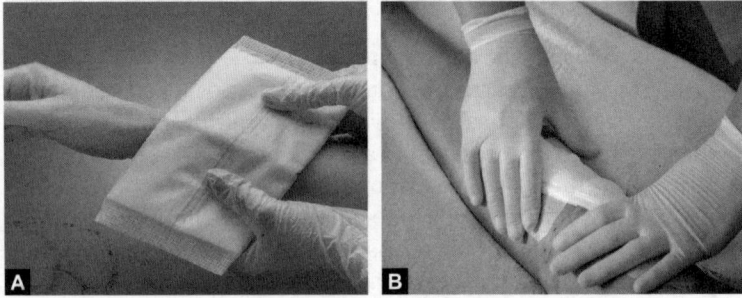

Figs. 14.16A and B: (A) Applying sterile dressing over a wound; (B) Applying tape to secure dressing.

- Replace all articles.
- Wash hands.
- Assist patient in a comfortable position.
- Record the procedure and any mention any abnormal findings.

BURN DRESSING

Articles Required

- Dressing pack
- Sterile bandages in a bin
- Sterile dressing pads in a bin
- Sterile vaseline gauze
- Silver sulfadiazine 1%
- Sterile normal saline
- Cheatle forceps

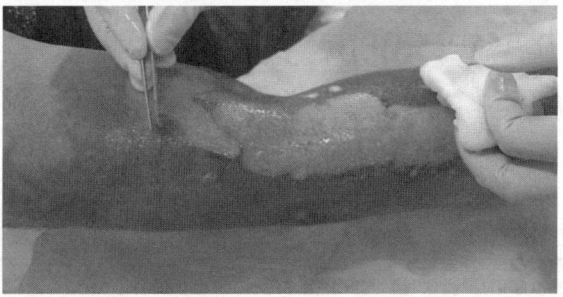

Fig. 14.17: Removing wound debris in burns using tweezers.

- Adhesive tape and scissors
- Sterile scissors
- Sterile sheets
- Receptacle for waste

Steps of Procedure

- Identify the patient and explain the procedure.
- Administer analgesics if prescribed.
- Maintain the room temperature at 24°C (80°F) and humidity at 40–50% using portable humidifiers if accessible.
- Gently, remove the previous dressings. Soak the dressings with normal saline if necessary.
- Assess the wound and its surrounding area.
- Wear mask and cap.
- Wash hands and don gloves and gown.
- If debris, loose eschar are present in the wound, use sterile scissors and tweezers to remove it **(Fig. 14.17)**.
- Clean the wound using normal saline and pat dry with sterile dry guaze.
- Apply the prescribed tropical medicine to the wound and cover with a bandage over the dressing pad.
- Replace articles and send reusable articles for autoclaving.
- Remove gown, mask, cap and gloves.
- Wash hands.
- Record the procedure and note all observation.

CHAPTER 15

Health Assessment

INTRODUCTION

Health assessment is an essential functions of nursing care, it acts as a foundation for quality nursing care and intervention by identifying the needs and strength of the patients. Health assessment are essential to patient safety because a lack of nursing assessments can put patients at risk. Timely and appropriate holistic nursing assessment is a fundamental skill that all nurses should show in any field of nursing practice.

HISTORY TAKING

History taking is the systematic gathering of information or data about the patient's physical state, as well as his or her psychological, social, and sexual functions, from the patient and other relevant sources.

PURPOSES

- To collect health-related patient information.
- To establish therapeutic nurse-patient relationship.
- To identify healthcare priorities.
- To plan appropriate interventions.

COMPONENTS OF HISTORY COLLECTION

Biographic Data

This includes all information related to demographics profile of patient:
- Name
- Age
- Sex
- Date of birth
- Address
- Religious beliefs

- Marital status
- Next of kin information
- Education
- Occupation
- Per capita income
- Nationality

HEALTH AND ILLNESS PATTERN

Chief Complaint or Presenting Problem

Collecting present complaints/chief complaints of the patient's helps the nurse in planning an action. The patient may have one or more chief complaints and related complaints must be listed together while unrelated complaints separately. Data can be collected from patient and family members, friends, roommates, primary care physician, or any other reliable source. Chief complaints gathered from the patient must includes character, onset, location, duration, severity, pattern and associated factor. PQRST can be used to assess each symptom:

PQRST

- **P** = Provocative or palliative: What makes the symptom(s) better or worse?
- **Q** = Quality: Describe the symptom(s).
- **R** = Region or radiation: Where in the body does the symptom occur? Is there radiation or extension of the symptom(s) to another area of the body?
- **S** = Severity: On a scale of 1–10, (10 being the worst) how bad is the symptom(s)? Another visual scale may be appropriate for patients that are unable to identify with this scale.
- **T** = Timing: Does it occur in association with something else (i.e., eating, exertion, movement)?

Past Medical History

The past medical history must include information about the patient's childhood illnesses and immunizations, accidents or traumatic injuries, hospitalizations, surgeries, psychiatric or mental illnesses, allergies, chronic illnesses and home medications or supplements that were taken. For women, include history of menstrual cycle, how many pregnancies and how many births.

Family History

Family history assists in identifying health risks and predisposing factors linked with the patient's current and future health conditions. Examine and record the prevalence of heart disease, diabetes, hypertension, kidney disease, tuberculosis, alcoholism or drug addiction, and genetic conditions in the family.

Family Tree

Family tree is a genealogical tree/pedigree tree, representing family structure, ties and relationships, and also health and social problems in a family using standardized symbols **(Fig. 15.1)**. This is helpful in identifying the genetic link of patient present illness within the family.

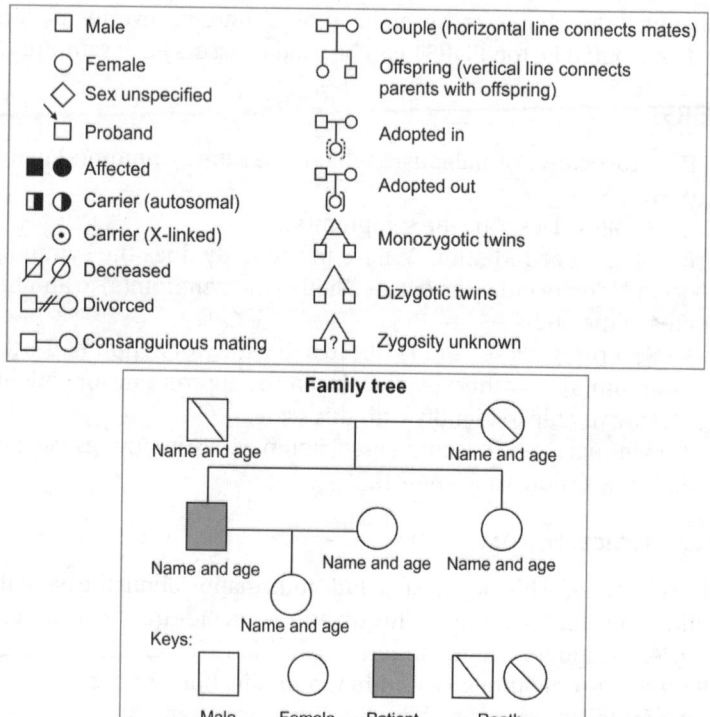

Fig. 15.1: Family pedigree symbols and chart.

Personal History

Personal history includes relevant information about the patient as a person. Elements of personal history includes patient's lifestyle or high-risk behaviors (if any), personal hygiene practices, dietary pattern, sleep patterns, elimination pattern (bowel/bladder), unhealthy practices—substance abuse, smoking, alcoholism, etc.

Obstetrical History (Female Patient)

Menstrual history, history of pregnancy—type of delivery, number of live birth, history of complication or previous abortion, etc.

PHYSICAL EXAMINATION

Physical examination is a routine examination of the body from head to toe that helps in determining the health status of the patients. The following techniques are used in physical examination:
- Inspection
- Auscultation
- Palpation
- Percussion

Inspection
Inspection begins during the initial contact with the patient. It is the systematic visual observation of the patient's color, shape, size, symmetry, position, movements and the senses to detect smell, hearing, and odors **(Fig. 15.2)**. It focuses on:
1. Overall appearance of health or illness.
2. Signs of distress.
3. Facial expression and mood.
4. Body size.
5. Grooming and personal hygiene.

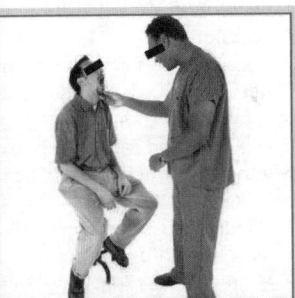

Fig. 15.2: Inspection.

Auscultation
Auscultation process is done by listening to sounds generated within the body using stethoscope **(Fig. 15.3)**. The heart (circulation of blood), lungs (breath sounds) and abdomen (bowel sounds) are auscultated for pitch sound, loudness, quality and duration.

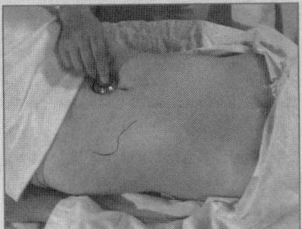

Fig. 15.3: Auscultation.

Palpation

Palpation is an assessment approach that makes the use of the sensation of touch. It is used to determine the size and position of the organs, body temperature, turgor, texture, moisture, vibrations, size, position, consistency, masses and fluid. During palpation keep the following points in mind:
- Keep the hands warm and fingernails short.
- Use gentle touch.
- Palpate tender areas at the last.
- To measure temperature use the dorsum surface of the hand.
- The palmar surface is used to measure the texture, shape, fluid, size, consistency, pulsation and vibration.
- Wear gloves whenever necessary.
- Light palpation is performed by depressing the fingertips about half an inch (Fig. 15.4A) and is used to assess surface irregularities.
- Deep palpation is performed to locate organs and masses by depressing 1.5–2 inches with the fingertips (Fig. 15.4B).

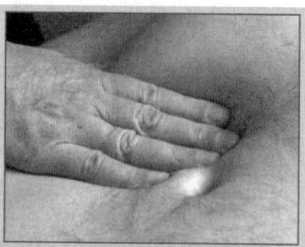

Fig. 15.4A: Light palpation.

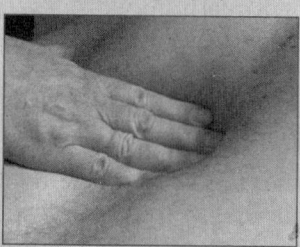

Fig. 15.4B: Deep palpation.

Percussion

Percussion is performed by tapping the fingers on the body in order to determine the state of the internal organs based on the sounds produced. It helps to determine whether the structure is air filled, fluid-filled or solid.
- Direct percussion: Tapping directly by using fingertips (Fig. 15.5A).
- Indirect percussion: It involves the use of two hands and it is done by placing the hands to the area to be percussed and the finger creating vibrations that allows discrimination among five different tones (Fig. 15.5B).

Percussion produced five sounds:
1. Percussion of abdomen: Tympanic.
2. Hyperinflated lung tissue: Hyper-resonant
3. Normal lung tissue: Resonant
4. Liver: Dull
5. Bone: Flat

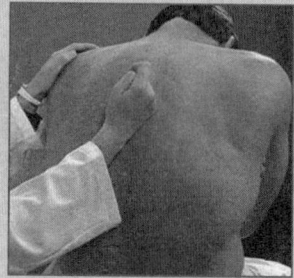

Fig. 15.5A: Direct percussion.

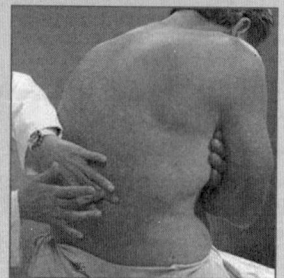

Fig. 15.5B: Indirect percussion.

HEAD TO TOE EXAMINATION

Preprocedure Steps

- Explain the procedure and its purpose to the patients.
- Provide privacy and comfort.
- Wash hands before touching the patient.
- Before using any equipment, ensure that it is in good working condition.
- Ask relevant questions.
- Maintain active listening.
- Proceed in a systematic and organized manner.

General Appearance

Assess for patient's general well-being, emotional status, level of orientation, level of consciousness, general appearance, hygiene, mobility, and gait.

Skin

- Observe skin-related problems such as ecchymosis, macule, papules, hair loss, and excessive hair growth.
- **Inspection:** Skin color, rashes, bruises, blisters, itching, lump or masses, inflammation, color of nails, capillary refill, hair pattern, pallor and any other abnormalities present **(Figs. 15.6A to F)**.
- **Palpation:** Skin turgor, texture (pale, cool, moist), temperature, moisture, edema.

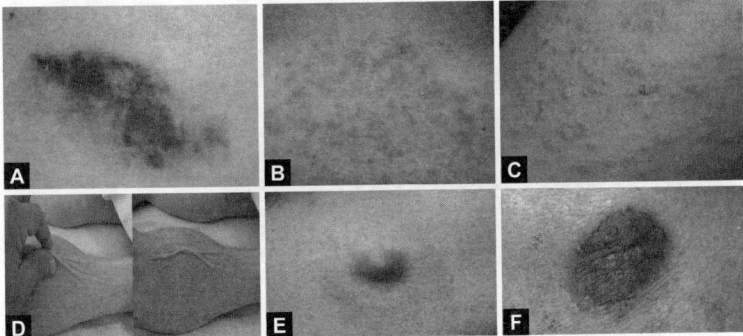

Figs. 15.6A to F: Some abnormal findings of skin related problems: (A) Bruises; (B) Skin rashes; (C) Pruritic skin; (D) Decrease skin turgor; (E) Lump; (F) Macule.

Head and Neck

- ❖ **Head:** Ask for presence of headache and any other associated complaints. History—head injuries, surgery, seizures.
- ❖ **Eyes:** Ask for presence any pain, ptosis, exophthalmos, itching, dryness in the eyes. History—eye surgery, use of any visual aids and duration.
  - **Inspection:** Pupillary response, any deformity, color of sclera, discharge and drainage **(Figs. 15.7A to C)**, check for visual acuity using Snellen chart.
- ❖ **Ear:** Ask for presence of any complaints related to ear such as vertigo. History—use of hearing aids.
  - **Inspection:** Pull pinna of ear upward and backward, using otoscope inspect external canal for discharge, impacted cerumen **(Fig. 15.8A)**, inflammation, masses for foreign bodies.
  - **Palpate:** Palpate the mastoid process for tenderness or deformity. Preauricular and postauricular lymph nodes for enlargement **(Fig. 15.8B)** and tenderness.
- ❖ **Nose:** Ask for presence of cold, history of epistaxis, history of nasal surgery.
  - **Inspection:** Nasal structures for colour and swelling, nasal septum deviation or perforation **(Fig. 15.9)**, discharge, turbinates, patent airways.

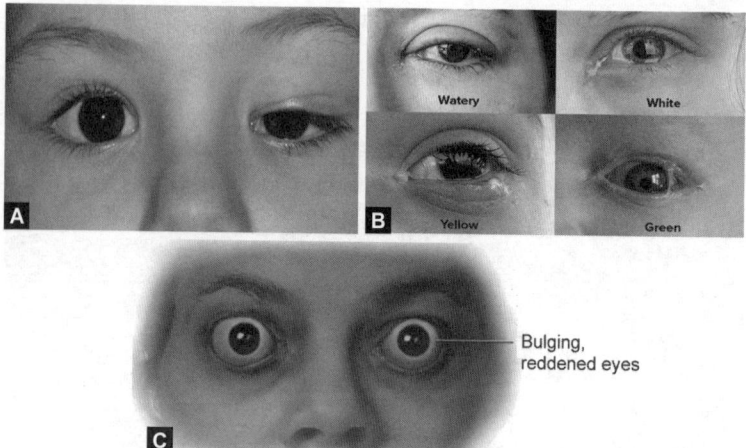

Figs. 15.7A to C: Some eye-related abnormalities. (A) Ptosis; (B) Discharge from eyes; (C) Exophthalmos.

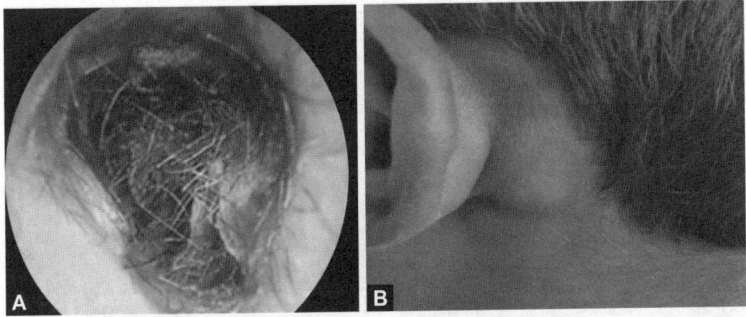

Figs. 15.8A and B: Some abnormal findings of ears: (A) Impacted cerumen; (B) Postauricular lymph nodes enlargement.

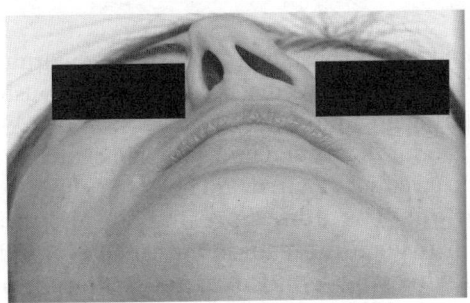

Fig. 15.9: Nasal septum deviation.

- **Palpation:** Palpate sinuses (upward press under both eyebrows with thumb in case of frontal sinus; upward press under maxilla for maxillary sinus) and ask patient for any discomfort or pain.
- ❖ **Face and lips:** Inspect for symmetry, chapped lip, cheilosis.
- ❖ **Mouth:** Inspect for oral hygiene, loose tooth, gum bleeding, dental caries, and other abnormalities.
- ❖ **Neck:**
  - **Inspection:** Inspect for symmetry, scar, and lesions.
  - **Palpation:** Palpate for neck for the presence of any lumps, lymph node swelling **(Fig. 15.10A)**, or any abnormal pulsation, jugular vein distension **(Fig. 15.10B)**.

Thorax and Lungs

- ❖ Ask patient for any history of respiratory diseases such as COPD, asthma, pneumonia and any previous treatment or surgery undertaken.

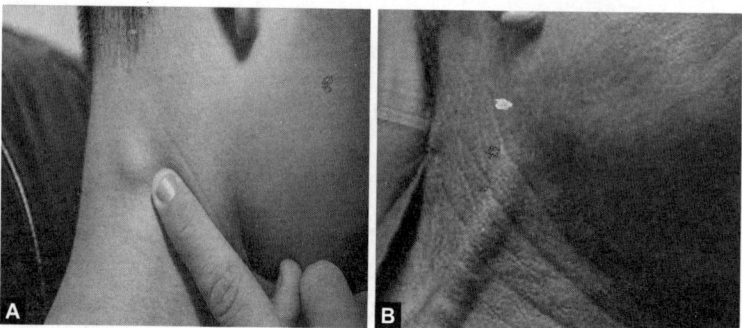

Figs. 15.10A and B: Some abnormal findings of the neck: (A) Swollen lymph nodes; (B) Jugular vein distension.

- **Inspection:** Inspect chest for asymmetry or deformity, abnormal pattern of breathing, abnormal breathing sounds, use of accessory muscles during breathing.
- Inspect posterior thorax and lungs for skin changes, alignment of spine, lump swelling, symmetry of posterior chest.
- **Auscultation:** It is done by using the diaphragm of the stethoscope to identify breath sounds such as crackles, rhonchi, rales and wheezing, etc. During auscultation of **posterior chest**—auscultate from top to bottom on both sides and **anterior chest**—auscultate from side to side and top to bottom **(Fig. 15.11)**.
- **Percussion:** Resonant lung sound which changes to dull sound towards the diaphragm.

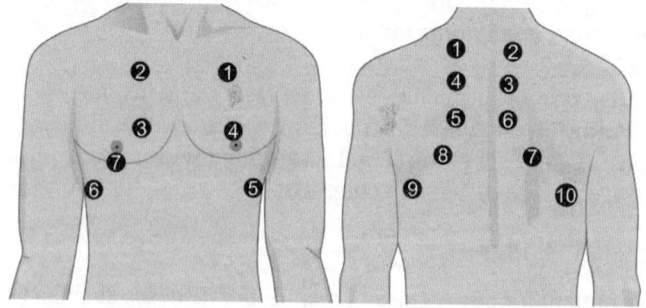

Fig. 15.11: Accurate area for auscultation anteriorly and posteriorly.

Abdomen

- Ask patient for any history associated with gastrointestinal problems, abnormal bowel patterns, dietary habits, any past treatment undertaken.
- **Inspection:** Inspect the abdomen for shape, abdominal distension, hernias, lesion, scars, hernias, rashes, masses, distended veins.
- **Auscultation:** Auscultate for hypoactive or hyperactive bowel sounds in all quadrants of the abdomen for 1 minute (**Fig. 15.12**).
- **Palpation:** Palpate all quadrants of the abdomen masses or lump, pain or tenderness.
- **Percussion:** Percuss all quadrants in clockwise direction for tympani or dullness.

Genitals

Females

- Ask for the presence of any vaginal discharge, itching, warts, sores or lumps, urinary incontinence on coughing, obstetrical history, menstrual history.
- **Inspection:** Conduct vaginal examination

Males

- Ask for urinary incontinence, frequency and characteristic of urination, etc.
- **Inspection:** Conduct rectal and testicular examination.

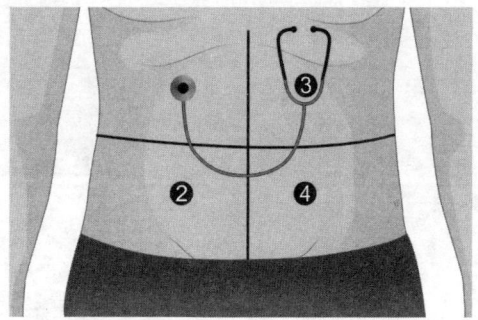

Fig. 15.12: Area of auscultation for abdomen.

Upper and Lower Extremities

- ❖ Ask patient for any complaints of muscle, joint pain, any past history of treatment related to joints, muscles, etc.
- ❖ Assess for handgrip strength bilaterally, bilaterally for plantar flexion and dorsiflexion of the feet against resistance and compare.
- ❖ **Inspection:** Skin color of the extremities, swelling, abnormal movements, skin integrity, and bilateral symmetry.
- ❖ **Palpation:** Temperature, pain, capillary refill, pulses of the femoral, popliteal, pedal, and posterior tibial **(Figs. 15.13A to F)**.

Vital Signs

Refer Chapter 2 for vital signs.

Height and Weight

Purposes

- ❖ To obtain baseline data about patient health status.
- ❖ To calculate body mass index (BMI).
- ❖ For estimation of child's growth.
- ❖ For routinely screening patients' nutritional status.
- ❖ To assess fluid balance in patients.

Articles Required

- ❖ **Weighing machine:**
  - Mechanical or digital weighing scales (adults and children).
  - Conventional beam balance or digital balance (infants)

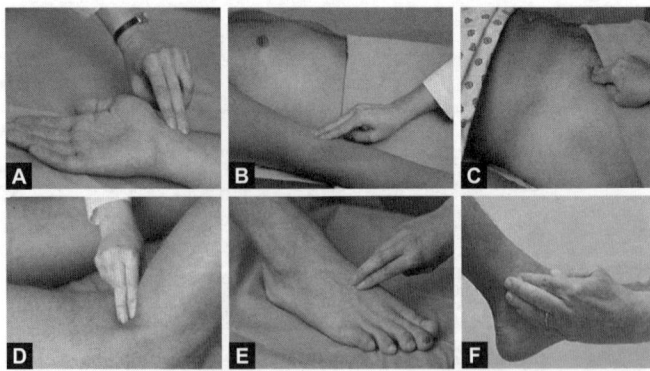

Figs. 15.13A to F: Palpation of pulses in upper and lower extremities.

Health Assessment

- ❖ **Height:**
  - Measuring tape and ruler (adults)
  - Stadiometer (children)
  - Measuring tape or infantometer (infants)

Steps of Procedure

Checking Weight using Digital Weighing Scales

- ❖ Wash hands.
- ❖ Assess whether patient can stand independently or need assistance.
- ❖ Check that the weighing machine is in good working order.
- ❖ Explain the procedure to the patient.
- ❖ Bring the weighing machine near the patient, turn on the scale and set it to zero.
- ❖ Instruct patient to remove shoes and step on the scale **(Fig. 15.14)**.
- ❖ After the digital numbers stop fluctuating, read the weight.
- ❖ Instruct the patient to take a step down and assist the patient in returning to the bed or chair.
- ❖ Wash hands.
- ❖ Record the date, time and weight of the patient.

Measuring Height using Measuring Tape and Ruler

- ❖ Wash hands.
- ❖ Assess whether patient can stand independently or need assistance.
- ❖ Vertically fasten the measuring tape to the wall.
- ❖ Instruct patient to remove the shoes and stand against the wall, Check that the floor is not carpeted and that it is flat.
- ❖ Instruct patient to stand straight, arms at the side and shoulders are level.

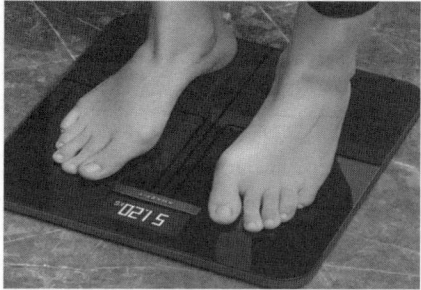

Fig. 15.14: Checking weight on digital weighing scales.

- ❖ The height is measured in inches or centimeters with a ruler placed horizontally on the head at a 90° angle to the measuring tape **(Fig. 15.15)**.
- ❖ Instruct/assist patient in returning to the bed or chair.
- ❖ Replace all articles.
- ❖ Wash hands
- ❖ Record the date, time and height.

Measuring Length of Infant using Infantometer

- ❖ Wash hands.
- ❖ Explain the procedure to the mother/attendant.
- ❖ Remove any bulky clothing.
- ❖ Place a clean sheet on the measuring board or infantometer.
- ❖ Place the infant on his or her back in the middle of the infantometer.
- ❖ Ensure that the infant's head is directly against the measuring board.
- ❖ Grasp the knees together and stretch the legs till fully extended and flat against the infantometer or measuring board.

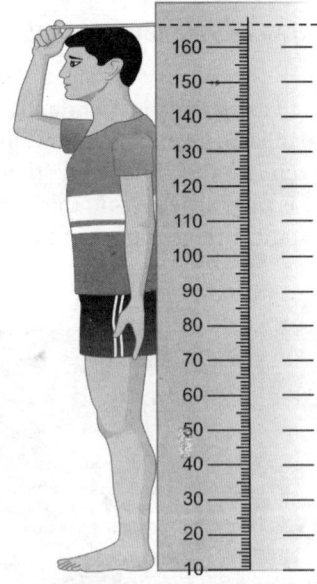

Fig. 15.15: Ruler placed horizontally on the head at a 90° angle to the measuring tape.

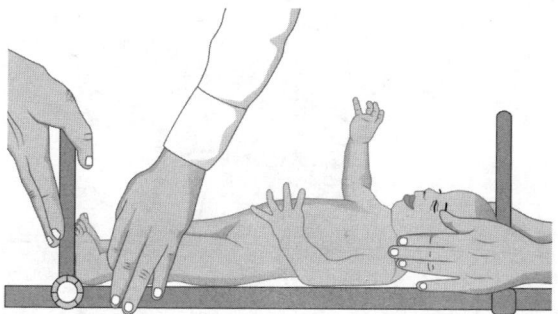

Fig. 15.16: Measuring length of infant on infantometer.

- Adjust the infantometer's length to the baby's length by bringing the end to the baby's feet **(Fig. 15.16)**.
- Note and record the readings.

Measuring Height of Child using Stadiometer (Fig. 15.17)

- Explain the procedure to the mother/attendant.
- Assist the child to stand on the stadiometer.
- Ensure that the child head is in the midline, eyes parallel to the ceiling or floor.
- Place the ruler of the stadiometer on top of the head of the child.
- Read the measurement and record.

Measuring Weight of Infant

- Explain procedure to the mother or attendant.
- Before weighing the infant make sure the weighing scale is clean.
- Set the digital display of the weighing scale at zero.
- Place a thin-clean sheet on the pan where the infant will be placed.
- Remove the clothing's of the infant and place a naked infant on the platform of the weighing scale **(Fig. 15.18)**.
- Ensure to hold the infant lightly while weighing to prevent from fall.

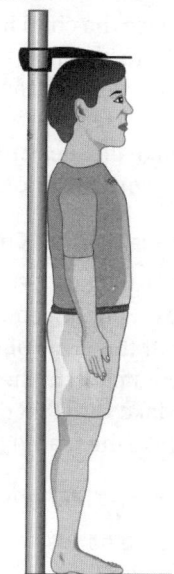

Fig. 15.17: Measuring height of child using stadiometer.

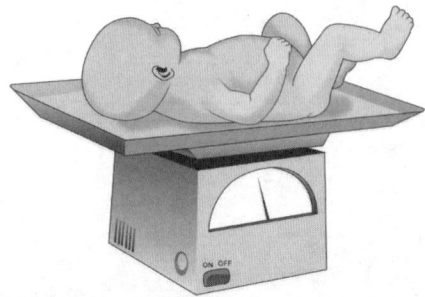

Fig. 15.18: Measuring weight of infant.

- Read the weight.
- Lift the baby from the pan and assist the mother in dressing the baby.
- Record the finding.

Measuring Head Circumference (Fig. 15.19A)

- Wash hands.
- Explain procedure to the mother or attendant.
- Place the child in sitting or supine position.
- Wrap the measuring tape across the forehead slightly above the eyebrows anteriorly and around the occipital protuberance posteriorly.
- Take the measurement at the midpoint of the tape.
- Record the findings.

Measuring Chest Circumference (Fig. 15.19B)

- Wash hands.
- Explain procedure to the mother or attendant.
- Lift the arms of the infants and wrap the measuring tape across your chest at the nipple level.
- Make sure that the tape is not wrap too tightly.
- Take the reading at the end of exhalation and maintain record.

Measuring Mid-arm Circumference (Fig. 15.19C)

- Wash hands.
- Explain procedure to the mother or attendant.
- Straighten the child arm and locate the midpoint of the upper arm by placing tape vertically from the acromion process and to the olecranon process.

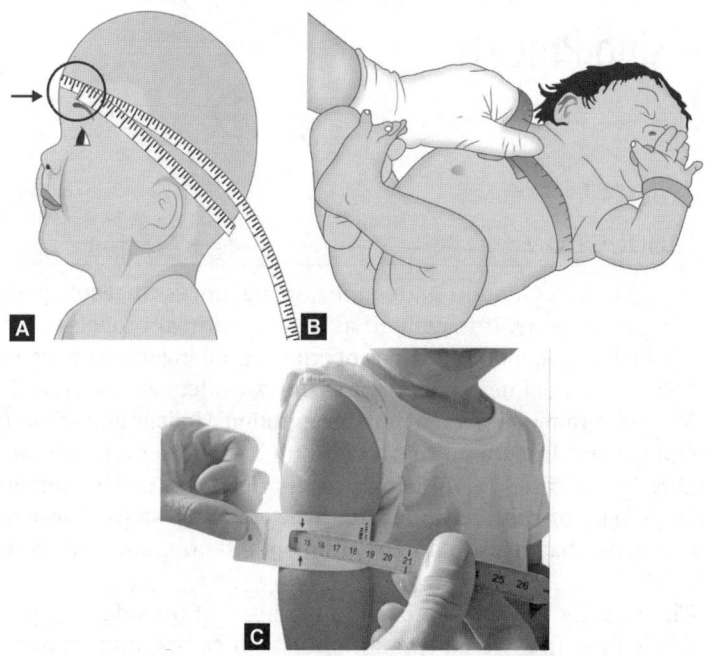

Figs. 15.19A to C: (A) Measuring head circumference; (B) Measuring chest circumference; (C) Measuring mid-arm circumference.

- Mark the midpoint.
- Measure the mid-arm circumference at the marked midpoint.
- Read the measurement and record the findings.

CHAPTER 16

Nursing Process

INTRODUCTION

In 1958, Ida Jean Orlando started the nursing process that still guides nursing care today. It is defined as a systematic approach to care using the fundamental principles of critical thinking, client-centered approaches to treatment, goal-oriented tasks, evidence-based practice (EDP) recommendations, and nursing intuition. Holistic and scientific postulates are integrated to provide the basis for compassionate, quality-based care. The nursing process functions as a systematic guide to patient-centered care with five sequential steps. These are assessment, diagnosis, planning, implementation, and evaluation **(Fig. 16.1)**.

The nursing process is crucial to the heart of nursing care plan, and it is time that we all (practitioners, educators, and students) become adept in using the nursing care plan as a vehicle to promote documentation and growth of nursing practice. The nursing process is a means for nurses to demonstrate accountability and responsibilities to clients as professionals.

PURPOSES

- ❖ To identify a patient's health status and actual or potential healthcare problems or needs.
- ❖ To establish plans to meet the identified needs.
- ❖ To deliver specific nursing interventions to meet those needs.

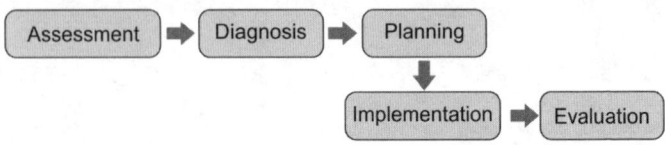

Fig. 16.1: Five sequential steps of nursing process.

CHARACTERISTICS (FIG. 16.2)

- Cyclic
- Dynamic nature
- Patient centered
- Focus on problem-solving and decision-making
- Interpersonal and collaborative style
- Universal applicability
- Use of critical thinking and clinical reasoning

ASSESSMENT

Assessment is the first step and involves critical thinking skills and data collection; subjective and objective. Subjective data involves verbal statements from the patient or caregiver. Objective data is measurable, tangible data such as vital signs, intake and output, and height and weight.

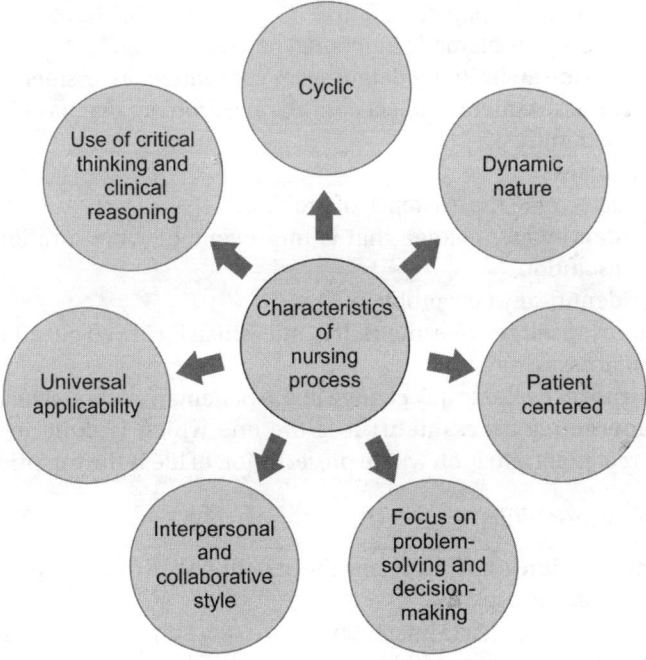

Fig. 16.2: Characteristics of nursing process.

Data may come from the patient directly or from primary caregivers who may or may not be direct relation family members. Friends can play a role in data collection. Electronic health records may populate data and assist in assessment.

Critical thinking skills are essential to assessment, thus the need for concept-based curriculum changes.

Purposes

- Gather data about patient (individual, family, or community)
- Use a data diagnosing, identifying, outcomes, planning and implementing, etc.

Types of Assessment

- **Initial assessment:** It is performed when the patient enters a healthcare facility.
  Purposes:
  - Evaluate the patients' status
  - Identify problematic functional patterns
  - Provide an in-depth database for subsequent assessment
- **Focus assessment:** Collect data about a problem that has already been identified.
  Purposes:
  - Determine the existence of problem
  - Identify any change that is improvement, deterioration, or resolution
  - Identify any new problem
- **Time lapsed reassessment:** It is, one which is carried out after the initial assessment.
  Purpose: Evaluate any change in the patients' functional health.
- **Emergency assessment:** It is the one which is done in life-threatening situation where preservation of life is the top priority.

Assessment Skills

- **Observation** is not just seeing the patient, but also the use of smell, hearing, and touch.
- **Interviewing** means interaction with patient and communication, to gather data by questioning.
- **Physical examination** is a systematic method of collection of data, using the sense of sight, hearing, smell, and touch, and to

detect health problem. The various techniques used are inspection, palpation, percussion, and auscultation.

- **Intuition** is defined as the use of insight instinct and clinical experience to make clinical judgments about the patient.

Activities

- Collection of data
- Validation of data
- Organization of data
- Analyzing of data
- Recording/documentation of data

 Clinical Pearls

Types of data
Subjective data: Symptoms or covert cues are the patient's feelings and statements
Objective data: Signs or overt cues are observable perceptible and measurable data
Source of data
- **Primary data:** From the patient
- **Secondary data:** Family member's health records, laboratory tests and diagnostic procedures, health team members, and literature's review
- **Documenting data** is permanent part and medical record.
- **Validation of data** is the process of confirming the accuracy of data collected.

DIAGNOSIS

The formulation of a nursing diagnosis by employing clinical judgment assists in the planning and implementation of patient care.

The North American Nursing Diagnosis Association (NANDA) provides nurses with an up-to-date list of nursing diagnoses. A nursing diagnosis, according to NANDA, is defined as a clinical judgment about responses to actual or potential health problems on the part of the patient, family, or community.

Nursing diagnosis provides the basis for selection of nursing interventions to achieve outcomes for which the nurse is accountable.

Purposes

- To identify the healthcare needs and prepare a nursing diagnosis
- To diagnose in nursing
- It intends to analyze information and derive useful meaning from it.

Components

- **Diagnostic label:** It is total name of the nursing diagnosis. It describes the essence of the problem using as few words possible, e.g., stress incontinence.
- **Qualifier:** Words used to give additional meaning in a nursing diagnosis. For example, impaired, intermittent, infective, increased, dysfunctional deficient, decreased, acute, and chronic.
- **Definition** describes the characteristics of the human response under consideration.
- **Risk factors** are identifiable intrinsic and extrinsic characteristic of the patient, e.g., risk for infection.
- **Related factors:** They describe the conditions, circumstances, or etiologies that contribute the problem, e.g., fluid volume deficit related to vomiting.

PLANNING

The planning stage is where goals and outcomes are formulated that directly impact patient care based on EDP guidelines. These patient-specific goals and the attainment of such assist in ensuring a positive outcome. Nursing care plans are essential in this phase of goal setting. Care plans provide a course of direction for personalized care tailored to an individual's unique needs. Overall condition and comorbid conditions play a role in the construction of a care plan. Care plans enhance communication, documentation, reimbursement, and continuity of care across the healthcare continuum.

Goals should be:
- Specific
- Measurable or meaningful
- Attainable or action-oriented
- Realistic or results-oriented
- Timely or time-oriented

IMPLEMENTATION

Implementation is the step that involves action or doing and the actual carrying out of nursing interventions outlined in the plan of care. This phase requires nursing interventions such as applying a cardiac monitor or oxygen, direct or indirect care, medication administration, standard treatment protocols, and EDP standards.

EVALUATION

This final step of the nursing process is vital to a positive patient outcome. Whenever a healthcare provider intervenes or implements care, they must reassess or evaluate to ensure the desired outcome has been met. Reassessment may frequently be needed depending upon overall patient condition. The plan of care may be adapted based on new assessment data.

The nursing process is summarized in the **Figure 16.3**.

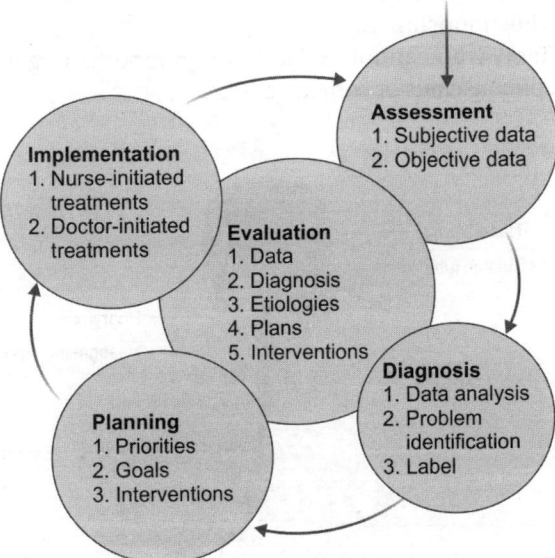

Fig. 16.3: Summary of nursing process.

CHAPTER 17

Nasogastric Tube Insertion and Feeding

DEFINITION

Nasogastric tube feeding (gastric gavage) is an artificial method of administering fluids and nutrients through a tube that has been passed into the esophagus and stomach through the nose, mouth, or through an opening made on the abdominal wall **(Fig. 17.1)**.

PURPOSES

- ❖ To provide adequate nourishment.
- ❖ To patient who cannot feed themselves.
- ❖ To administer medication.
- ❖ To provide nourishment.
- ❖ To patients who cannot be fed through mouth, surgery in oral cavity, unconscious or comatose state.

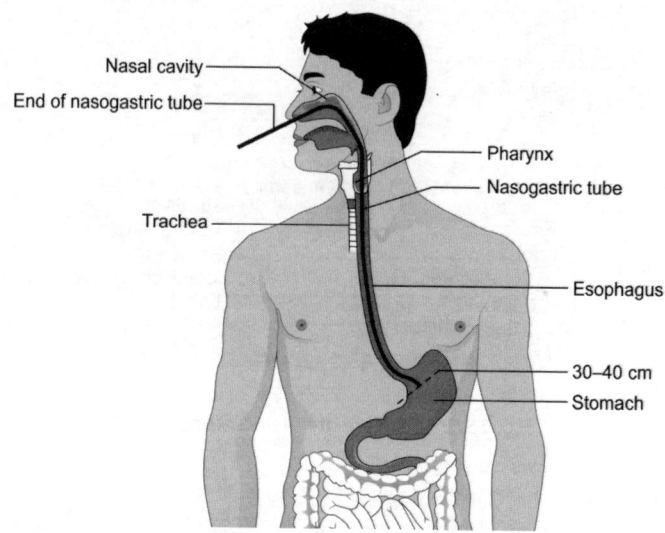

Fig. 17.1: Nasogastric tube placement.

TYPES OF TUBES

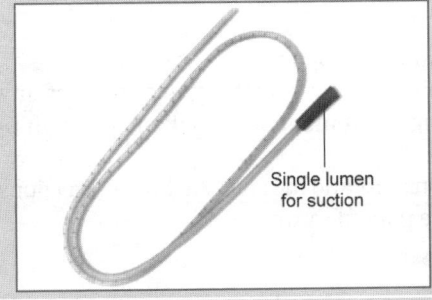

Levin's tube
Is a single-lumen multipurpose plastic tube that is commonly used in nasogastric intubation.

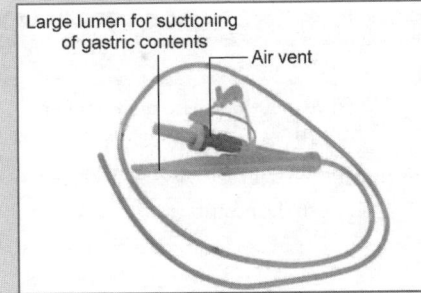

Salem tube
A double-lumen tube with a "pigtail" used for intermittent or continuous suction.

GENERAL INSTRUCTIONS

- Tube feeding is given only by a doctor's prescription.
- If the patient is conscious patient, explain the procedure to get cooperation.
- Remove dentures if any to prevent dislodging and blocking the respiratory tract.
- Avoid introducing air into the stomach during each food.
- Pinch tube before the fluid runs into the stomach completely from the tube to avoid air entry.
- All articles used for feeding should be clean. The food has to be handled and stored under hygienic conditions.
- Every time before giving the feed ensure the positioning of the tube.
- Feeding may be given 2–3 hourly and it should not exceed 150–300 mL per feed; total amount between 2,000 and 3,000 mL in 24 hours.
- Intake output recorded accurately.
- Observe for complications, e.g., asphyxia, electrolyte imbalance, distension, diarrhea, etc.
- Frequent mouth care to be provided to prevent complications of neglected mouth.

ADMINISTERING TUBE FEEDING

Preliminary Assessment

- Identify the client with name and bed no.
- Check the doctor's orders for any specific precautions if any, regarding the tube feeding, movement of the patient, positioning of the patient, etc.
- Assess the level of consciousness and the ability to follow directions.
- Arrange the articles in the patient's unit.

Articles Required

Article	Purpose
A tray containing:	
Feeding cup with water Kidney tray	To give mouthwash before and after the feed
Mackintosh and towel	To protect the garments and bed linen
Cotton tipped applicators Saline or soda bicarb solution Levine tube or Ryle's tube in a bowl of ice Lubricant such as water-soluble jelly or glycerine or liquid paraffin	To clean the nostrils
Adhesive plaster and scissors	To fix the tube in position
Rag pieces in a container	To wipe the secretions
Paper bag	To collect the wastes
Clean syringe or a funnel in a tray	To aspirate the gastric contents and to give the feeding
A glass of feed in a bowl of warm water	To give the feed at the body temperature
Ounce glass	To measure the fluid intake
A bowl with water	To test the location of the tube
Clamp	To clamp the tube to prevent leakage of gastric contents
Suction apparatus	To clear the airway in case of unconscious or seriously ill client who vomits and aspirates the fluid into the respiratory tract

Preparation of Patient and Unit

- Explain the procedure to the patient.
- Provide a safe and comfortable position for the patient.
- Place the mackintosh and face towel across the chest and under the chin to protect the garments and the bed linen.
- Allow the patient to adjust the kidney tray according to his convenience or keep the kidney tray next to the patient ready to use if he vomits.
- Remove the dentures, if any, and place it in a bowl of clean water. Arrange the articles conveniently on the bedside locker.
- Give a guaze piece in the patient's hand to wipe the face and lips when necessary.
- Give a mouth wash and help them to clean the teeth.
- Clean the nostrils, if there is secretion or crust formation, using swab stick dipped in saline or soda-bicarb solution.

Steps of Procedure

- Wash hands
- Take the tube and expel the water from the tube and check the tube for patency.
- Measure distance on the tube from the bridge of the nose to the ear lobe plus the distance from the ear lobe to the tip of the xiphoid process of the sternum. Mark the distance of the tube **(Fig. 17.2)**.
- Lubricate the tube for about 6–8 inches with the lubricant, using a guaze piece. Lubricant should be applied to the minimum.
- Hold the tube coiled in the right hand and introduce the up into the left nostril.
- Instruct the patient to swallow while inserting the tube. Insert the tube till the marking.
- Check the placement of the tube in the stomach.
  - Aspirate for gastric contents with a syringe.
  - Ask the client to hum or speak.
  - After the tube is in place, tape it to the side of the face and wait for sometime before giving the feed.
- Before giving the feed, pour some water through the funnel and lower the funnel slowly, to expel the air. Then give the feed and the medicines kept ready for the client. When the feed is finished, pour a little water, and clamp the tube firmly to prevent leakage of fluids.

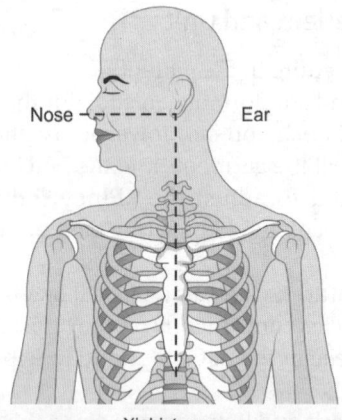

Place the tip of the nasogastric tube at the tip of the nose, then measure from the nose to the ear lobe and down to the tip of the xiphisternum

Fig. 17.2: Measuring the distance of nasogastric tube.

After Care of Patient and Articles

- Provide mouth wash.
- Clean the face and hands and dry them.
- Remove the mackintosh and towel.
- Make the patient comfortable in bed.
- Take all articles to the utility room.
- Discard the waste and clean the articles with soap and water.
- Dry them.
- Replace them into their proper places.
- Wash hands.
- Record the time, date, amount of feed, the nature of the feed, the reaction of the client if any, in the nurses record as well as in the intake and output chart.
- Remove the tube when the tube feeding is to be stopped.

Chapter 18

Bed Bath

INTRODUCTION

Bed bath is an essential part of nursing care for patients confined to bed. The time of bed bath depends entirely on the prevailing circumstances, weather or according to the wishes of the patients or according to the advice of doctors. Bed bath provides the patients physical comfort, and psychological support in encouraging the establishment of rapport between patient and nursing staff.

DEFINITION

Bed bath means bathing a patient who is confined to bed and who does not have the physical and mental capability to perform self-bath. Examples include unconscious patients, bedridden patients, postsurgery patients, etc.

PURPOSES

- ❖ To clean the body from greasy material and dirt of perspiration or sweating.
- ❖ To prevent multiplication of pathogenic organisms on the skin surface.
- ❖ To prevent bedsores.
- ❖ To accelerate blood circulation over skin surface.
- ❖ To improve general muscle tone.
- ❖ To have better aesthetic sense for self, relatives and neighboring patients.

ARTICLES REQUIRED

- ❖ Basin
- ❖ Jug or mug with warm water
- ❖ Bedpan/urinal
- ❖ Bath towel
- ❖ Bath blanket

- Wash clothes
- Soap
- Clean bed linen
- Clean patient's dress for change
- Table to keep all materials at bedside
- Talc powders and lotions as required
- Laundry bag
- Bedside screen

STEPS OF PROCEDURE (FIG. 18.1)

- All the materials are kept on the table on bedside ready for use.
- The patient should be informed about the bath and convenient time should be selected suiting both to nursing staff and patient.
- Encourage participation from patients or relatives.
- Close windows and doors, if in a single room.
- Place the bedside screen.
- Offer bedpan/urinal if needed.
- Position patient close to the side of the bed or close to nurse.
- Raise the bed high.
- Wash hands and wear gloves.
- Loosen top bedding at sides and foot.
- Place articles within your reach.
- Cover patient with bath blanket while removing top sheet.
- Check temperature of the water by pouring water on the inner aspect of the palm of the patient.

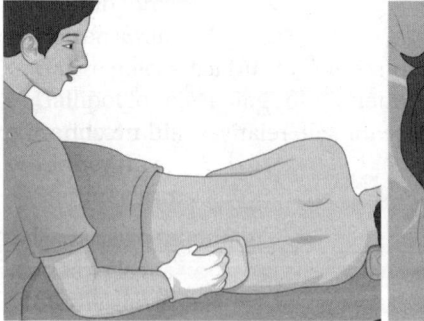
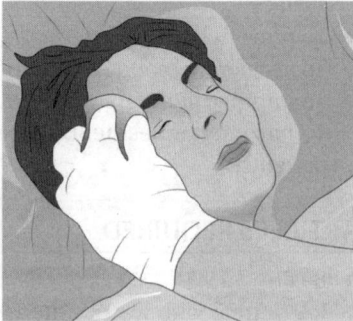

Fig. 18.1: Bed bath.

Bed Bath

- Place face towel under the chin, wash face, eyes and ears with soapy wash, cloth over hands, tucking in loose corners.
- Eyes should be protected from soap or lathers. If at all eyes come in contact with soap it should be rinsed properly with plain water.
- Uncover the forearm and place towel lengthwise under the arm.
- Wash, rinse well and dry the armpit. The same procedure is done for forearm.
- Cover the chest with bath towel and turn bath blanket down to abdomen. Wash chest thoroughly after removing the bath towel.
- Uncover abdomen area. Wash and rinse down to pubic area. Make sure that umbilical area is cleaned properly. Dry well.
- Draw cover up and remove bath towel from chest.
- Uncover far leg and drape with bath blankets arranging bath towel underfoot. Flex knee, wash leg, rinse and dry well. The feet can be immersed in basin, if required.
- Repeat the same procedure for the other leg.
- The water in basin should be changed in between when dirty, cold or soapy.
- Now turn the patient on side with back towards you. Wash back, rinse and dry by wiping with dry towel from neck to buttocks.
- The pressure areas are observed for any bedsores.
- The genitals of patients also require cleaning. If the patient cannot do himself then cleaning procedure is applied as cleaning other parts of body with soap water and drying by wiping with towel. The junction area of thigh and hip should be sprinkled with talc powder.
- Assist patient in wearing gown or dress.
- The patient can be asked to rinse his mouth, if he can do it.
- Arrange dirty linen in one place. Remove bath basin, powder, etc.
- Make bed as described for an occupied patient.
- Adjust the patient's position, head and knee and other bed garments according to his comfort and as per doctor's advice.
- Comb the patient's hair.
- All bathing items are kept tidy and in proper place.
- The soiled clothes are collected in laundry bag and sent for washing.
- Wash hands.
- Record procedure.
- Replace articles.
- Record the procedure in patient's chart with date and time.

CHAPTER 19

Hair Washing

INTRODUCTION

Though the care of hair seems to be a purely personal hygiene but for a hospitalized patient it is part of the nursing job. A fully conscious patient in perfectly walkable condition and with normally functioning head can take care of his own hair. But it becomes essential as a nursing care when the patient is unconscious or semiconscious or otherwise unable to take care of his/her hair.

DEFINITION

Hair washing is the process of cleansing hair of dandruff, grime, nits, lice, flakes, dryness, and irritation with water and shampoo/soap.

PURPOSES

- To provide an aesthetic sense for patient and for attending persons and neighboring patient.
- To keep hair clean and dry.
- To accelerate blood circulation to hair roots over scalp.
- To clean hair after application of drugs for removal.

ARTICLES REQUIRED

- Two separate jugs for cold and hot water
- Shampoo/liquid soap
- Wash basin
- Bucket for collection of dirty water
- Two mackintosh
- Wash cloth to protect eyes
- Cotton to plug ears from entry of dirty water
- Oil, comb and brush
- Two towels
- Bath blanket
- Bucket

- Clean linen
- Newspaper
- Small jug or mug to pour water over hair
- Kidney tray and paper bag
- Hot water bottle in winter filled with hot water

HAIR WASH PROCEDURE (FIG. 19.1)

- Check for any specific instruction to be followed during hair washing.
- Assess the general condition of the patient hair, scalp and the amount of shampoo to be used.
- Ask patient for any specific shampoo preference.
- Keep all items ready on bedside table.
- Inform the patient about the procedure.
- Wash hands.
- Assist the patient to take comfortable position may be sitting or lying depending on the patient condition.
- Move the patient's head at the edge of the bed and place pillow under the head.
- Place mackintosh under patient's shoulder keeping the head down. Mackintosh should form a trough to carry dirty water into bucket.
- Plug patient's both ears with cotton.
- Place the washed cloth over patient's eyes to prevent contact of dirty water which causes irritation to eyes and is a avoidable discomfort.
- Mix hot and cold water to 40°–42°C (lukewarm water) and pour slowly over scalp to wet the hair.

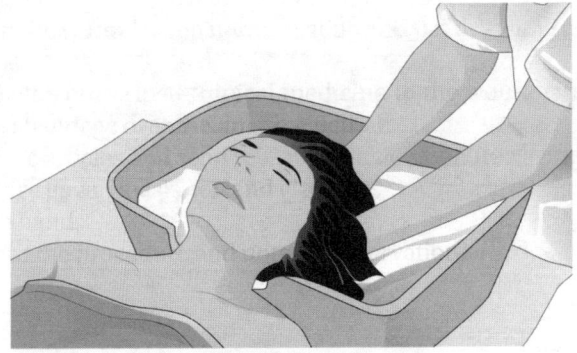

Fig. 19.1: Hair wash.

- Apply shampoo or liquid soap and massage the scalp really well.
- Rinse the hair thoroughly. Repeat washing and rising until hair is clean.
- Squeeze off water from the hair, wipe the scalp with towel and dry the hair.
- Discard the cotton plugs used to plug ears.
- Reposition patient in proper alignment.
- Clean the comb and brush.
- Apply oil or if required as per wishes of the patient.
- Comb hair gently starting at the ends going upward towards head, leave the patient comfortable and tidy.
- Change linen if wet or soiled.
- Take all articles to the utility room and clean them. Disinfect towels, mackintosh, basin and bucket.
- Wash hands.
- Record the procedure in chart with date and time.

CHAPTER 20

Care of Pressure Points and Back Care

PRESSURE POINTS

Pressure sores, also known as pressure ulcers or bedsores, are localized areas of damage to the skin and underlying tissues due to prolonged pressure and/or shear forces on the skin. They typically develop in areas with bony prominences and are commonly seen in individuals who are immobile or have limited mobility.

Common Sites of Pressure Points

The sites of pressure points depend on the position of patient in bed.

The pressure points in **supine position** are back, occiput, scapula, sacral region, elbow, and heels **(Fig. 20.1)**.

In **side-lying position** the pressure points are the ears, acromion process of shoulder, ribs, greater trochanter of hip, medical and lateral condyle of knee, malleolus of the ankle joint **(Fig. 20.2)**.

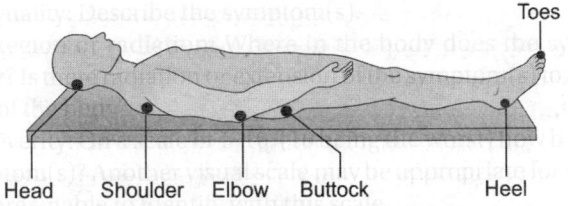

Fig. 20.1: Pressure points in supine position.

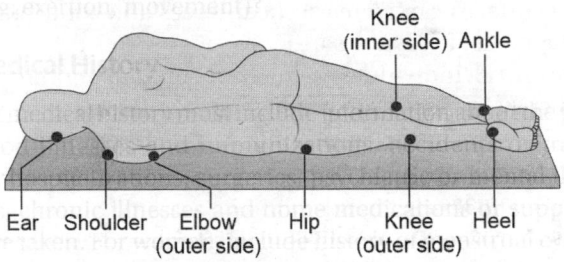

Fig. 20.2: Pressure points in side-lying or lateral position.

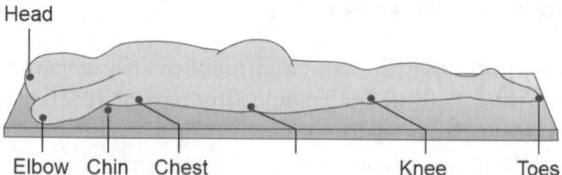

Fig. 20.3: Pressure points in prone position.

In **prone position**, the pressure points are the ears, cheek, acromion process, ribs, breasts (in female)/genitalia (in male) knees, and toes **(Fig. 20.3)**.

Purposes of Care of Pressure Sores

- To improve circulation
- To facilitate healing
- To prevent infection
- To prevent further damage
- To treat bedsores

Causes of Pressure Sores

- **Prolonged pressure:** Sustained pressure on the skin and underlying tissues can impede blood flow and lead to tissue damage. When a person remains in one position for an extended period, such as sitting or lying in bed without movement or repositioning, it can result in pressure sores.
- **Friction and shear:** Friction occurs when the skin rubs against a surface, such as bedding or clothing. Shear refers to the sliding of skin layers against each other. These forces can cause damage to the underlying tissues, especially when combined with pressure. For example, sliding down in bed or being pulled or dragged across surfaces can increase shear forces and contribute to the development of pressure sores.
- **Immobility:** Individuals who have limited mobility or are completely immobile are at a higher risk of developing pressure sores. The inability to change positions or shift body weight can lead to prolonged pressure on specific areas, increasing the likelihood of tissue damage.
- **Reduced sensation:** Conditions that result in decreased or impaired sensation, such as spinal cord injuries, peripheral neuropathy, or certain neurological disorders, can prevent individuals from feeling

discomfort or pain caused by pressure. This lack of sensation makes it difficult for them to recognize the need to change positions or relieve pressure.
- **Moisture and incontinence:** Excessive moisture or prolonged exposure to moisture, such as from perspiration, urine, or fecal incontinence, can weaken the skin and make it more susceptible to damage. Moisture can also contribute to the breakdown of the skin's natural protective barrier, increasing the risk of pressure sores.
- **Poor nutrition and hydration:** Inadequate nutrition and hydration can compromise the skin's integrity and reduce its ability to withstand pressure. Poor nutrition can lead to malnourishment and impaired tissue healing, while dehydration can affect the skin's elasticity and overall health.
- **Medical devices:** The use of medical devices, such as oxygen masks, orthopedic braces, or urinary catheters, can create pressure points and increase the risk of pressure sores if proper precautions and monitoring are not followed.
- **Advanced age:** Older adults are generally more susceptible to developing pressure sores due to factors such as thinner skin, reduced mobility, and underlying health conditions that may affect tissue healing and resilience.

Risk Factors

- Acutely ill patients
- Elderly bedridden patients
- Obese patients
- Sedated patients who have spinal cord injuries
- Paralyzed patients
- Neurological patients with lack of sensation
- Edematous patients
- Malnourished patients
- Agitated patients with restraints
- Postoperative patients with limited movements
- Diabetic patients

Signs and Symptoms of Pressure Ulcers

- Redness, heat, tenderness, and discomfort in the area
- The area becomes cold to touch and insensitive.
- Local edema
- Later, the area becomes blue, purple of mottled.

- Due to continued pressure that circulation is cut off, the gangrene develops, and affected area is sloughed.

The signs and symptoms of pressure ulcers may depend on the stage of the ulcer's development. Here are the common signs and symptoms to watch for:

- **Redness:** Persistent redness over a specific area of skin that does not fade when pressure is relieved may indicate the initial stage of a pressure ulcer. The redness may appear as a patch of irritated or discolored skin.
- **Discoloration:** The affected area may exhibit changes in skin color, such as darker or lighter patches compared to the surrounding skin.
- **Pain or discomfort:** Pressure ulcers can be painful or tender, particularly in the early stages. However, in some cases, individuals with reduced sensation may not experience pain or discomfort.
- **Swelling:** The area around the pressure ulcer may become swollen or edematous.
- **Warmth:** The skin over the pressure ulcer may feel warmer to the touch compared to the surrounding skin
- **Skin texture changes:** As the pressure ulcer progresses, the skin may become dry, scaly, or flaky. It may also feel unusually firm or spongy to the touch.
- **Blistering:** In more severe cases, fluid-filled blisters or sacs may develop on the surface of the pressure ulcer. These blisters may be fragile and prone to rupture.
- **Skin breakdown:** With further progression, the skin can break down, exposing the underlying tissue. The ulcer may appear as an open wound or crater-like depression. The wound bed may contain necrotic (dead) tissue, slough, or eschar (black, dry, or leathery tissue).
- **Drainage:** Pressure ulcers may produce various types of wound drainage, including serous fluid (clear, watery), serosanguinous fluid (pale red or pink), or purulent fluid (thick, yellow, green, or foul-smelling), depending on the presence of infection.
- **Undermining or tunneling:** In advanced cases, pressure ulcers may develop channels or tunnels beneath the skin surface.

 Clinical Pearls

Pressure ulcers can rapidly progress and deepen, leading to more severe complications, including infection, cellulitis, abscess formation, or involvement of deeper tissues, such as muscles and bones. Therefore, early detection and prompt intervention are crucial in managing pressure ulcers.

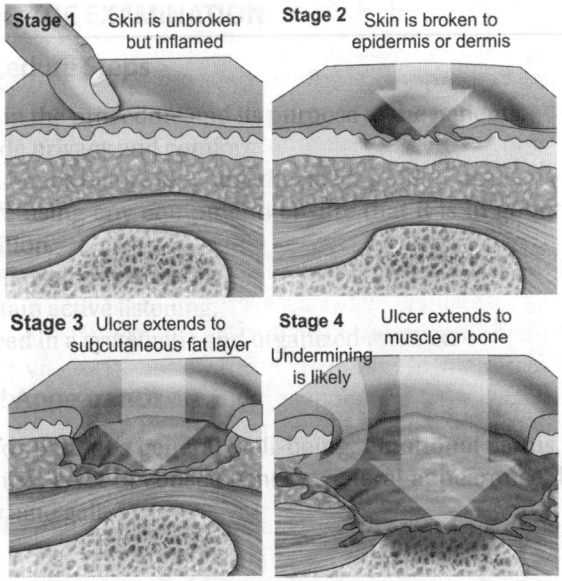

Fig. 20.4: Stages of pressure sores.

Stages of Pressure Sore (Fig. 20.4)

Clinical Manifestations According to the Stage

- **Stage 1:** The area looks red and feels warm to the touch. With darker skin, the area may have a blue or purple tint. The person may also complain that it burns, hurts, or itches.
- **Stage 2:** The area looks more damaged and may have an open sore, scrape, or blister. The person complains of significant pain and the skin around the wound may be discolored.
- **Stage 3:** The area has a crater-like appearance due to damage below the skin's surface.
- **Stage 4:** The area is severely damaged, and a large wound is present. Muscles, tendons, bones, and joints can be involved. Infection is a significant risk at this stage.

Prevention of Pressure Sores

Preventing pressure ulcers is crucial in maintaining the skin's integrity and overall health. Some key strategies for preventing pressure ulcers.
- **Regular skin assessment:** Conduct regular skin assessments to identify areas of vulnerability or early signs of pressure damage.

Examine bony prominences, such as the heels, sacrum, hips, and elbows.

- **Pressure redistribution:** Utilize pressure-reducing devices and support surfaces, such as specialized mattresses, cushions, and pads, to distribute pressure more evenly and reduce the risk of developing pressure ulcers.
- **Repositioning:** Encourage regular changes in position to relieve pressure on specific areas. For individuals who are immobile or have limited mobility, establish a repositioning schedule based on their risk assessment, generally every two hours.
- **Moisture management:** Keep the skin clean and dry to minimize the risk of skin breakdown. Promptly address any moisture sources, such as perspiration, urine, or fecal incontinence, by using absorbent pads, moisture-wicking clothing, and proper hygiene practices.
- **Nutritional support:** Ensure adequate nutrition and hydration to promote healthy skin. A well-balanced diet with sufficient protein, vitamins, and minerals is essential for maintaining skin integrity and facilitating tissue healing.
- **Skin care:** Practice gentle and thorough skin cleansing using mild soap and warm water. Avoid aggressive rubbing or scrubbing that can damage the skin. Apply moisturizers or barrier creams to keep the skin hydrated and protected.
- **Education and awareness:** Educate patients, caregivers, and healthcare professionals about the importance of pressure ulcer prevention. Teach proper positioning techniques, skin care practices, and the recognition of early signs of pressure damage.
- **Support surfaces and equipment:** Choose appropriate support surfaces and equipment, such as pressure-relieving mattresses, cushions, and wheelchair pads, based on the individual's specific needs and level of risk.
- **Encourage mobility and exercise:** Promote regular movement and exercise within the individual's capabilities. Physical activity helps improve circulation, muscle strength, and overall tissue health.
- **Collaborative care:** Work as a multidisciplinary team, involving nurses, physicians, physical therapists, occupational therapists, nutritionists, and other healthcare professionals, to develop and implement a comprehensive pressure ulcer prevention plan tailored to the individual's needs.

Nursing Responsibilities

- Report to the senior nursing officer or supervisor and the physician the early symptoms of a bedsore so that steps may be taken as early as possible to prevent further damage.
- Whenever possible, take off the pressure from the decubitus ulcers by placing the patient on pillows or foam cushions or change the position of the patient.
- Prevent the ulcerated area from becoming infected, follow strict aseptic technique.
- A cleaning agent is used to clean the ulcerated area, e.g., normal saline.
- Apply all the possible measures for the healing of the wound.
  - Heat is applied by an electric bulb (no watt). This is placed from 45 to 60 cm away from the wound and is left in place for 10 minutes.
  - Application of a few drops of insulin which has healing effect. The wound is then exposed to air to dry.
- Application of waterproof ointment like zinc oxide on the surface of wound that will prevent infection of underlying tissues.
- If slough is present, clean with hydrogen peroxide diluted with distilled water. If it is loose, physician may cut off the slough.
- If required physician may prescribe antibiotics.

BACK CARE

Scientific form of massaging the back using different massaging strokes to provide cutaneous stimulation and thus promote comfort.

Purposes

- To prevent pressure sores.
- To stimulate blood circulation to back.
- To detect pressure sores at an early stage.
- To maintain the cleanliness and dryness of the skin and reduce the chance of infection.
- To reduce muscle tension and enhance physical comfort.
- To relieve insomnia.

Contraindications

Back care is contraindicated in patients with:
- Rib fracture
- Burns

- ❖ Immediate postoperative period after coronary artery bypass graft
- ❖ Spinal injuries
- ❖ Surgeries on back

Preparation of Articles

Article	Purposes
Mackintosh with draw sheet	To prevent linen soiling
A small tub or bath basin	To take warm water
Sponge cloth 2	One to apply soap on skin and other soap off the skin
Soap dish with soap	To clean the skin
Spirit/oil	To massage the back
Powder	To smoothen the skin and prevent friction
Towel	To dry the skin
Bath sheet	To provide privacy

Preparation of Patient

- ❖ Identify the need for back care in patient.
- ❖ Explain the procedure to the patient.
- ❖ Draw curtains, close doors, and windows.
- ❖ Put the patient on his abdomen or on his side and bring him to the edge of the bed near you.
- ❖ Put a bath sheet on the patient. Remove blankets, etc.
- ❖ Expose the patient's back from shoulders to buttocks.
- ❖ Spread rubber sheet lined with cloth alongside the patient's side.

Steps of Procedure

- ❖ Wash your hands.
- ❖ Expose patient's back, shoulders, upper arms, and buttocks. Cover rest of the body with bath sheet.
- ❖ Wash back with mild soap using soapy sponge cloth, followed by washing off the soap with wet sponge cloth, from shoulders to buttocks using long circular movements.
- ❖ **Massaging:** Provide massage with oil/lotion/powder according to the season or patient preference.
  - Take oil/powder in your palm and spread it all over the back.
  - Do **effleurage/stroking:** Following the direction of venous stream long, firm, slow, rhythmic, and sweeping movement

should be done with palm. Small surface area like neck can be reached by finger **(Fig. 20.5)**.

- Do **petrissage:** This is considered as deeper massage technique than effleurage. Here with the help of thumb, fingers or palm large grasping of the skin, subcutaneous tissue, and muscles from is done. It should be following rhyme and equality in application of pressure. In between two kneading the caregiver can roll the muscle **(Fig. 20.6)**.

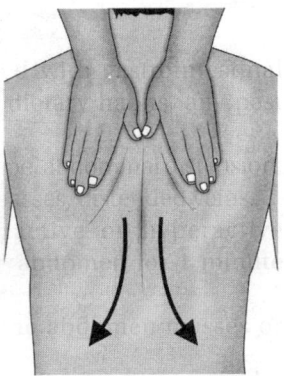

Fig. 20.5: Effleurage.

- Do **friction:** Deep massage by using palm, finger, or thumbs in circular motion in defined small part of the back. Controlled pressure uses to be applied **(Fig. 20.7)**.
- Do **vibration:** Fine vibrating movements should be given by fingertips, produced by contraction and relaxation of the muscles of forearm **(Fig. 20.8)**.
- Do **tapotements:** Light, stimulating, and repetitive massages are produced via wrist, fists, fingers, sides of the hands **(Fig. 20.9)**. Different types of tapotement techniques are:
  - Perform **hacking**: Stretched the elbow, keep the palms face to face in little right angle and do very quick and sharp striking **(Fig. 20.10)**.

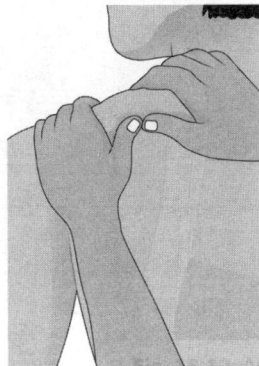

Fig. 20.6: Petrissage.

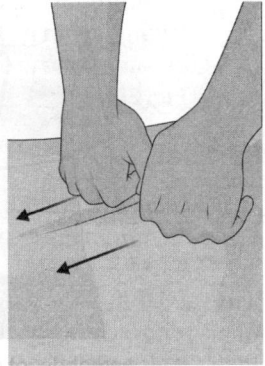

Fig. 20.7: Friction.

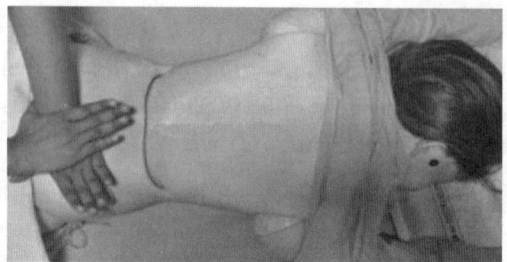

Fig. 20.8: Vibration.

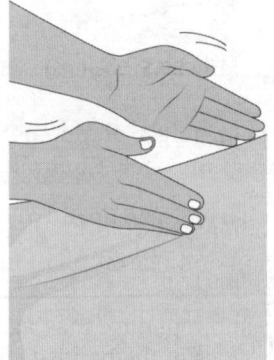

Fig. 20.9: Tapotement.

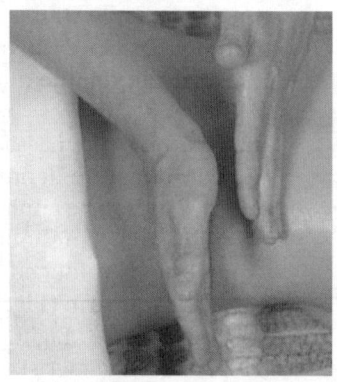

Fig. 20.10: Hacking.

- Perform **cupping**: Stretched the elbow and make a cup shape with hand, create vacuums, and try to produce cupping sound striking against the surface of the back. May produce redness **(Fig. 20.11)**.

After Care

- ❖ Assist patient to put the clothes.
- ❖ Provide comfortable position after giving back care.
- ❖ Do evaluation of the patient's satisfaction after providing back care.
- ❖ Replace all articles.
- ❖ Do hand washing.

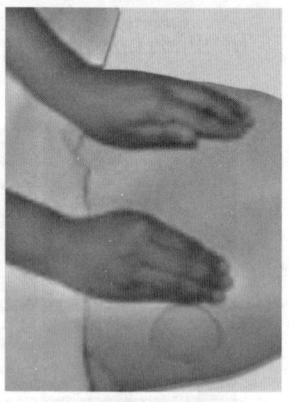

Fig. 20.11: Cupping.

CHAPTER 21

Oral Hygiene

INRODUCTION

In practical sense, the care of mouth is not routinely a part of nursing for a patient who can take care of himself and is fully conscious and able to clean his mouth. But it is certainly essential for bedridden patient who cannot properly clean his mouth. Dirty mouth causes discomfort and loss of appetite. It may lead to monilial or candidial infection, parotitis, septic ulceration of gums and fauces, gastroenteritis and even inhalation pneumonia.

DEFINITION

Oral hygiene is the practice of keeping patient's teeth and oral cavity clean through regular oral hygiene practices.

PURPOSES

- ❖ To keep mouth clean and refreshed.
- ❖ To avoid foul breath and foul odor while talking.
- ❖ To help in keeping teeth in good condition.
- ❖ To prevent and treat mouth infections.
- ❖ To help increase in appetite and stimulate flow of saliva.
- ❖ To prevent infection of salivary glands.
- ❖ To remove sores and prevent their formation.

ORAL CARE OF CONSCIOUS PATIENTS (FIG. 21.1)

Articles Required

- ❖ Toothbrush and paste
- ❖ Mackintosh
- ❖ A jug of water for mouth wash
- ❖ A bowl for collection of waste dirty water
- ❖ Towel
- ❖ Emollient

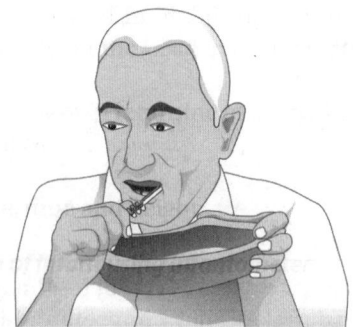

Fig. 21.1: Oral care of conscious patient.

- Kidney tray
- Tongue-brush, if required.

Steps of Procedure

- For such patient who can take care of his teeth, place everything ready for use in front of the patient or on side.
- Assess patient self-care abilities.
- Wash hands and wear gloves.
- Assess the patient's oral cavity for presence of any infection.
- Place the patient in comfortable position.
- Place the mackintosh in front of the patient on his lap in sitting position.
- Apply toothpaste and hand over the toothbrush.
- Allow him to clean his teeth and mouth himself by moving the bristles up and down by stroking it gently.
- Use the backside of the toothbrush to clean tongue.
- Rinse the mouth thoroughly with water and ask patient to discard out in kidney tray.
- Repeat the procedure till mouth is clean.
- Wipe the patient's mouth and apply emollient on the lips.
- After cleaning, place the cleaning items tidy in its place in bedside locker, if provided.

ORAL CARE OF UNCONSCIOUS PATIENTS (FIG. 21.2)

Articles Required

- Glass or feeding cup
- Mouthwash solution

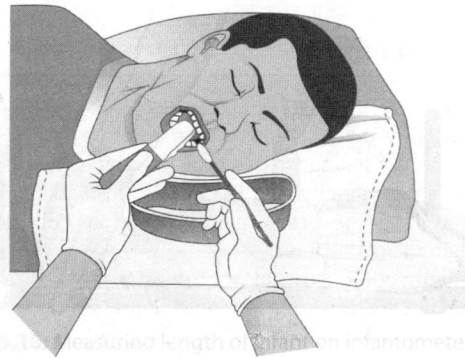

Fig. 21.2: Oral care of unconscious patient.

- Jug of water
- Gauge pieces in bowl
- Kidney tray
- One artery forceps
- Thumb forceps
- Applicator
- Emollient
- Mackintosh
- One small towel
- Clean gloves
- Tongue depressor
- Mouth gag to open mouth in unconscious or semiconscious patient.

Steps of Procedure

- Assess the oral hygiene of patient.
- Assess for the presence of gag reflex.
- Bedside screen is placed for privacy.
- Raise the bed according to the comfortable working level.
- Place patient in comfortable position with head turning towards you.
- Bring the tray to the bedside.
- Place the towel and mackintosh under the patient head to protect the bed from soiling.
- Place a towel under the chin spreading over the chest of the patient.
- Raise the side rails of the bed from both sides.
- Wash hands and wear clean gloves.

Clinical Pearls

Care of dentures
- The artificial dentures should be cleaned twice daily.
- The denture are scraped in clean warm water with brush.
- Nowadays denture cleaning fluid is also available in different packs marketed in various brand names by various companies which are equally good and hygienic.
- The patient should clean his mouth after removal of denture. After cleaning, the denture is placed conveniently.

- Lower the side rails on the working side.
- Insert a padded tongue depressor to separate the upper and lower teeth.
- Take a swab firmly holding by an artery forceps dipped in mouth wash solution, squeeze it well against the side of the bowl inside and out and then swab the teeth gums. The swabs are changed one after another as per requirement.
- Clean chewing surface first and then inner and outer surface from gum to crown. The lower teeth must be clean from both sides followed by upper teeth.
- Gently clean the roof of the mouth, gums and inner side of cheeks with a swab.
- The inside of the teeth and tongue cleaned in the same manner using water.
- Wipe the mouth and dry.
- Apply emolient over the lips, if required.
- Place the patient in same position prior to the procedure.
- Raise the side rails and lower the bed.
- Remove and keep all items tidy in proper place.
- Special care should be taken to remove sores and crusts very gently to avoid bleeding underneath mucous membrane.

CHAPTER 22

Perineal Care

INTRODUCTION

The region between the anus and the vaginal opening is referred to as the perineum. Because the perineum region is prone to infection due to its proximity to the sites of urine and fecal excretion, it is critical for nurses to provide perineal care for hospitalized patients. Perineal care is required more frequently in certain situations, such as diarrhea, fecal or urine incontinence, vaginal bleeding or discharge.

DEFINITION

Perineal care means care of perineum of a female patient. It means cleaning the area, to prevent contamination in an aseptic technique.

PURPOSES

- To prevent contamination and sepsis (pus formation).
- To clean and remove the discharge.
- To prevent foul smell from the area.
- To assist better and quick healing of wound.
- To relieve from itching, scratching and providing comfort.

INDICATIONS

- Postnatal
- Bedridden patient
- Vaginal infection
- Episiotomy cases
- Incontinence of urine or stool
- Patients with indwelling catheter
- Patients who have undergone rectal or genital surgery

ARTICLES REQUIRED

- Disposable gloves
- Soap dish with soap

- Wash basin with warm water
- Cotton swabs
- Sanitary pad or napkin
- Sponge holding forceps
- Mackintosh
- Bedpan
- Kidney tray
- Wash cloths
- Towel
- Bedsheet
- Bedside screen
- Toilet tissues or diaper wipes

STEPS OF PROCEDURE

Preliminary Assessment

- Explain to the patient regarding the procedure.
- Ask the patient to empty the bladder.
- Collect all the materials required on a table near the bed.
- Wash your hands and wear gloves.
- Put the bedside screen for privacy.

Female Genital Care

- Ask the patient to lie on her back with her knees flexed and spread out.
- Place the top linen or bed sheet towards the foot side of bed and fold patient's gown above the genital area.
- Put the back of the patient on the mackintosh.
- Remove all old soiled dressings carefully. Care should be taken while removing dressing sticking to the stitches otherwise with forceful removal of dressing from stitches, the stitch may be removed which is a bad procedure.
- Assess for any signs of inflammation, infection, discharge or lochia.
- If there is any presence of fecal material, remove by using a toilet tissue. Clean the buttocks and anus from front to back using a tissue.
- Dry the area thoroughly after cleaning.
- Change the gloves
- Test the temperature of solution by pouring a drop or two over the genitalia from pubis down towards the vagina and rectum.
- Stand on right side of the patient and lower the side rails.

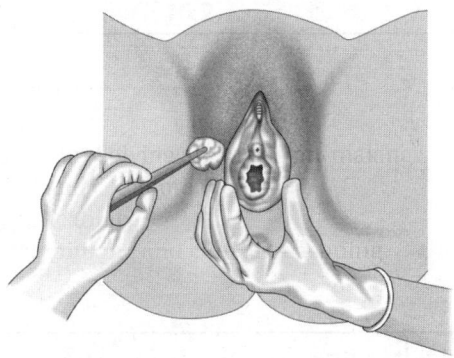

Fig. 22.1: Female genital care.

- Now take sterile cotton swab with a sponge holder and soak it with sterile solution, never dip the swab in the solution.
- Retract the labia from thigh using nondominant hand **(Fig. 22.1)**. Using cotton swab gently clean the labia majora with dominant hand from perineum to rectum. Change the cotton swab and repeat the same on the opposite side.
- Expose the urethral meatus and vaginal orifice using nondominant hand, clean downward gently from pubic area towards rectum using dominant hand.
- Clean the vulva and labia minora gently from top to down.
- Use two or three sponges by discarding 1st one and changing one after another.
- Dry the area with sterile dry sponges.
- Take care of episiotomy stitches while sponging the stitch area. Put sterile pad over vulva. if any.
- Remove the bed pan.
- Ask the patient to turn to one side, clean the buttock and back with unsterilized cotton.
- Remove the mackintosh and ask patient to lower the legs and resume comfortable position.
- Record the amount and type of vaginal discharge, the condition of perineum and condition of stitches, if any.

Male Genital Care

- Instruct the patient to lie in the supine position.
- Position the gown to cover the chest. Fold the top part bath blanket/sheet just below the penis **(Fig. 22.2)**.

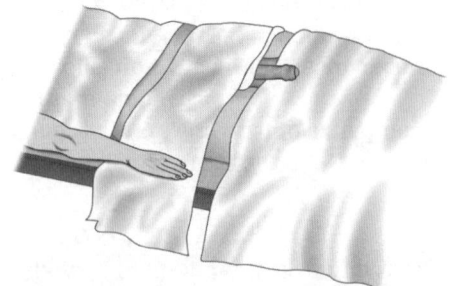

Fig. 22.2: Covering a male patient for genital care.

- Wash the upper thigh and dry the area using a towel.
- Place a bath towel underneath it as you slowly raise the penis.
- If the patient hasn't been circumcised, firmly grasp the shaft of the penis and retract the foreskin.
- Take cotton swab/wash cloths and soak it with sterile solution, never dip the swab in solution.
- Using a circular motion cleanse the urethral meatus, from outward to inward **(Fig. 22.3)**.
- Change cotton swab/wash cloths after one stroke. Dry with dry sponges/clean cloth.
- Return the foreskin to its original position.
- Instruct patient to spread legs apart and clean the shaft of the penis in a firm downward position. Dry with a sterile dry sponges/clean cloth.

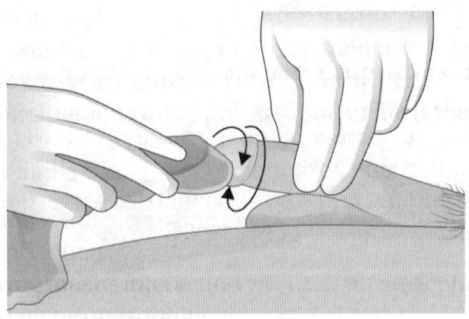

Fig. 22.3: Male genital care.

- Gently lift the scrotum and cleanse it using a cotton swab. Dry it by using a dry sterile sponges/clean cloth.
- Remove the gloves.
- Assist patient to comfortable position and cover him/her with top sheet.
- Remove bath blanket, dispose of all soiled bed linen, and return unused articles to storage area.
- Record procedure and mention any abnormal findings.

CHAPTER 23

Urinary Catheterization

INTRODUCTION

The word, catheterization means "introduction of a catheter", into a hollow or tubular organ having fluid in it. Urinary catheter can be inserted through the urethra or through the suprapubic region into the bladder and allowing urine to drain out. This procedure is considered as an effective management for bladder dysfunctions.

DEFINITION

Urinary catheterization is an aseptic procedure in which a hollow tube is inserted through the urethra into the bladder to drain or collect urine.

TYPES (FIG. 23.1)

Intermittent Catheterization

Inserting a catheter through the urethra into the bladder and removing it once the bladder has been cleared. It is a catheter-based treatment for a brief period of time.

Purposes
- For collecting sterile urine specimen.
- To empty bladder before surgery or delivery.

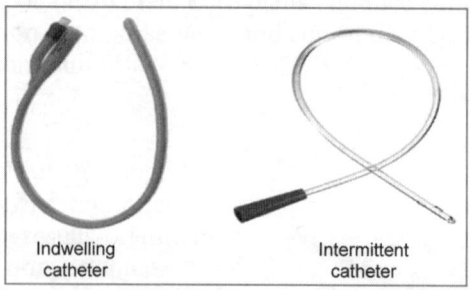

Fig. 23.1: Types of catheter.

- To relieve bladder distension.
- To measure residual urine.
- To decompress the bladder.

Indwelling Catheterization

Catheter is inserted through the urethra into the bladder and left in place for a period of time. It is used in cases where continuous evacuation of bladder content is required.

Purposes

- To monitor urine output after surgery.
- To prevent urinary obstructions.
- To provide urine elimination in case of acute and chronic urinary retention.
- To promote healing perineal ulcers or incision where urine may cause further skin breakdown.

ARTICLES REQUIRED

- A sterile tray.
- Sterile perineal care set/tray.
- Indwelling/straight Catheters/Foley's catheter.
- Sterile cotton swabs.
- Small bowl.
- Sterile kidney tray.
- Sterile gloves.
- Sterile gauze pieces.
- Sterile towel.
- Artery forceps.
- Dissecting forceps.
- Sterile syringe (20 mL) and distilled water.

A Clean Tray Containing

- Light source or torch.
- Disposable gloves (2 nos.)
- Sponge holding forceps.
- Antiseptic solution.
- Distilled water or normal saline.
- Lubricant jelly.
- Adhesive tape and scissors.
- Uro bag.

- ❖ Paper bag.
- ❖ Bedpan.
- ❖ Specimen bottle.
- ❖ Mackintosh.
- ❖ Draw sheet.
- ❖ Bed side screen.
- ❖ Unsterilized kidney tray.

STEPS OF PROCEDURE

Preliminary Assessment

- ❖ Explain the procedure to the patients.
- ❖ Assess the patient condition regarding mobility, pathological condition and awareness.
- ❖ Place all equipment's near the bedside table.
- ❖ Put the bedside screen to maintain privacy.
- ❖ Wash hands and don the clean gloves.

Female

- ❖ Position the patient in modified dorsal recumbent position with knees flexed and thighs externally rotated.
- ❖ Place mackintosh and draw sheet under hip.
- ❖ Keep all articles ready in place:
    - Open sterile tray without touching the inside of the tray.
    - Open the cover of the prepackaged catheter and place it in the tray.
    - Open the lubricant and squeeze the required amount out on a sterile gauze (Discard the first drop).
- ❖ Clean the perineal area using perineal care set (Refer chapter 22 for perineal care procedure).
- ❖ Put on the sterile gloves.
- ❖ Open sterile specimen bottle and place it in the sterile tray.
- ❖ Take the 20 mL sterile syringe and filled it with distilled or normal saline. Check the balloon by inflating it. Deflate the balloon and place it in the sterile tray with syringe attached to it (only for indwelling catheter).
- ❖ Apply the lubricant at the tip of the catheter and place it in the sterile tray.
- ❖ Separate labia minora with two fingers of left hand by means of sterile sponges and expose to see the urethral meatus (Use flashlight if necessary).

Urinary Catheterization

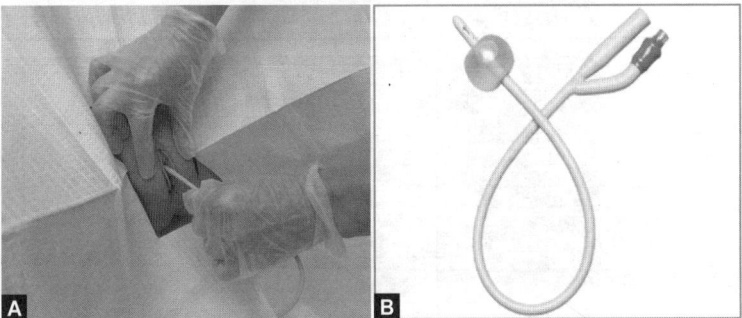

Figs. 23.2A and B: (A) Insertion of urinary catheter in female; (B) Inflated balloon of catheter.

- Clean the meatus using antiseptic solution (If recommended). Take sterile cotton swabs dipped in antiseptic solution and clean perineal area from clitoris towards anus using one swab for each wipe.
- Using the dominant hand, hold the catheter 3" to 4" from tip. Instruct patient to take a deep breath and insert the catheter gently **(Fig. 23.2A)** for 2.5–5 cm till urine starts flowing in the kidney tray.
- When urine starts flowing hold the catheter by left hand fingers to avoid slipping out.
- If a sterile urine sample is required, discard few mL of urine in unsterilized kidney tray then collect in sterilized bottle.
- When urine flow stops, remove the catheter and put it in unsterilized kidney tray (For intermittent catheterization).
- Inflate the balloon with distilled or normal saline (For indwelling catheterization) **(Fig. 23.2B)**.
- Connect the catheter with the uro bag and tie it to the bed below the level of bladder.
- Using adhesive tape fix the catheter to the thigh.
- Clean and replace all articles.
- Record the procedure in patient's chart.
- The sterile specimen should be labelled properly before sending to laboratory.
- When removal of catheter is required never forget to remove the injected water by a syringe first through its thinner end.
- When the water is withdrawn, then gently remove the catheter which comes out easily. If there is still difficulty, then see that some water may be left in bulb. So, try again to remove water by withdrawing through a syringes.

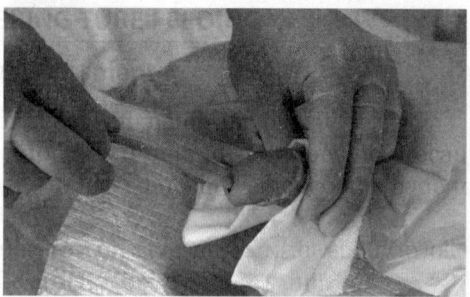

Fig. 23.3: Insertion of urinary catheter in male.

Male

- Position the patient in supine position with thighs slightly abducted.
- Place mackintosh piece over thighs under penis.
- Put a sterile towel over mackintosh.
- The foreskin or prepuce or penis is retracted back using dominant hand to expose the urethral meatus.
- With the dominant hand clean the area with antiseptic solution by using sterile swab in backward direction from meatus. Use one swab for each wipe.
- Clean the area using sterile saline in the same manner.
- Instruct patient to take a deep breath, with dominant hand insert the lubricated catheter for 15–25 cm **(Fig. 23.3)**, until urine begins to flow.
- Do not use force while inserting the catheter.
- When urine starts flowing hold the catheter by left hand fingers to avoid slipping out.
- When urine flow stops, remove catheter and put it in unsterilized kidney tray (For intermittent catheterization).
- Inflate the balloon with distilled or normal saline (For indwelling catheterization).
- Connect the catheter with the uro bag and tie it to the bed below the level of bladder.
- Using adhesive tape fix the catheter to the thigh.
- Clean and replace all articles.
- Record the procedure in patient's chart.

CHAPTER 24

Assisting with Bedpan

INTRODUCTION

Bedpans are used to treat elimination issues in patients who are unable to leave their bed to use the restroom. Bedpans come in a variety of sizes and are a ubiquitous piece of medical equipment in hospitals. Nurses play an essential role in assisting patients with bedpan usage.

DEFINITION

Bedpan is a shallow toilet pan made of steel or plastic used by bedridden patient for urination or defecation.

PURPOSES

- To facilitate bowel and bladder elimination.
- For specimen collection.
- For bowel and bladder training.
- To give perineal wash.

ARTICLES REQUIRED

- Bedpan with lid.
- Clean gloves.
- Mackintosh.
- Draw sheets.
- Towels.
- Bedside screen.
- Water and mug.
- Tissue paper.
- Soap with soap dish K-basin and towel.

STEPS OF PROCEDURE

- Assess the patient's level of consciousness and understanding.
- Assess the patient's level of limitations in movements and positions that he can assume.

Assisting with Bedpan

- ❖ Check for any special instructions from the physician.
- ❖ Explain the procedure to patients and relatives, ask relatives to assist in case if assistance is required.
- ❖ Wash hands and wear gloves.
- ❖ Place mackintosh over the bed to prevent the bed from getting wet.
- ❖ Place the bedside screen near the bed.
- ❖ Dry the bedpan, pour water in the bedpan just enough to cover the bottom part. Keep the bedpan within reach.
- ❖ Remove the top sheet just enough to give space to put the bedpan under the patient buttocks.
- ❖ Elevate the height of the bed as needed.
  - *If lower limbs movement is not restricted:*
    - Instruct patient to flex the knees and weight of the body resting on the back or legs.
    - Instruct the patient to raise the buttocks and slide the bedpan under the buttocks at a count of three **(Fig. 24.1A)**.
  - *If lower limbs movement is restricted:* Position the patient in side-lying position, place the bedpan against the buttocks **(Fig. 24.1B)** and roll the patient onto the bedpan in supine position.
- ❖ While placing the bedpan make sure the smooth, wider flat area is beneath the buttocks **(Fig. 24.2)**.
- ❖ Elevate the bed in semi-Fowler's position or support patient back with pillows.
- ❖ Cover the patient with a bed linen and raise the side rails. Leave the patient alone if possible and keep call bell within reach.

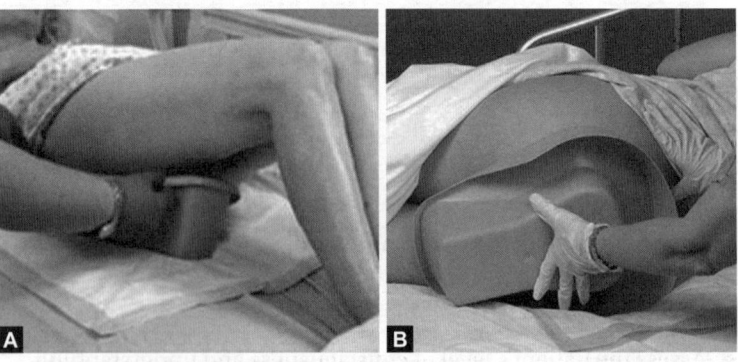

Figs. 24.1A and B: Placing of bedpan for hospitalized patient. (A) For unrestricted lower limbs patient; (B) For restricted lower limbs patient.

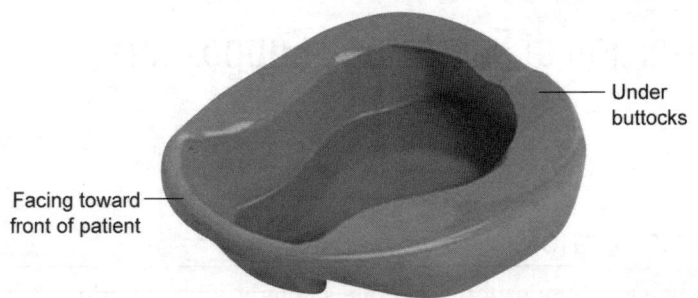

Fig. 24.2: Bedpan.

- If the patient is able to clean himself, provide tissue to wipe it clean.
- If a patient is unable to clean himself, provide perineal care and anal care.
- Remove the bedpan carefully, close the lid and put it away from the bed.
- Provide soap and water to patients for handwashing.
- Remove the mackintosh. Change linen if wet.
- Cover the patient with a top sheet and instruct patient to assume comfortable position.
- Place the bed in the same position as before the procedure.
- Send bedpan to utility room. Clean and replace all articles.
- Wash hands and record the procedure.

CHAPTER 25

Insertion of Enema and Suppository

INTRODUCTION

Enema and suppositories operate similarly, with the primary goal of softening the hardened stools. Enema is more effective than suppositories because it contains more medication with each use and can reach farther, whereas suppositories have fewer side effects, are considered safer, and can be used for a longer period of time.

ENEMA

An enema is the introduction of fluid into rectum mostly either to empty lower bowel or to introduce a medicinal substance for its general or local effect or for diagnostic purpose.

Types of Enema

See **Fig. 25.1**.

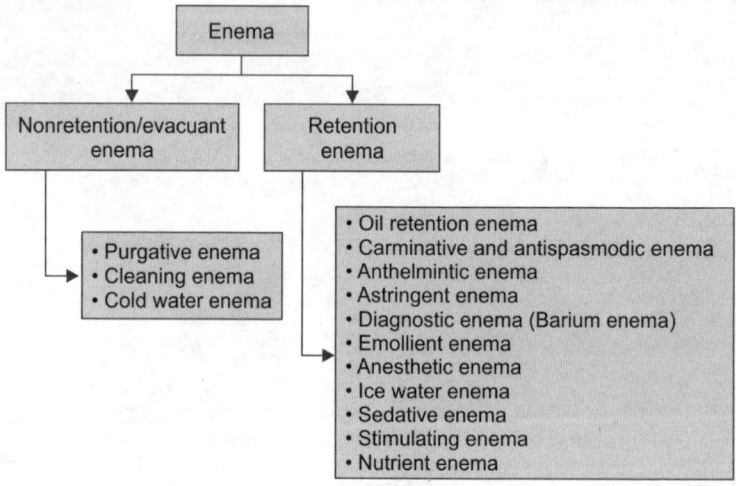

Fig. 25.1: Types of enema.

Insertion of Enema and Suppository

Purposes

- Cleaning of lower bowel.
- For emptying purpose—soap solution enema.
- For diagnostic purpose—barium enema.
- For introducing drug/substance—retention enema.
  - Cold enema to reduce temperature.
  - Coffee enema to stimulate patient.
  - Sedative enema to quite patient.
  - Starch or opium enema for soothing irritated mucosa of colon.
  - Carminative enema for relieving gases and distention.
  - Check shelling enema to stimulate peristalsis.
  - Starch to check diarrhea.
  - Nutrient enema of glucose or saline to provide fluid or other nutrients.
  - Hypertonic enema to destroy parasites.
  - Anesthetic enema for anesthesia purpose (not used nowadays).
  - Oxytocic enema to stimulate uterine contraction and labor.

Evacuant Enema/Cleansing Enema

Articles Required

- Large tray.
- Enema-can with rubber tubing.
- Disposable gloves.
- Rectal catheter.
  - Adult size: 22–30 Fr.
  - Child size: 12–18 Fr.
- Bath thermometer.
- Solution of soap or disposable enema solution packet.
- Lubricant solution or Vaseline.
- Towel.
- Clean sheet.
- Bowl.
- Toilet tissues/clean gauze
- Enema/IV stand.
- Bedpan with cover.
- Bed side screen.
- Bowl of cotton swabs.
- Forceps.

- ❖ Kidney tray
- ❖ Mackintosh

Solutions Used

Solution

- ❖ Hypertonic: Sodium phosphate and fleet enema.
- ❖ Hypotonic: Tap water.
- ❖ Isotonic: Physiological saline (one tsp. of table salt in 500 mL of tap water).
- ❖ Others: 3–5 mL of concentrated soap solutions in 1,000 mL of water.

Amount Used with Different Age Group

Amount

- ❖ Adult: 750–1,000 mL.
- ❖ Adolescent: 500–750 mL.
- ❖ School age: 300–500 mL.
- ❖ Toddler: 250–300 mL.
- ❖ Infant: 150–250 mL.

Steps of Procedure

- ❖ Identify the patient and review physician's order.
- ❖ Explain the procedure and purpose to the patient.
- ❖ Arrange all articles near the bedside.
- ❖ Wash hands and don gloves.
- ❖ Place the bedside screen near the bedside.
- ❖ Instruct the patient to lie in a side-lying/Sim's position. Provide assistance if necessary.
- ❖ Place the bedpan next to the bedside so that it is easily accessible.
- ❖ Cover the patient with a clean sheet and expose only the anal area.
- ❖ Place the mackintosh beneath the patient's buttocks and hips.
- ❖ Check the temperature of the solution using bath thermometer or use inner wrist.
- ❖ Open the clamp of the tubing and remove air by elevating the tubing and allowing the solution to fill the tubing. Clamp the tubing.
- ❖ Apply lubricant or Vaseline to the tip of the tube.
- ❖ Locate the anus by spreading the buttocks.
- ❖ With one hand, hold the tube in place and Instruct patient to take a deep breath.

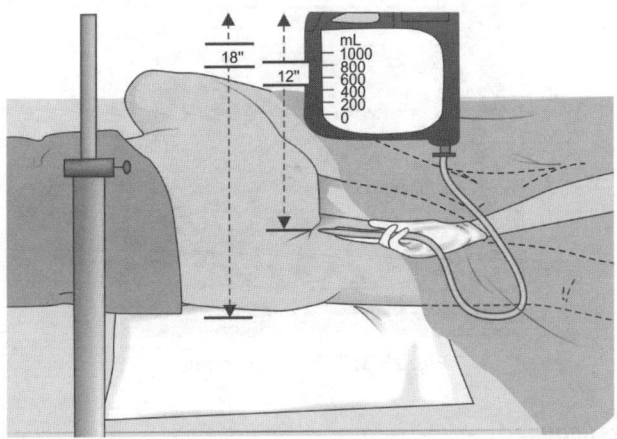

Fig. 25.2: Inserting tip of rectal tube.

- Insert the tip of the tube into the anus **(Fig. 25.2)** for 7.5–10 cm (adults), 5–7.5 cm (children), 2.5–3.7 cm (infant).
- Raise the enema can by suspending it from the IV stand.
- Open the clamp and allow solution to enter slowly.
- Stand near the patient and observe for any signs of cramping or pain. In case of any cramping lower the can or clamp the tubing for 30 seconds.
- After all the solution is instilled clamp the tube.
- Gently withdraw the tube from the anus.
- Place the clean gauze/toilet tissue at the anal end of the tubing and remove it slowly.
- Instruct patient to retain the solution for at least 5–10 minutes.
- Provide bedpan to the patient or assist to position on bedpan if necessary.
- Observe the expelled fecal material or solution for presence of mucus, blood or any abnormalities.
- Discard used items in appropriate places.
- Remove gloves and wash hands.
- Clean and replace reusable articles.
- Record the procedure and mention any abnormal findings.

Proctoclysis

Proctoclysis enema is a laxative or bowel cleanser medication used for the treatment of constipation.

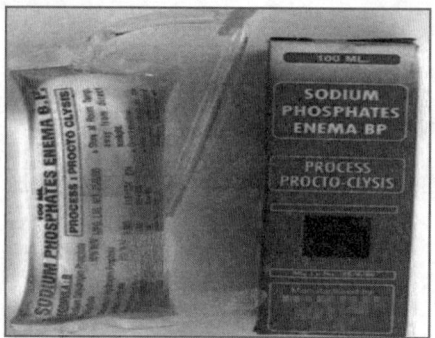

Fig. 25.3: Prepacked enema.

Articles Required

- Packet of enema (prepacked) **(Fig. 25.3)**.
- Clean gloves.
- Soap and water.
- Mackintosh.
- Kidney tray.
- Lubricant jelly or Vaseline.
- Toilet tissue/clean gauze.
- Beside screen.
- Bedpan.

Steps of Procedure

- Identify the patient and review physician's order.
- Explain the procedure and purpose to the patient.
- Arrange all articles near the bedside.
- Wash hands and don gloves.
- Place the bedside screen near the bedside.
- Instruct the patient to lie in a side-lying/Sim's position. Provide assistance if necessary.
- Place the bedpan next to the bedside so that it is easily accessible.
- Cover the patient with a clean sheet and expose only the anal area.
- Place the mackintosh beneath the patient's buttocks and hips.
- Remove the cap of the rectal tube and apply lubricant as needed.
- Locate the anus by spreading the buttocks.
- Instruct patient to take a deep breath and insert the tip of the prepacked enema into the anus **(Fig. 25.4)** for 7.5–10 cm (adults), 5–7.5 cm (children), 2.5–3.7 cm (infant).

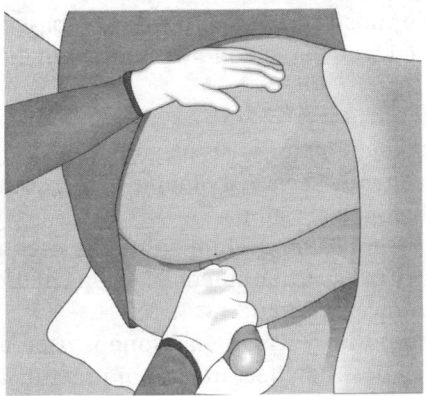

Fig. 25.4: Insertion of prepacked enema.

- Hold the enema bottle/pouch in upward direction and squeezed it till emptied.
- Place the clean gauze/toilet tissue at the anal end of the tubing and remove it slowly.
- Instruct patient to retain the solution till the urge to defecate occurs.
- Provide bedpan to the patient or assist to position on bedpan if necessary.
- Observe the expelled fecal material or solution for presence of mucus, blood or any abnormalities.
- Discard used items in appropriate places.
- Remove gloves and wash hands.
- Clean and replace reusable articles.
- Record the procedure and mention any abnormal findings.

SUPPOSITORIES

Suppository is a form of rectal medication mainly for local effects and sometimes for general effects. Usually, it is solid at room temperature. When introduced it melts at body temperature and produces 'local effect.

Types of Suppositories

- **Glycerin suppository:** This is an evacuant suppository used for starting defecation reflex. It acts as hygroscopic agent slowly causing evacuation by withdrawing fluid from tissue.

Insertion of Enema and Suppository

- **Bisacodyl Suppository:** This procedure is based on peristalsis in large bowed by reflex action by contact with mucosal nervous plexus.
- **Retained Suppository:**
  - *Aminophylline suppository* is given for retention in rectum to produce general effects of aminophylline by way of absorption in case of bronchial asthma.
  - *Anesthetic suppository:* Thiopentone is used sometimes as suppository to cause anesthetic effect in children as alternate route to intravenous route.
  - *Steroid suppository:* Hydrocortisone is used as suppository to produce desired effect in case of proctitis and ulcerative colitis.

Purposes

- To induce peristaltic movement.
- To empty the bowel to relieve constipation.
- To relief from pain.
- To reduce body temperature.

Articles Required

- Rectal suppository.
- Clean gloves.
- Mackintosh.
- Kidney tray.
- Lubricant jelly or Vaseline.
- Toilet tissue/clean gauze.
- Bedpan.
- Bed side screen.

Steps of Procedure

- Identify the patient and review physician order.
- Explain the procedure to the patient.
- Arrange all articles near the bedside.
- Wash hands and don gloves.
- Place the bedside screen near the bedside.
- Instruct/assist patient to lie in a side-lying/Sim's position.
- Cover the patient with a clean sheet and expose only the anal area.
- Place the mackintosh beneath the patient's buttocks and hips.

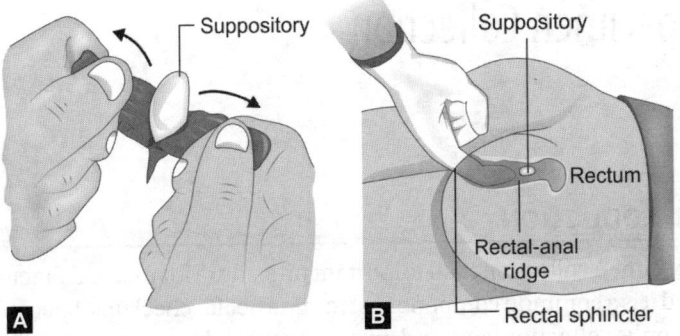

Figs. 25.5A and B: (A) Suppository; (B) Insertion of suppository.

- Inspect the rectal area for presence of any bleeding and palpate the rectal walls to determine whether the rectum if filled with feces.
- Open the suppository from package **(Fig. 25.5A)**, take the suppository and lubricate the rounded end.
- Instruct patient to take a deep breath, using the dominant hand insert the suppository into the anus, pass the internal sphincter muscle nearly 10 cm (5 cm in children and infants) into rectum or approximately one index finger length **(Fig. 25.5B)**.
- Withdraw the finger and apply pressure over area and hold buttocks together for short time.
- If the suppository is for evacuation of bowel put bed pan under buttock as the patient may desire at any time to pass stool. If the suppository is retained instruct the patient to retain it for 20–30 minute till it completely melts to cause desired effect even if he feels to pass stool.
- Instruct patient to lie flat on the bed for 5 minutes.
- After 5 minutes, evaluate the patient's condition to check if the suppository is in place and if the patient is experiencing any anal or rectal discomfort/pain.
- Remove gloves and wash hands.
- Discard and replace all articles.
- Record the procedure.

CHAPTER 26

Specimen Collection

INTRODUCTION

Specimen collection is an important procedure for medical diagnosis and it is a common component of routine health checkups. Specimen/sample collection go hand-in-hand with laboratory test assisting medical professionals to rule out diagnosis and treatment plans according to the results obtained. Some of the sample collection may include urine, stool, blood, throat swab, cerebrospinal fluid, biopsy etc.

DEFINITION

Specimen collection may be defined as collection of sample for laboratory analysis for the purpose of diagnosis, treatment and monitoring disease.

URINE SPECIMEN FOR ROUTINE EXAMINATION

Purposes

- To measure protein, hormones, minerals and other chemical compounds.
- To identify the presence of bacteria.
- To identify presence of any abnormalities such as red blood cells, white blood cells, casts, pH, sugar, albumin, and specific gravity.
- To rule out presence of drugs, alcohol.

Articles Required

- Wide mouth urine sample container (use sterile container for culture).
- Laboratory requisition form.
- Soap and water.
- Bedpan or urinal.
- Clean gloves.

Steps of Procedure

- ❖ Identify the patient.
- ❖ Explain the procedure to the patient.
- ❖ Instruct the patient to wash the external genitalia with soap and water. For female patients, separate the labia and clean. For male patients, retract the foreskin and clean the glans penis.
- ❖ Hand over the labelled container to the patient. The container must be labelled with patient name, age, sex, date and time.
- ❖ Instruct patient not to contaminate the inside of the container and lid.
- ❖ Instruct the patient to collect 100–120 mL of midstream urine **(Fig. 26.1A and B)**.
- ❖ **In 24 hour urine collection:** Instruct the patient to begin collecting urine at 6 AM and continue until 6 AM the next day. Save all collected urine in a large labelled container.
- ❖ **For culture:** Instruct patient to collect only midstream urine into the sterile container **(Fig. 26.1A and B)**.
- ❖ **For catheterized patients:** Clamp the collection tube for 30 minutes before taking sample, withdraw the required amount of urine using sterile needle and syringe from the catheter sampling port.

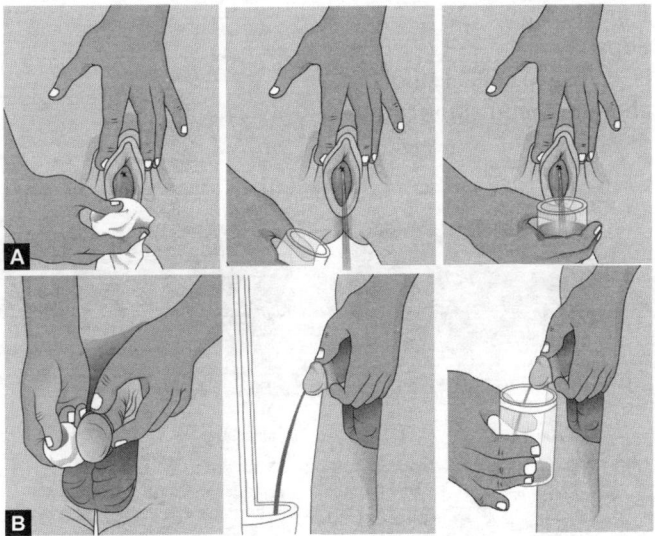

Figs. 26.1A and B: (A) Collection of midstream urine in female; (B) Collection of midstream urine in male.

- Instruct patient to place the specimen container in sample collection area.
- Wear gloves and place the urine container in sample collection bag/box and send it to the laboratory along with the laboratory requisition forms.
- Urine specimen must be send to the laboratory within 30 minutes (15 minutes for culture) or immediately place it in the refrigerator.
- Remove gloves and wash hands.
- Record the date, time and procedure.

STOOL SPECIMEN FOR ROUTINE AND CULTURE

Purposes

- To identify stool color, consistency, shape, odor, mucus and pH.
- To test for presence of any abnormalities.
- To detect presence of bacteria, viruses and parasites.
- To help in the diagnosis of gastrointestinal disorders.

Articles Required

- Stool specimen container (spatula attached) **(Fig. 26.2)**
- Fecal swab
- Clean gloves
- Bedpan
- Plastic bag to collect stool
- Laboratory requisition form

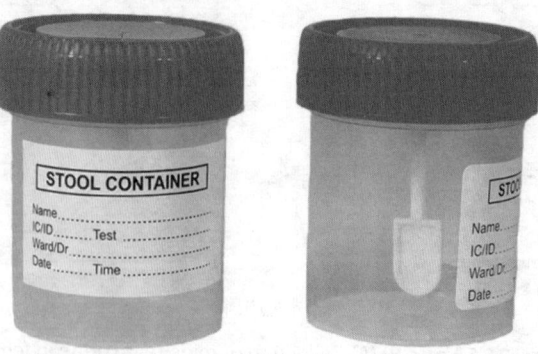

Fig. 26.2: Stool sample container.

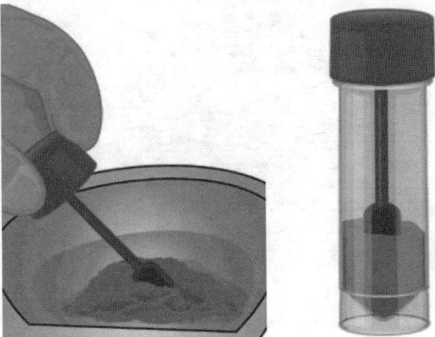

Fig. 26.3: Stool sample in sample container.

Steps of Procedure

- Check the physician order and identify the patient.
- Explain the procedure to the patient.
- Labelled the stool specimen container with patient name, age, sex, date and time.
- Handover the container to the patient.
- Instruct patient to defecate in a dry bedpan (assist if necessary) and not to urinate in the pan.
- Use two bedpans in case of bedridden patients. One for sample collection and other for cleaning.
- Instruct patient to keep the bedpan on the side.
- Wear gloves and collect the stool sample in the sample container (Fig. 26.3)
    - *Routine examination:* Formed stool: 2 cm, diarrheal stool: 20–30 mL.
    - *Culture analysis:* Formed stool: 1cm, diarrheal stool: 10–15 mL.
- Place the stool specimen container in a plastic bag and send it to the laboratory with the requisition form.
- Wash and dry hands.
- Replace all the articles.
- Record the procedure with date and time of sample collection.

THROAT SWAB SPECIMEN FOR CULTURE

Articles Required

- Cotton tipped applicators in sterile packed test tube.
- Tongue depressor.

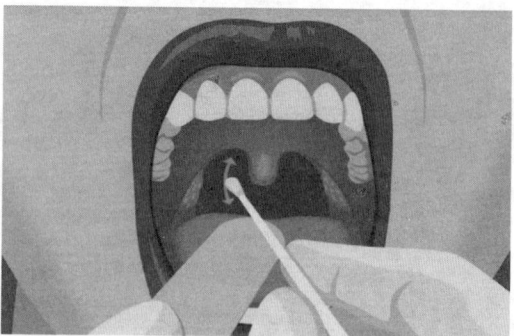

Fig. 26.4: Collecting throat swab specimen.

- Laboratory requisition form.
- Flashlight.
- Clean gloves.
- Clean gauze.

Steps of Procedure

- Check the physician order and identify the patient.
- Explain the procedure to the patient.
- Wash hands and wear gloves.
- Have the patient sit comfortably in chair or bed and instruct patient to sit in upright position (assist if necessary).
- Ask patient to tilt his head back and open his/her mouth saying "Ahhh". Hold the tongue using a tongue depressor.
- Assess the back of the throat for any inflammation using a flashlight.
- Rub the cotton tipped applicator over the tonsil areas from side-to-side. Ensure the cheek, teeth and gums are untouched **(Fig. 26.4)**.
- Place the cotton tipped applicator inside the culture tube immediately.
- Immediately send the specimen to the laboratory immediately along with the requisition form.
- Remove gloves and wash hands.
- Replace all the articles.
- Record the procedure with date and time.

WOUND SWAB FOR CULTURE

Articles Required

- Cotton tipped applicators in sterile packed test tube.
- Culture swab container.

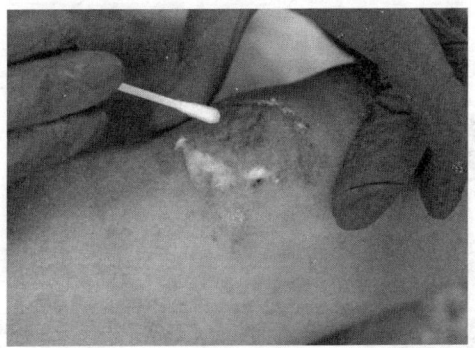

Fig. 26.5: Collecting wound swab.

- Laboratory requisition form.
- Bedside screen.
- Clean gloves.

Steps of Procedure

- Check the physician order and identify the patient.
- Explain the procedure to the patient.
- Check that the culture swab container is label correctly. Mention the anatomic part from where the exudate is obtained.
- Have the patient sit comfortably in a chair or bed and instruct patient to sit in upright position (assist if necessary).
- Place bedside screen if necessary to provide privacy.
- Wash hands and wear gloves.
- Using one hand expose the wound area and on the other hand collect exudate from the wound using cotton tipped applicators **(Fig. 26.5)**.
- Ensure that exudate is collected from the center of the wound moving towards the periphery in circular motion.
- After an adequate amount of exudate is collected, put it in the culture swab container.
- Send it to the laboratory along with the requisition form.
- Record the procedure.

BLOOD SAMPLE COLLECTION FOR ROUTINE EXAMINATION

Articles Required

- Syringes (10 mL)
- Tourniquet

Specimen Collection

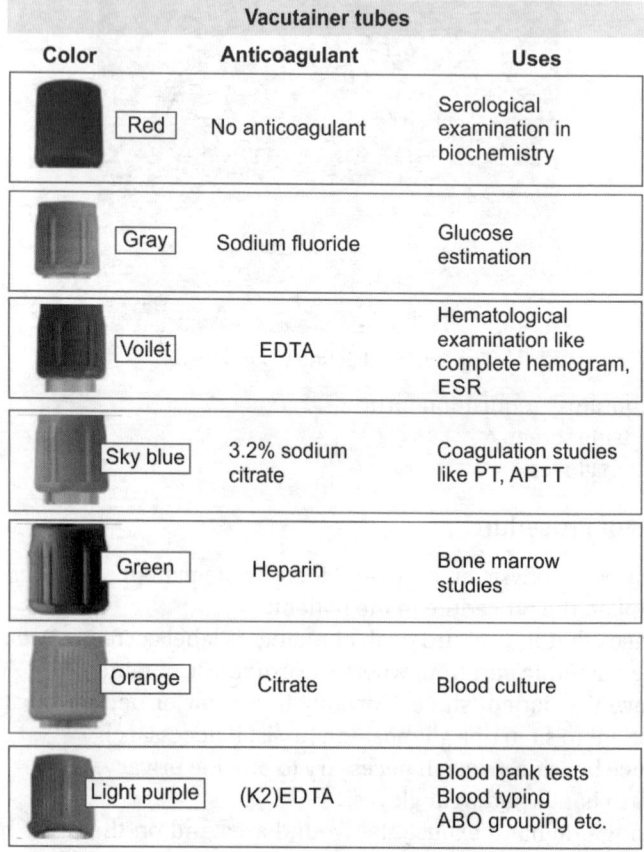

Fig. 26.6: Blood sample container.

- Clean gloves
- Alcohol swabs
- Blood sample container **(Fig. 26.6)**
- Laboratory requisition form
- Dry gauze
- Adhesive tape

Steps of Procedure

- Check the physician order and identify the patient.
- Explain the procedure to the patient.

Specimen Collection

- Wash hands and wear gloves.
- Have the patient sit comfortably in a chair or bed and instruct patient to sit in upright position (assist if necessary).
- Instruct patient to extend his/her arm and examine the vein. Inspect the antecubital fossa or forearm. Palpate the vein and select the vein which is straight and clear.
- Instruct patient to hold the arm straight with fist clenched and apply tourniquet 5–15 cm/4–5 fingers width just above the selected site.
- Apply alcohol swab at the selected site from center to periphery in a circular motion. Ensure that it covers an area of 2 cm or more.
- Hold the patient's arm with one hand and insert the thumb below the venipuncture site to secure the vein.
- Insert the needle smoothly along the vein and obtain the blood sample by pulling back on the plunger of the syringe **(Fig. 26.7A)**.
- After the required amount of blood sample is collected release the tourniquet.
- Apply gentle pressure to the site with a dry gauze and gently withdraw the needle **(Fig. 26.7B)**.
- Instruct patient to hold the gauze in place, with the arm extended and raised.
- Remove the needle carefully and gently eject blood sample to the appropriate container/sample tube.
- Invert the tube gently several times to mix the blood with the anticoagulant, if applicable.
- Apply adhesive tape at the puncture site.
- Label the sample container/tube and send it to the laboratory along with requisition forms.
- Dispose materials in appropriate places. Ensure the needle is disposed at puncture proof container.

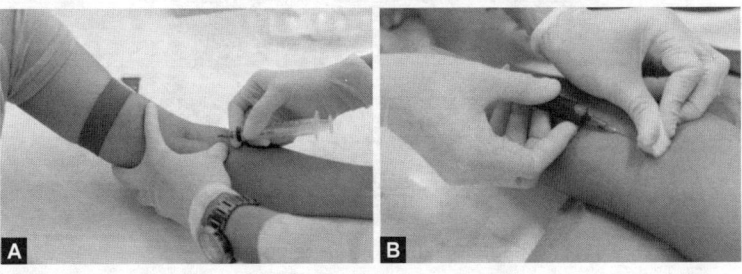

Figs. 26.7A and B: (A) Collecting blood sample; (B) Withdrawing the needle.

- Remove gloves and wash hands.
- Record the procedure.

BLOOD SAMPLE COLLECTION FOR CULTURE

Articles Required

- Syringes (10 mL)
- Tourniquet
- Povidone-iodine solution
- Sterile gloves
- Alcohol swabs
- Blood culture bottles **(Fig. 26.8)**
- Laboratory requisition form
- Dry gauze
- Adhesive tape

Steps of Procedure

- Check the physician order and identify the patient.
- Explain the procedure to the patient.
- Wash hands and wear gloves.
- Have the patient sit comfortably in a chair or bed and instruct patient to sit in upright position (assist if necessary).

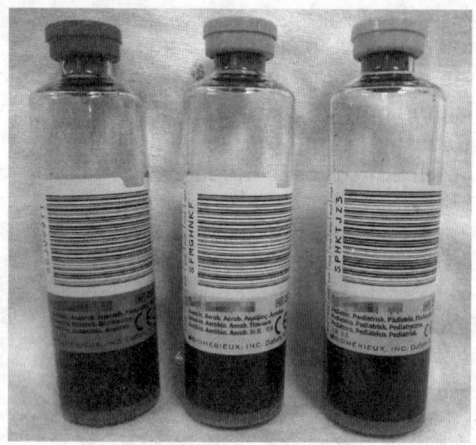

Fig. 26.8: Blood culture bottles.

- Instruct patient to extend his/her arm and examine the vein. Inspect the antecubital fossa or forearm. Palpate the vein and select the vein which is straight and clear.
- Instruct patient to hold the arm straight with fist clenched and apply tourniquet 5–15 cm/4–5 fingers width just above the selected site.
- Apply alcohol swab at the selected site from center to periphery in a circular motion. Ensure that it covers an area of 2 cm or more.
- Cleanse the site again with povidone-iodine from center to periphery and leave it for 1 minute, then clean the site with alcohol swab.
- Hold the patient's arm with one and insert the thumb below the venipuncture site to secure the vein.
- Insert the needle smoothly along the vein and obtain the blood sample by pulling back on the plunger of the syringe **(Figs. 26.7A and B)**.
- After the required amount of blood sample (10 mL) is collected release the tourniquet.
- Apply gentle pressure to the site with dry gauze and gently withdraw the needle.
- Instruct patient to hold the gauze in place, with the arm extended and raised.
- Remove the needle carefully and replace it with a fresh sterile needle.
- Remove the metal cap of the culture bottle and inject blood sample into the bottle without touching the sides.
- Invert the tube gently several times to mix the blood and culture media.
- Apply adhesive tape at the puncture site.
- Label the culture sample bottles and send it to the laboratory along with requisition forms.
- Dispose materials in appropriate places. Ensure the needle is disposed at puncture proof container.
- Remove gloves and wash hands.
- Record the procedure.

CHAPTER 27

Oxygenation

INTRODUCTION

Oxygen is administered in order to maintain adequate tissue oxygenation with less cardiopulmonary effort. Oxygen therapy may be needed in different situation such as in emergency, acute illness and chronic illness. Oxygen can be administered in various ways using different oxygen delivery devices.

DEFINITION

Oxygenation is the process of administering oxygen to a patient via inhalation in order to deliver an appropriate amount of oxygen to bodily tissues or cells.

PURPOSES

- ❖ To reduce or prevent hypoxemia and hypoxia.
- ❖ To relieve dyspnea.
- ❖ To increase oxygen saturation in tissue.
- ❖ To increase oxygen levels in the blood.

SOURCE OF OXYGEN

- ❖ Oxygen cylinder
- ❖ Oxygen wall outlets

TYPES OF OXYGEN DELIVERY SYSTEM (TABLE 27.1 AND FIG. 27.1)

High flow delivery method:
- ❖ Ventilators
- ❖ CPAP/BiPAP drivers
- ❖ Face mask or tracheostomy mask with an Airvo 2 humidifier
- ❖ Nasal prong (High flow)
- ❖ Oxygen tent

Oxygenation

Table 27.1: Oxygen delivery devices with flow rate, concentration and indication.

Device	Flow rate (Liters/min)	Oxygen (%)	Indications
Nasal Cannula	1–6	24–44	• Non severe respiratory distress • Need for supplement oxygen at home • Low oxygen requirement • Sedation for procedure
Simple face mask	5–10	35–60	• Moderate oxygen requirement • Sedation for procedure • Mouth breathing • For aerosolized medications
Face tent	5–15	<40	• Moderate oxygen requirement • Discomfort with tight fitting mask
Venturi mask	2–15	25–60	High oxygen requirement
Nonrebreather mask	10–15	95	High supplemental oxygen requirement
High flow nasal cannula	15–60	21–100	Hypoxemic respiratory failure

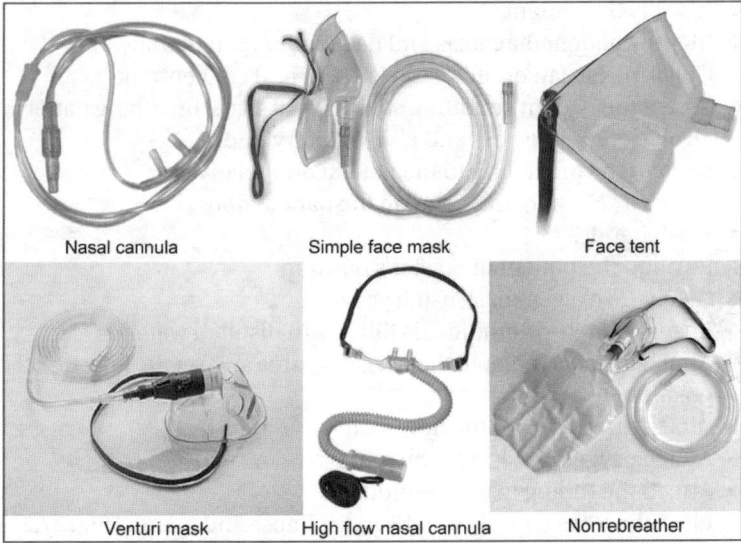

Fig. 27.1: Different types of oxygen delivery system.

Low flow delivery method:
- Simple face mask
- Non re-breather mask (NRBM)
- Nasal prongs (Low flow)
- Tracheostomy mask
- Ambu bag
- Tracheostomy HME connector
- Isolette—neonates (usually for use in the neonatal intensive care unit only)

ADMINISTRATION OF OXYGEN BY MASK METHOD

Articles Required

- Simple oxygen mask
- Oxygen source
- Flow meter
- Gauze pieces
- Humidifier with distilled water
- "No smoking" sign

Steps of Procedure

- Identify the patient.
- Identify patient diagnosis and need for oxygen therapy.
- Check physician order for device, rate and concentration.
- Assess the patient condition such as vital signs, breathing pattern, level of consciousness and all laboratory findings.
- Explain the procedure to the patient and relatives.
- Attach a "No smoking" sign on the patient door.
- Wash hands.
- Position the patient in Fowler's position.
- Clean the oxygen mask using gauze.
- Ensure that the humidifier is filled with distilled water.
- Attach the flow meter to the oxygen source and set the flow in "off" position.
- Attach humidifier to the flow meter.
- Attach oxygen mask with the tubing.
- Attach the tubing to the humidifier.
- Place the oxygen mask over the patient nose and mouth (**Fig. 27.2**).

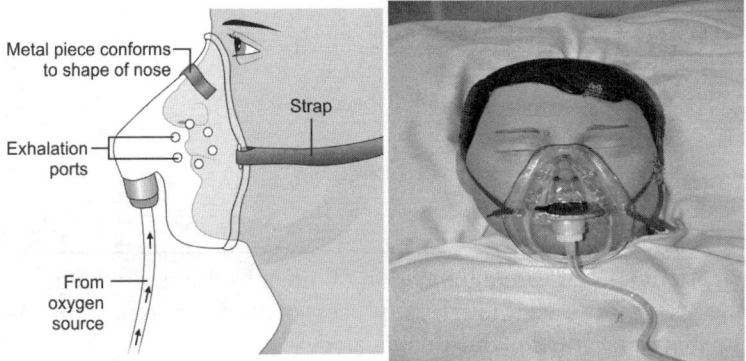

Fig. 27.2: Administration of oxygen with simple face mask.

- Ensure the fittings of the mask by shaping the metal band on the mask to bridge of the nose.
- Place the elastic band around the patient head and adjust it as required.
- Apply gauze pad behind the patient head and ears where the elastic band passes.
- Regulate the flow rate according to the physician prescription.
- Assess patient condition and the oxygen device frequently.
- If the oxygen is to be administered continuously, remove the mask and dry the skin every 2–3 hours.
- Do not put powder around the mask.
- Wash hands.
- Record the procedure.

CHAPTER 28

Steam Inhalation

DEFINITION

Steam inhalation is the inhalation of moist heat into the lungs via the respiratory tract through the process of deep breathing. Inhaling steam can be either plain or medicated.

PURPOSES

- To relieve inflammations of the upper respiratory tract in conditions such as sinusitis, nasal catarrh.
- To relieve inflammations in lower respiratory tract like bronchitis.
- To soften the thick bronchial secretion and easy expectoration.
- To promote easy absorption of oxygen.
- To provide antiseptic action of respiratory tract.

TYPES

- Nelson's inhaler
- Electric steamer

STEAM INHALATION: NELSON'S INHALER

Articles Required

A tray containing:
- Nelson's inhaler **(Fig. 28.1)**.
- Bath towel.
- Face towel.
- Sputum cup.
- Tincture Benzoin (if prescribed).
- Inhaler mouthpiece.
- Gauze piece.
- Cotton.
- Boiling water.
- Cardiac table.

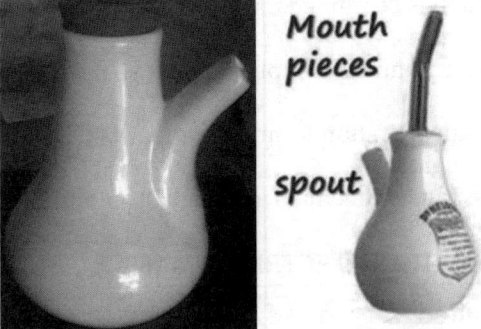

Fig. 28.1: Nelson's inhaler with parts.

- Bedside screen.
- Kidney tray.

Steps of Procedure

- Check physician's order.
- Explain the procedure to the patient.
- Switch off the fan, close windows and doors to prevent draught.
- Wrap the inhaler in a warm towel or put it in a bowl of hot water.
- Pour boiling water into the inhaler and fill to a level below the spout.
- Place sterile mouthpieces and close the inhaler tightly.
- Make sure that the spout is in the opposite direction to the patient.
- Cover the mouthpiece with a gauze piece and plug the spout with a cotton ball.
- Cover the inhaler with a towel and take it to bed side of the patient.
- Instruct the patient to sit in high Fowler's or sitting position.
- Place the inhaler in front of the patient on the cardiac table with spout opposite to the patient direction.
- Wrap the mouthpiece in a piece of gauze. Remove cotton plug and discard it into the kidney tray.
- Instruct the patient to place lips in the mouthpiece and take a deep breath.
- Instruct patient to breath out air through nose after removing the lips from the mouthpiece.
- Observe the patient during the procedure.
- Alternately place the inhaler close to the patient's mouth. Then place a large towel over his head and bring it down extended over the inhaler so that he gets all the steam.

- The inhalation is continued for 15–20 minutes as long as patient gets the vapors.
- Once the stated time is completed, remove the inhaler from the patient.
- Wipe off all perspiration from the patient's face and encourage patient to cough.
- Instruct the patient to remain in bed for 30 minutes.

STEAM INHALATION: ELECTRIC STEAMER

Articles Required

Same as in Nelson inhalation except an electric steamer (**Fig. 28.2**) is required in place of Nelson inhaler.

Steps of Procedure

- Explain the procedure to the patient.
- Check whether the electric steamer is functioning and ensure that electric points are working at the bedside.
- Instruct the patient to sit in high Fowler's or sitting position.
- Place the electric inhaler on the cardiac table.
- Spread a cotton blanket over tip of the screen and extend it halfway down to bed in front. The patient should not be entirely covered in.
- Switch on the electric inhaler.
- Instruct the patient to inhale by mouth and exhale through the nose for 15–20 minutes.

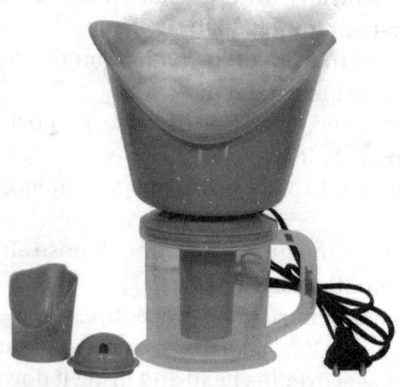

Fig. 28.2: Electric steam inhaler.

- Once the stated time is completed, remove the inhaler and place the patient in a comfortable position.
- Keep the sputum cup with disinfectant near the bedside and encourage the patient to cough.
- Wipe off all perspiration from the patient face using a face towel.
- Observe the patient for 1 hour and cover him/her to prevent chilling.

After Care Procedure for Steam Inhalation
- Take all articles to the utility room for cleaning.
- Empty the inhaler.
- Wash the inhaler with warm soapy water and then rinse with clean water.
- Wash the mouthpieces with soap and water and send for autoclaving.
- Dry all articles and replace them.
- Wash hands.

CHAPTER 29

Chest Physiotherapy

DEFINITION

The term "chest physiotherapy" or "chest physical therapy" refers to a collection of interventions intended to enhance respiratory function, promote lung expansion, strengthens the respiratory muscles, and eliminate the respiratory secretions **(Fig. 29.1)**.

The technique includes postural drainage, chest percussion, chest vibration, turning, deep breathing exercises, and coughing acts. It is usually done in conjunction with other treatments include suctioning, nebulizer treatments, and the administration of expectorant drugs to rid the airways of secretions.

This technique is used in impaired mucus clearance conditions like chronic obstructive pulmonary disease (COPD), bronchitis, and cystic fibrosis. The main goal of this therapy is to help the patient to clear excessive mucus secretions in order to prevent complications like mucus plugs, infections and atelectasis.

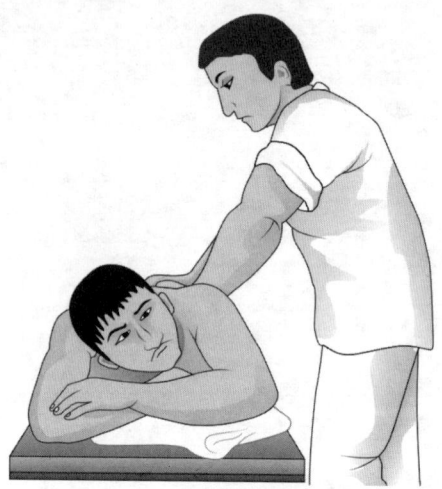

Fig. 29.1: Chest physiotherapy.

Chest Physiotherapy

PURPOSES

- To clear mucus and secretions from the lungs and improve respiratory function.
- To facilitate the removal of retained or profuse airway secretions.
- To optimize lung compliance and prevent it from collapsing.
- To promote oxygen exchange in the lungs, improve circulation, and reduce inflammation in the airways.
- To decrease the work of breathing.
- To reduce the risk of lung infections.
- To optimize the ventilation-perfusion ratio/improve gas exchange.

INDICATIONS

- **Chronic Obstructive Pulmonary Disease (COPD):** This is a lung disease that causes breathing difficulties. Chest physiotherapy helps to remove mucus and secretions from the lungs, which can improve breathing.
- **Cystic fibrosis:** This is a genetic disease that affects the lungs, pancreas, and other organs. Chest physiotherapy helps to remove mucus from the lungs, which can reduce the risk of lung infections and improve lung function.
- **Bronchiectasis:** This is a condition in which the airways in the lungs become damaged and widened. Chest physiotherapy helps to remove mucus from the airways, which can reduce the risk of lung infections and improve breathing.
- **Pneumonia:** This is a lung infection that can cause breathing difficulties. Chest physiotherapy helps to remove mucus from the lungs, which can reduce the risk of complications and speed up recovery.
- **Neuromuscular disorders:** People with neuromuscular disorders, such as muscular dystrophy, may have difficulty clearing mucus from their lungs. Chest physiotherapy can help to remove mucus from the lungs.

CONTRAINDICATIONS

- **Hemoptysis:** Coughing up of blood from the respiratory tract. Chest physiotherapy can exacerbate this condition, so it is generally contraindicated.

- **Active tuberculosis:** People with active tuberculosis should not undergo chest physiotherapy, as it can increase the risk of spreading the infection to others.
- **Recent surgery or trauma to the chest:** People who have had recent surgery or trauma to the chest should avoid chest physiotherapy, as it can cause pain and discomfort.
- **Fractured ribs:** Fractured ribs can cause further pain and discomfort.
- **Severe respiratory distress:** Severe respiratory distress can exacerbate their symptoms.

TECHNIQUES OF CHEST PHYSIOTHERAPY

Postural drainage involves positioning the patient in a way that allows gravity to help move mucus from different parts of the lungs towards the mouth. This is typically done by placing the patient in different positions for 10–15 minutes, such as lying on their back with their head and shoulders elevated, sitting up with their arms crossed over their chest, or lying on their stomach with their head turned to one side. By changing the position of the body, mucus can be directed towards the mouth and more easily coughed out **(Fig. 29.2)**.

Each position in postural drainage is followed by **percussion** over the lung area to be drained **(Fig. 29.3)**. Percussion is a technique where the chest is gently tapped with a cupped hand or a mechanical device to help loosen mucus in the lungs. The tapping helps to break up the mucus and make it easier to cough out **(Fig. 29.4)**.

Vibration is a technique where a mechanical device is used to vibrate the chest wall, which helps to loosen mucus in the lungs. The vibration can help to break up the mucus and make it easier to cough out **(Fig. 29.5)**.

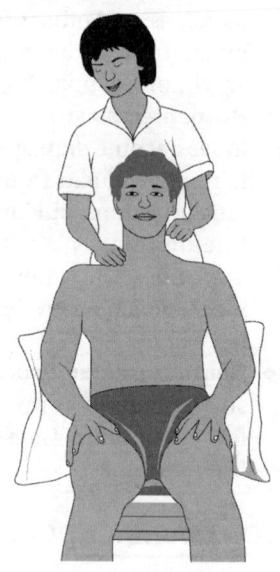

Fig. 29.2: Postural drainage.

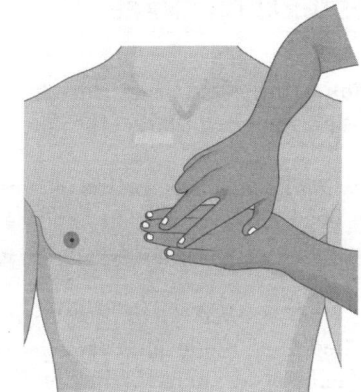

Fig. 29.3: Percussion.

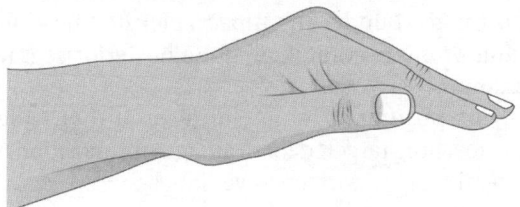

Fig. 29.4: Cupped hand.

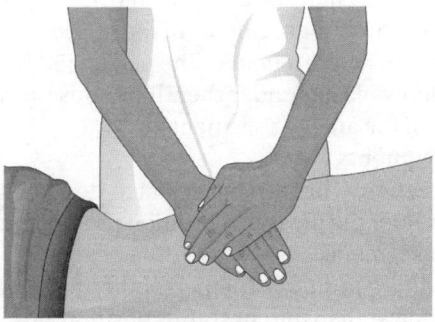

Fig. 29.5: Vibration.

Overall, these techniques are used together in chest physiotherapy to help clear mucus from the lungs and improve respiratory function.

POSITIONS IN POSTURAL DRAINAGE

❖ **Upper lobes**
  • *Sitting position:* The person sits upright, leaning slightly backward. This position helps target the apical segments of the upper lobes.
  • *Supine position with head elevated:* The person lies flat on their back with the head elevated at a 30 to 45-degree angle. This position aids in draining the posterior segments of the upper lobes.

❖ **Middle lobes**
  • *Supine position with the bed tilted:* The person lies flat on their back with the bed tilted or elevated at a 30 to 45-degree angle. This position facilitates drainage of the middle lobe.

❖ **Lower lobes**
  • *Prone position:* The person lies face down with a pillow or support placed under the hips to elevate them slightly. This position promotes drainage of the posterior segments of the lower lobes.
  • *Side-lying position:* The person lies on their side with the uppermost lung targeted for drainage. This position helps drain the lateral segments of the lower lobes.

❖ **Anterior segments**
  • *Fowler's position:* The person sits upright at a 45-degree angle with the knees bent and supported. This position aids in draining the anterior segments of the lungs.
  • *Supine position with a pillow:* The person lies flat on their back with a pillow placed under their hips. This position facilitates drainage of the anterior segments.

❖ **Posterior segments**
  • *Prone position:* The person lies face down with a pillow or support under the hips. This position promotes drainage of the posterior segments.
  • *Trendelenburg position:* The person lies flat on a surface with the head lower than the chest. This position aids in draining the posterior segments.

Note

The specific positions and techniques used in postural drainage should be determined by a healthcare professional based on the individual's condition, specific lung segments to be targeted, and overall assessment. The duration and frequency of each position should also be guided by

Left and Right Upper Lobes

To drain the secretions of anterior apical bronchi **(Fig. 29.6)**.

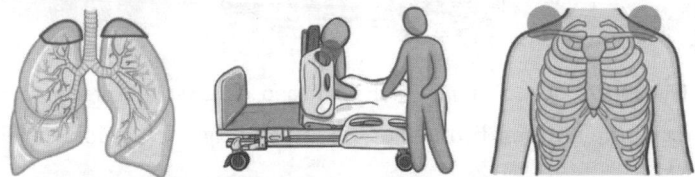

Fig. 29.6: Anterior apical bronchi drainage.

To drain the secretions of posterior apical bronchi **(Fig. 29.7)**.

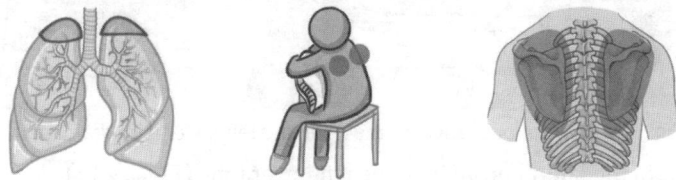

Fig. 29.7: Posterior apical bronchi drainage.

To drain the secretions of anterior part of the upper lobes **(Fig. 29.8)**.

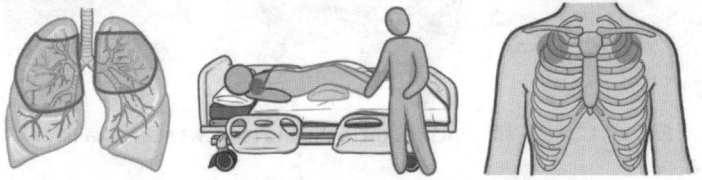

Fig. 29.8: Anterior part of the upper lobes.

To drain the lingula, which is a projection in the lower part of the left upper lobe and the right middle lobe **(Fig. 29.9)**.

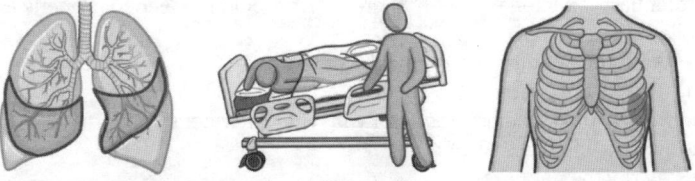

Fig. 29.9: Lingula and right middle lobe drainage.

Lower Lobes

To drain the superior bronchi of the right and left lower lobes (**Fig. 29.10**).

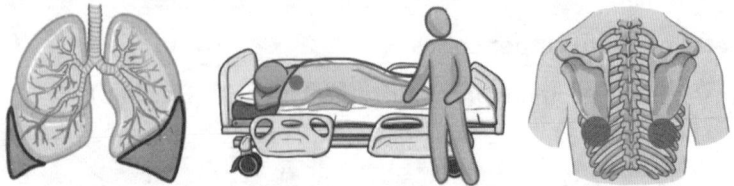

Fig. 29.10: Superior bronchi of the right and left lower lobe drainage.

To drain the anterior bronchi of the left and right lower lobes (**Fig. 29.11**).

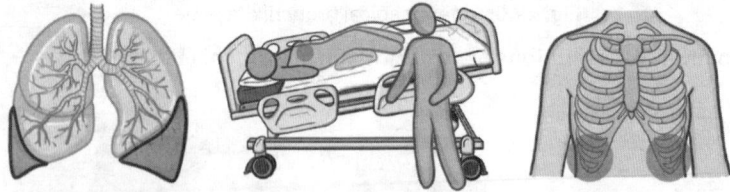

Fig. 29.11: Anterior bronchi of the right and left lower lobe drainage.

To drain the lateral bronchi of the left lower lobe (**Fig. 29.12**).

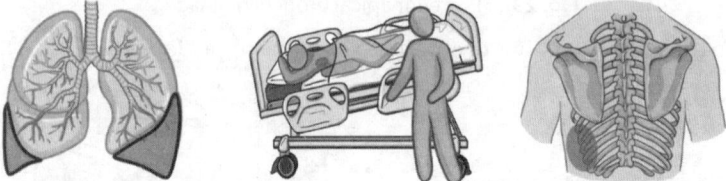

Fig. 29.12: Lateral bronchi of the right and left lower lobe drainage.

 Note

Postural drainage and chest physiotherapy (CPT) are usually done after bronchodilators are given. Remember use of nebulizer equipment is the potential for bacterial growth. Therefore, it should be cleaned properly as follows:
- Wash the nebulizer daily in soap and water
- Rinse it with water
- Soak it for 20–30 minutes in 1:1 with vinegar-water solution
- Rinse it again with water
- Air dry the nebulizer

STEPS OF PROCEDURE

Before the Procedure

- Identify the patient and check the physician's order.
- Explain the procedure to the patient.

During the Procedure

- Wash hands.
- Instruct the patient to perform the diaphragmatic breathing.
- Position the patient for postural drainage as per the physician's order.
- Cover the area with towel to reduce the discomfort.
- Do percussion that helps in dislodging the mucus plugs and mobilizes the secretions into main bronchi stem and trachea.
- Do vibration.
- Instruct patient to perform abdominal breathing.
- Vibrate for 5 exhalations over affected lung area. After 3–4 vibrations encourage the patient to cough/huff and expectorate sputum.
- Allow patient to rest.
- Auscultate the breath sounds to detect the presence of crackles/rhonchi which indicates mucus in bronchi.
- Repeat percussion and vibration according to patient's tolerance.

After Procedure

- Wash hands.
- Assist patient to comfortable position.
- Encourage patient to practice oral hygiene to lessen the bad taste or odor of the secretions they spit out.
- Document the procedure.

NORMAL RESULTS

The patient is responding positively to chest physiotherapy, if some may show:

- Improved vital signs.
- Improved chest X-ray.
- Increased volume of sputum secretions.
- Changes in breath sounds.
- Increased oxygen in the blood as measured by arterial blood gas patient reports of eased breathing.

Oral Suctioning

DEFINITION

Oral suctioning is the process of removing secretions from the oral cavity and pharynx.

PURPOSES

- To remove secretions that obstruct the airway.
- To facilitate ventilation.
- To obtain secretions for diagnostic purposes.
- To prevent infection that may result from accumulated secretions.

ARTICLES REQUIRED

- Appropriate size sterile suction catheter 12–18 Fr **(Fig. 30.1)**.
- Portable or wall suction unit with connecting tubing and Y-connector.
- Sterile water/normal saline in a sterile bowl.
- Clean disposable gloves.
- Face mask.
- Oral airway if indicated.
- Towel.

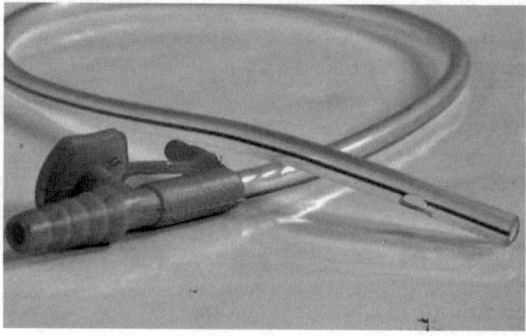

Fig. 30.1: Suction catheter.

PREPARATION OF PATIENT AND UNIT

- ❖ Explain the procedure to the patient.
- ❖ Instruct the patient and his family about the safety precautions.
- ❖ Assemble articles in the patient's unit.
- ❖ Assess for signs and symptoms indicating the presence of upper airway secretions: gurgling respirations, restlessness, drooling, etc.
- ❖ Explain to the patient that suctioning will stimulate the cough, gag, or sneeze reflex.
- ❖ Place a towel across patient's chest.
- ❖ Turn on suction and adjust to appropriate pressure.

Clinical Pearls

Normal Suction Pressure (Figs. 30.2A and B)
- ◂◂ Wall unit:
  - ➢ Adult: 100–120 mm Hg
  - ➢ Child: 95–110 mm Hg
  - ➢ Infant: 50–95 mm Hg.

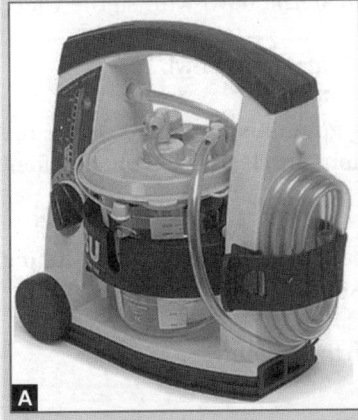
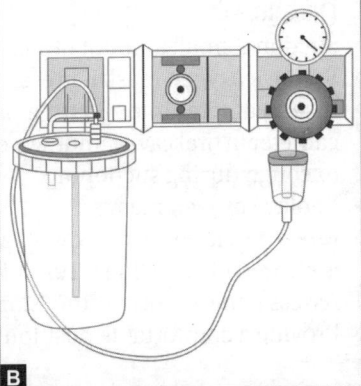

Figs. 30.2A and B: (A) Portable unit suction; (B) Wall mount suction.

- ◂◂ Portable unit:
  - ➢ Adult: 10–15 mm Hg
  - ➢ Child: 5–10 mm Hg
  - ➢ Infant: 2–5 mm Hg

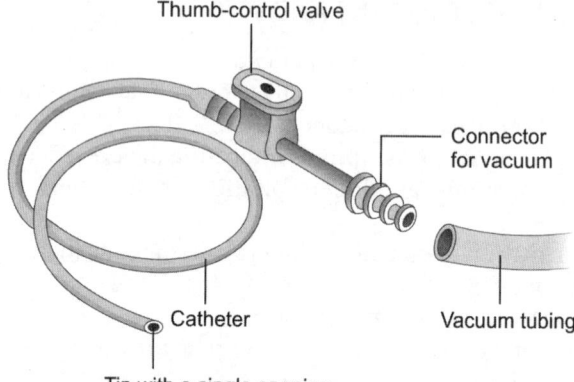

Fig. 30.3: Method of connecting suction catheter.

STEPS OF PROCEDURE

- Wash hands
- Wear clean gloves.
- Connect one end of connecting tubing to the suction machine and other to suction catheter, fill sterile bowl with sterile water **(Fig. 30.3)**.
- Suction a small amount of sterile water from bowl.
- Remove oxygen mask if present.
- Insert catheter into mouth along gum line to pharynx. Move the catheter in oral cavity until secretions are cleared. Encourage client to cough during suctioning.
- Replace oxygen mask.
- Rinse the catheter in a bowl of clean water until connecting tubing is cleared of secretions. Turn off suction.
- Assess patient's respiratory status.
- Provide a comfortable position to the patient.

AFTER CARE

- Wash and rinse used articles and dispose of the consumables.
- Wash hands.
- Document the procedure in nurses' record.

CHAPTER 31

Blood Transfusion

DEFINITION

Process of transferring blood or blood components into one's circulation intravenously.

BLOOD COMPONENTS

- **Blood plasma:** Watery liquid, straw colored extracellular matrix that contains dissolved substances.
- **Packed red blood cells:** They are prepared from whole blood by removing approximately 250 mL of plasma.
- **Fresh frozen plasma (FFP):** A blood product made from liquid portion of whole blood used to treat conditions of low blood clotting factors or other blood protein.

TYPES OF TRANSFUSION

See **Table 31.1**.

POSSIBLE COMPLICATIONS

- **Allergic reaction:** Rashes, flushing, hives, pruritis, laryngeal edema and dyspnea.
- **Febrile reactions:** Sudden chills, fever, flushing headache, and anxiety.
- **Delayed or acute hemolytic transfusion reaction:** Low back pain, tachypnea, hypotension.
- Post-transfusion purpura.
- **Circulatory overload:** Cough, dyspnea, distended neck veins, crackles, and elevated blood pressure.
- **Septic reaction:** Rapid onset of chills, vomiting, hypotension, and fever.

Table 31.1: Types of transfusion.

Blood product to be transfused	Indications	Contraindications	Transfusion time	Storage
Packed red blood cells	• Acute sickle cell crisis • Acute blood loss of >1,500 mL • Symptomatic anemia	Volume replacement	Completed within 4 hours of removal from controlled temperature storage	• 1–6° C in temperature controlled storage device • Transportation time not to exceed 24 hours • Shelf life: 42 days from day of collection
Platelets	• Thrombocytopenia • Platelet function defect	• Heparin-induced thrombocytopenia (HIT) • Thrombotic thrombocytopenic purpura (TTP)	Over time period of 30–60 minutes	• 20–24° C • Shelf-life: 5 days from date of collection • Once opened expiry is 4 hours from the time of opening
Plasma (Contains all coagulation factors)	• Bleeding due to multiple clotting factor deficiencies • Inherited clotting factor deficiencies	• Single coagulation factor deficiency • Volume replacement alone	30 minutes	• 1–6° C for up to 5 days • Can be stored for up to 36 months at minus 25° C or below • Thawed units of FFP stored up to 24 hours at 4° C

Blood Transfusion

PURPOSES

- To restore circulating blood volume in surgery and acute blood loss.
- To correct platelet and coagulation factor deficiencies.
- To correct anemia.
- To treat acute sickle cell crisis.

ARTICLES REQUIRED

- Blood transfusion set.
- Blood/blood components—sterile in appropriate container.
- Cannula 18G.
- Alcohol.
- Sterile gauze.
- Tourniquet.
- Adhesive tape.
- Scissors.
- Infusion stand.
- Disposal bag/kidney tray.
- Disposable gloves.

STEPS OF PROCEDURE

Before the Procedure

- Identify the patient.
- Check for the physician's order.
- Explain the procedure.
- Written and informed consent.
- Obtain blood from blood bank according to the hospital policy.
- Encourage the patient to empty their bowel and bladder and assist to a comfortable position.

During the Procedure

- Ensure privacy.
- Wash and dry hands.
- Check vital signs and record.
- Wear gloves.
- Insert IV cannula preferably 18G if not already present in a large peripheral vein.

- ❖ Inspect the blood product.
  - ● Identification number
  - ● Blood group and type
  - ● Expiry date
  - ● Compatibility
  - ● Patient's name
- ❖ Start the infusion slowly at the rate of 25–50 mL/hour for the first 15 minutes. Observe the patient and check vital signs every 15 minutes for the first 30 minutes.
- ❖ Increase the infusion rate if there are no adverse reactions. The flow rate should be within the safe limits.
- ❖ Assess the patient every 30 minutes. In case any adverse reaction occur, immediately stop the transfusion and notify the physician.
- ❖ Complete the transfusion if no adverse reaction is observed.

After the Procedure

- ❖ Disconnect the tubing.
- ❖ Dispose of the blood bag.
- ❖ Wash hands.
- ❖ Document the procedure.
- ❖ Assist patient to comfortable position.

CHAPTER 32

Drug Dose Calculations

INTRODUCTION

Drug dose calculation is an essential aspect of medication administration in healthcare. It involves calculating the correct amount of medication based on a patient's specific factors, such as age, weight, medical condition, and other relevant patient information. Accurate drug dose calculations are crucial to ensure that patients receive safe and effective treatment, while minimizing the risk of adverse reactions or medication errors. Various formulas and techniques are used to calculate drug doses, and healthcare professionals are trained to apply these calculations accurately and appropriately. Understanding drug dose calculations is critical for healthcare professionals in all clinical settings, from hospitals to outpatient clinics and pharmacies.

DRUG DOSAGE CALCULATIONS

Drug dosage calculations are required when the amount of medication ordered (or desired) is different from what is available on hand for the nurse to administer.

$$\frac{\text{Amount DESIRED (D)}}{\text{Amount on HAND (H)}} \times \text{QUANTITY (Q)} = Y \text{ (Tablets Required)}$$

Examples

1. Tab Metoprolol, 50 mg PO, is ordered. Tab Metoprolol is available as 100 mg per tablets. How many tablets would the nurse administer?

   $$\frac{\text{Amount Desired (D)}}{\text{Amount on Hand (H)}} \times \text{Quantity (Q)} = Y \text{ (Tablets required)}$$

   $$\frac{50 \text{ mg}}{100 \text{ mg}} \times 1 = 0.5$$

   Therefore, the nurse would administer 0.5 (half) of a tab Metoprolol.

2. 1,200 mg of Tab potassium chloride is ordered. This medication is only available as 600 mg per tablet. How many tablets should the nurse give?

$$\frac{\text{Amount Desired (D)}}{\text{Amount on Hand (H)}} \times \text{Quantity (Q)} = Y \text{ (Tablets required)}$$

$$\frac{1{,}200 \text{ mg}}{600 \text{ mg}} \times 1 = 2$$

Therefore, the nurse would administer 2 tablets of potassium chloride.

3. Furosemide is available as 40 mg in 1 mL. 10 mg is ordered to be administered through an IV. What amount of furosemide should the nurse administer?

$$\frac{\text{Amount Desired (D)}}{\text{Amount on Hand (H)}} \times \text{Quantity (Q)} = Y \text{ (Tablets required)}$$

$$\frac{10 \text{ mg}}{40 \text{ mg}} \times 1 \text{ mL} = 0.4 \text{ mL}$$

Therefore, the nurse should administer 0.4 mL furosemide.

DOSAGE CALCULATIONS BASED ON BODY WEIGHT

Dosage calculations based on body weight are required when the dosage ordered and administered is dependent on the weight of the patient. For example, many pediatric drugs are ordered and given per weight (usually in kg).

Dosage calculations based on body weight are calculated in two main stages.

Stage 1: Using the formula below, calculate the total required dosage based on given the body weight.

Weight (kg) × Dosage Ordered (per kg) = Y (Required Dosage)

Stage 2: Apply the $\frac{D}{H} \times Q$ formula to calculate the actual amount of medication to be administered.

Example

Methylprednisolone 4 mg/kg is ordered for a child weighing 64.8 lb. Methylprednisolone is available as 500 mg/4 mL. How many milliliters of medication must the nurse administer?

Weight: 64.8 lb
Dosage ordered: 4 mg/kg
Available on hand: 500 mg/4 mL
Convert lb to kg:
 1 lb = 0.45 kg
 64.8 lb = 29.39 kg
Therefore, the infant's weight is 29.39 kg.
Weight (kg) × Dosage ordered (per kg) = Y (Required dosage)
29.39 kg × 4 mg/kg = 117.56 mg

$$\frac{\text{Amount Desired (D)}}{\text{Amount on Hand (H)}} \times \text{Quantity (Q)} = Y \text{ (Tablets required)}$$

$$\frac{117.56 \text{ mg}}{500 \text{ mg}} \times 4 \text{ mL} = 0.94 \text{ mL}$$

Therefore, the nurse must administer 0.94 mL of methylprednisolone.

CALCULATION OF INTRAVENOUS DRIP RATES

In these types of calculations, for a given volume, time period, and drop factor (gtts/mL), the required IV flow rate in drops per minute (gtts/min) is calculated.

$$\frac{\text{Volume (mL)}}{\text{Time (min)}} \times \text{Drop Factor (gtts/mL)} = Y \text{ (Flow Rate in gtts/min)}$$

Example

Calculate the IV flow rate for 250 mL of 0.5% dextrose to be administered over 180 minutes. The infusion set has drop factor of 30 gtts/mL.
Volume: 250 mL
Time: 180 min
Drop factor: 30 gtts/mL

$$\frac{\text{Volume (mL)}}{\text{Time (min)}} \times \text{Drop factor (gtts/mL)} = Y \text{ (gtts/min)}$$

$$\frac{250 \text{ mL}}{180 \text{ min}} \times 30 \text{ (gtts/mL)} = 41.66 \text{ (gtts/min)}$$

CALCULATION OF FLOW RATE FOR AN INFUSION PUMP

Infusion pumps do not have a calibrated drop factor. The flow rate depends on the volume of fluid ordered and the time of infusion.

$$\frac{\text{Volume (mL)}}{\text{Time (h)}} = Y \text{ (Flow Rate in mL/h)}$$

Example

1,200 mL D5W IV is ordered to infuse in 10 hours by infusion pump. Calculate the flow rate in milliliters per hour.

$$\frac{\text{Volume (mL)}}{\text{Time (h)}} = Y \text{ (Flow Rate in mL/h)}$$

$$\frac{120 \text{ mL}}{10 \text{ h}} = 120 \text{ mL/h}$$

DRUG CALCULATION CONVERSIONS

1 kilogram	1,000 grams	2.2 pounds			
1 pound	0.45 kg	16 ounces			
1 gram	1,000 mg	15–16 grains			
1 mg	1,000 mcg				
1 grain	60 mg				
1 liter	1,000 mL	1 quart	2 pints	4 cups	32 ounces
1 teaspoon	5 mL	60 drops			
1 tablespoon	3 teaspoons	15 mL			
1 ounce	2 tablespoons	30 mL			
1 cup	½ pint	8 ounces	240–250 mL		
1 pint	2 cups	16 ounces	480 mL		
1 quart	2 pints	4 cups	32 ounces	1 liter	1,000 mL
1 gallon	4 quarts	8 pints	16 cups	128 ounces	3,785 mL

OTHER DRUG CALCULATION FORMULA

1. **Fried's formula: Infant's dosage (<1 year):**

   $$\frac{\text{Infant's age in months}}{150 \text{ months}} \times \text{Average adult dose}$$

2. **Young's rule: Child dosage (1–12 years):**

$$\frac{\text{Child's age in years}}{\text{Child's age in years} + 12} \times \text{Average adult dose}$$

3. **Clark's rule:**

$$\frac{\text{Weight of the child in pounds}}{150 \text{ pounds}} \times \text{Average adult dose}$$

4. **Surface area rule:**

$$\frac{\text{Surface area of the child in (sq m)}}{1.73} \times \text{Average adult dose}$$

5. **Parenteral dosage:**

$$\frac{\text{Dose ordered}}{\text{Dose available}} \times \text{Quantity in hand (mL)} = \text{Volume to be given}$$

6. **Intravenous fluid flow rate:**

$$\frac{\text{Total volume to be infused (mL)}}{\text{Total time of infusion in minutes}} \times \text{drops factor} = \text{Flow rate/min}$$

7. **Insulin dosage:**

$$\frac{\text{What we want}}{\text{What we have}} \times \text{Number of divisions on the given syringe}$$

8. **Ordered dose of medication in Microgram/min:**

$$\frac{\text{Vol to be infused}}{\text{Wt (kg)} \times 60 \text{ min}} \times \text{concentration}$$

9. **Concentration:**

$$\frac{\text{Dose of medication (mg)}}{\text{Volume to be infused}} \times 1,000$$

Oral Medication Administration

INTRODUCTION

Oral route of medication administration is one of the most common and convenient ways of taking medications, as it is relatively easy and does not require any special equipment. When medication is taken orally, it passes through the digestive system where it is broken down and absorbed into the bloodstream and then distributed throughout the body to reach its target site of action.

DEFINITION

The oral route of medication administration refers to the administration of medications through the mouth, typically in the form of tablets, capsules, liquids or suspensions **(Fig. 33.1)**.

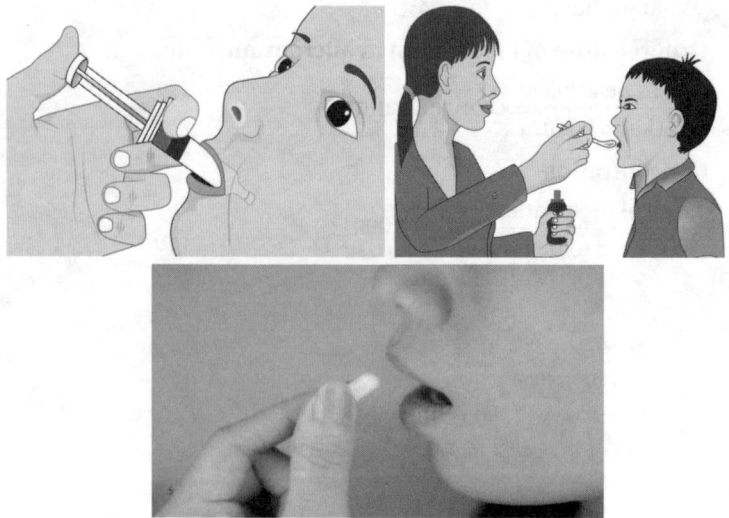

Fig. 33.1: Oral route of administering medications.

FORMS OF ORAL MEDICATIONS

Oral medications are available in various forms:
- Tablets
- Capsules
- Liquids
- Suspensions
- Powders
- Chewable tablets

PURPOSES

- To provide symptomatic treatment of a disease.
- To promote health and palliative treatment.
- To cure a disease.

ARTICLES REQUIRED

- Prescription order.
- Small tray.
- Medicine chart.
- Measuring device (Liquid medication): Medication cup, dropper.
- Pill cutter or crusher (If necessary).
- Container with drinking water.
- Spoon.

STEPS OF PROCEDURE

- Identify the patient.
- Review the medication order.
- Explain the procedure regarding medication administration, purpose and potential side effects.
- Perform hand hygiene: Wash hands with soap and water or use alcohol-based hand sanitizer.
- Check the label of drug on the containers.
- Prepare the medication: Depending on the medication form, prepare it as follows:
  - *Tablets or capsules:* Check the medication label for any specific instructions, such as whether it should be taken whole or can be crushed.

- *Liquid medications:*
  - Measure the prescribed dosage using an appropriate measuring device, such as a calibrated medication cup or oral syringe.
  - Shake the bottle well before measuring the medication.
- Instruct/Assist patient to sit in comfortable position. Ensure that the patient is in upright or semi-upright position.
- Avoid handling pills, tablets and capsules by tip of your fingers. Use a spoon or even the cap of a container to transfer the drug.
- Administer the medication:
  - Offer a glass of water.
  - Instruct patient to swallow the medication with the water in one fluid motion.
  - Ensure that the patient has swallowed the medication completely.
- Record the medication administration in patient's medical record including medication name, dosage, route of administration, date, time and any other relevant information.

CHAPTER 34

Topical Medication Administration

INTRODUCTION

Topical medications are commonly used to treat a wide range of conditions, such as skin infections, inflammation, pain, itching, burns, wounds, rashes, fungal infections, and more. When administering topical medications, it is important to follow proper procedures to ensure accurate dosage, appropriate application, and patient safety. Nurses must assess the patient's condition, prepare the medication, cleanse the application site, if necessary, apply the medication using the appropriate technique, educate the patient, and document the procedure **(Fig. 34.1)**.

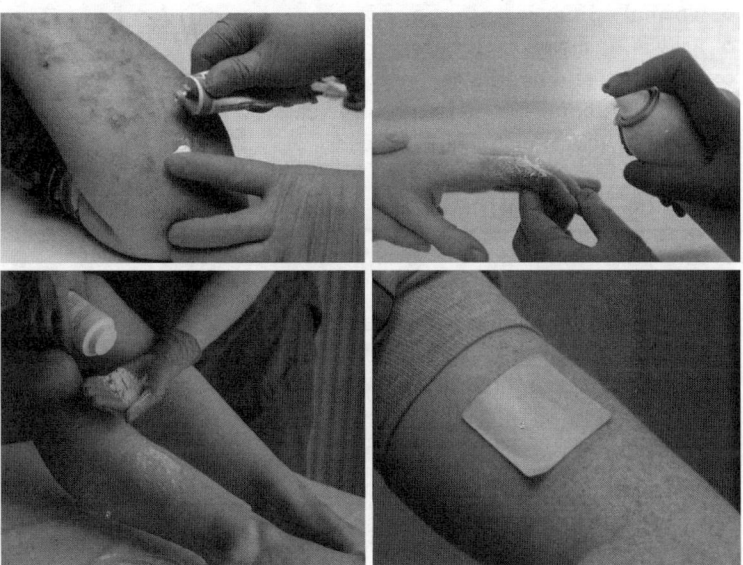

Fig. 34.1: Administration of different types of topical medication.

Topical Medication Administration

DEFINITION

Topical medication administration refers to the application of medications directly onto the skin or mucous membranes to treat localized conditions or provide systemic effects. These medications come in various forms, including creams, ointments, gels, lotions, solutions, sprays, patches, and foams.

PURPOSES

- To provide relief or treat the condition effectively.
- To provide relief at the site of application.

ARTICLES REQUIRED

- **Topical medication:** Creams, ointments, gel, lotions, solutions, sprays, patches, or foams.
- Disposable gloves.
- **Applicators:** Cotton balls, sterile swabs, brushes, spatulas, or specialized applicators with medication.
- Normal saline.
- Antiseptic cleanser (If necessary).
- Dressings and bandages.
- Soap or Alcohol-based hand sanitizer.
- Hand towels or disposable wipes.

STEPS OF PROCEDURE

- Identify the patient.
- Review the medication order.
- Check the medication label and expiry date.
- Explain the procedure regarding medication administration, purpose and potential side effects.
- Arrange all materials required near the patient bedside.
- Perform hand hygiene: Wash hands with soap and water or use alcohol-based hand sanitizer.
- Don gloves.
- Assess the site where the medication will be applied (infections, debris, rashes, skin integrity etc.).
- Clean the application site using normal saline if required and pat dry.
- Remove gloves.

- Apply the medication using the following techniques:
  1. **Paste, cream, ointment, or lotion**
     - Open the container and place the tube upside down on the table surface.
     - Apply clean gloves.
     - Place medication into gloved hands.
     - Apply the medication gently to the skin in the direction of hair growth.
     - Repeat as necessary till the entire area is applied.
  2. **Powder**
     - Apply clean gloves.
     - Clean and dry the area for application.
     - Apply a fine, thin layer of powder.
     - Ensure that the fine powder are spread all around the required area.
  3. **Suspension-based lotion**
     - Shake the container well before application.
     - Pour the lotion into a sterile gauze pad.
     - Apply the lotion in the direction of hair growth.
     - Repeat with new gauze till the entire area is covered.
  4. **Aerosol spray**
     - Shake the container before use.
     - Hold the spray 6 to 12 inches away from the affected area.
     - Apply the spray evenly to the affected area.
     - For applying to the head or neck, cover the patient's face with a towel.
  5. **Transdermal patch**
     - Remove old patches if available.
     - Clean and dry the area for application of the patch.
     - With each new application, rotate the sites.
     - Remove the wrapper from the patch and do not touch the adhesive surface.
     - Apply to the skin of selected site and press it firmly for at least 10 seconds.
- Dispose of supplies at appropriate places.
- Clean and replace articles.
- Perform hand hygiene.
- Document the procedure.

CHAPTER 35

Inhalational Medication Administration

INTRODUCTION

Inhalation medication administration is the delivery of medications directly to the respiratory system through inhalation. The medication can be delivered using various devices, including inhalers, nebulizers, and dry powder inhalers. It is important to note that the specific instructions for inhalational medication administration can vary depending on the type of device and medication prescribed. The nurse must ensure that inhalation medication is administered appropriately to ensure safe and effective treatment for patients with respiratory conditions.

DEFINITION

Inhalational medication administration refers to the process of delivering medications directly to the respiratory system through inhalation. It involves the use of inhalers, nebulizers, or dry powder inhalers to deliver the medication as a mist, aerosol, or dry powder that can be inhaled into the lungs. This method of administration is commonly used to treat respiratory conditions such as asthma, Chronic Obstructive Pulmonary Disease (COPD), and other lung diseases.

METHODS OF ADMINISTERING INHALATION MEDICATION

- **Inhalers:** Inhalers are handheld devices that deliver a measured dose of medication in the form of a mist or aerosol. There are different types of inhalers available, including metered-dose inhalers (MDIs), breath-actuated inhalers, and soft mist inhalers.
- **Nebulizers:** Nebulizers are devices that convert liquid medications into a fine mist or aerosol that can be inhaled. They are often used for patients who have difficulty using inhalers, such as young children or individuals with severe respiratory conditions.

Inhalational Medication Administration

- **Dry powder inhalers (DPIs):** DPIs deliver medication in a dry powder form, which is activated by the patient's inhalation. They are breath-actuated devices that release the medication when the patient inhales forcefully and deeply.

TYPES OF MEDICATION USED IN INHALATION

- **Bronchodilators:** To relax the airway muscles and open up the air passage.
- **Corticosteroids:** To reduce inflammation in the airways.
- **Anticholinergics:** To relax the airways and reduce mucus production.
- **Mucolytics:** Helps in thinning and clearing mucus from the airways.

ARTICLES REQUIRED

- Inhaler: Metered-dose inhaler (MDI).
- Spacer.
- Medication canister or cartridge.
- Handheld peak flow meter (optional).
- Tissue or disposable wipes.
- Clean water (if advised).

STEPS OF PROCEDURE

- Identify the patient.
- Review the medication order.
- Explain the procedure regarding medication administration, purpose and potential side effects.
- Perform hand hygiene: Wash hands with soap and water or use alcohol-based hand sanitizer.
- Remove the cap or cover from the inhaler.
- Shake the inhaler well if required.
- Check the inhaler:
  - Ensure that the inhaler is not expired.
  - Check the medication canister or cartridge to ensure it is not empty or damaged.
- Instruct/position the patient to sit in upright position.
- Instruct the patient to take a deep breath and exhale fully to empty the lungs.
- Device preparation (Metered-dose inhaler):

Inhalational Medication Administration

Metered-dose inhaler without spacer (Fig. 35.2A)	Metered-dose inhaler with spacer (Fig. 35.2B)
• Hold the inhaler in an upright position with the index finger on the top and thumb on the bottom • Shake the inhaler vigorously a few times • Instruct patient to open his/her mouth • Place the inhaler's mouthpiece between the patient's teeth, sealing the lips around it • Instruct patient to inhale slowly and deeply through his/her mouth while pressing down on the inhaler canister • Instruct patient to continue inhaling for 3–4 seconds till the lungs are full	• Connect the spacer to the inhaler **(Fig. 35.1)** • Shake the inhaler vigorously a few times • Hold the spacer with the mouthpiece towards the patient mouth/instruct patient to do so, if able • Instruct patient to press the canister to release one puff into the spacer • Then, instruct patient to take a slow deep breath in through the spacer mouthpiece

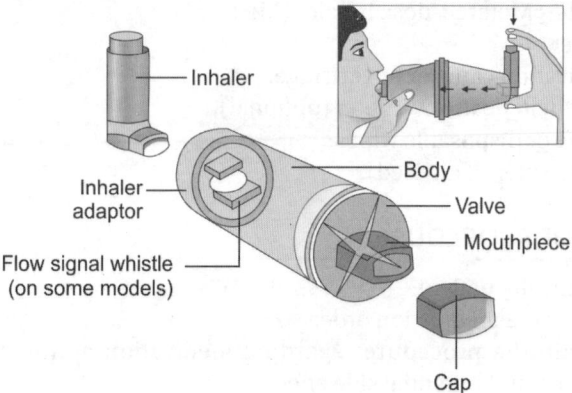

Fig. 35.1: Parts of inhaler with spacer.

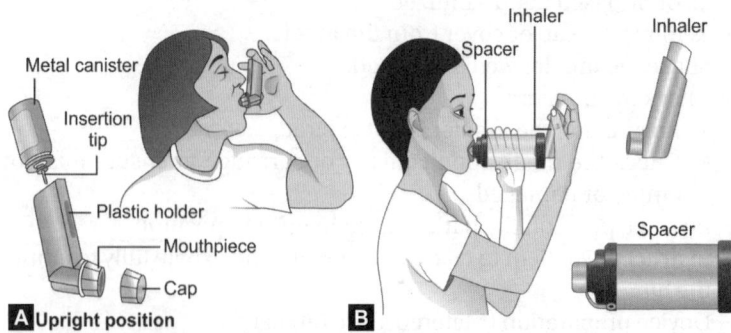

Figs. 35.2A and B: (A) Inhaler without spacer; (B) Inhaler with spacer.

- Instruct patient to hold breath for at least 10 seconds and exhale slowly, completely through his/her mouth.
- Repeat (if necessary). If it is prescribed to be taken for more than one puff wait for 30 seconds–1 minute and shake the inhaler before taking the next puff.
- Rinse mouth (if prescribed) to prevent oral thrush.
- Document the procedures.
- Disassemble the inhaler and rinse each part with warm water. Air dry the inhaler in well ventilated area.
- Reassemble the inhaler and store in a cool, dry place.

CHAPTER 36

Intradermal Injection Administration

INTRODUCTION

Intradermal injection administration is a specialized technique used to deliver medication or substances into the dermis layer of the skin. This method is commonly employed for diagnostic purposes, such as tuberculin skin testing, or for administering specific vaccines. By introducing medication or substances directly into this layer, intradermal injections facilitate a localized and targeted effect. Healthcare professionals who perform intradermal injections must receive appropriate training to ensure accurate placement and minimize complications. By mastering the skill of intradermal injection administration, nurses contribute to accurate diagnosis, effective treatment, and prevention of various diseases.

DEFINITION

An intradermal injection refers to the administration of a medication or substance into the dermis layer of the skin. The dermis is the layer of tissue located just below the epidermis, the outermost layer of the skin. Intradermal injections are typically used for diagnostic tests or specific vaccinations.

PURPOSES

- ❖ For conducting various test: Allergic testing, diagnostic testing, and sensitivity testing.
- ❖ To administer medications.
- ❖ To administer vaccine.
- ❖ For cosmetic purposes such as dermal fillers or skin rejuvenation treatments.

ARTICLES REQUIRED

- ❖ Syringe (1 mL or smaller).
- ❖ Needle (25–27 gauge).

Intradermal Injection Administration

- Medication to be administered.
- Alcohol swabs.
- Sterile cotton balls or gauze pads.
- Adhesive spot bandage.
- Clean gloves.

STEPS OF PROCEDURE

- Identify the patient.
- Review the medication order.
- Explain the procedure regarding medication administration, purpose and potential side effects.
- Assess the patient's arm for any contraindications, such as skin lesions or inflammation, and choose an appropriate injection site.
- Arrange all materials required near the patient's bedside.
- Perform hand hygiene: Wash hands with soap and water or use alcohol-based hand sanitizer.
- Prepare the medication by drawing the accurate prescribed dosage into the syringe.
  - If drug is in ampoule pour spirit on one cotton ball and clean the neck of the ampoule and the cutting file with spirit.
  - File the ampoule at the base of the neck and break top portion off holding the cotton ball over neck to protect fingers.
- Insert the needle carefully into the ampoule being careful that it does not touch the glass. Draw drug as per requirement.
- Instruct/assist patient to sit in a comfortable position.
- Select the appropriate site for injection: Inner aspect of the forearm.
- Don gloves.
- Clean the site for injection with alcohol swab in circular motion from center to periphery.
- Hold syringe using the dominant hand, while using nondominant hand to stabilize the patient's skin **(Fig. 36.1)**.
- Remove the needle cover and hold the needle at a 10–15-degree angle to the skin.
- Insert the needle steadily and quickly into the dermis at 15° angle. Aspirate and slowly inject the medication into the dermis **(Fig. 36.2)**.
- Withdraw the needle gently with minimal pressure at the same angle it was inserted. Do not massage or rub the site of injection.
- Using a cotton ball apply light pressure to the injection site and apply adhesive bandage over the injection site after 1–2 seconds.

Intradermal Injection Administration

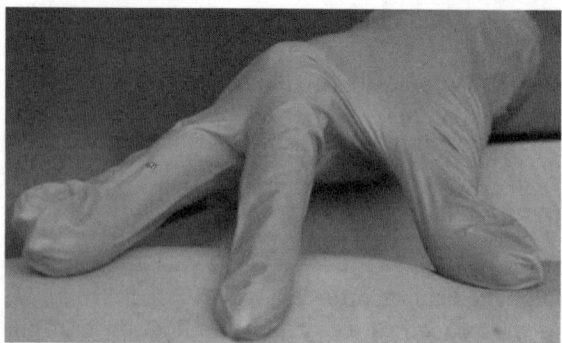

Fig. 36.1: Pulling the skin tight at the injection site.

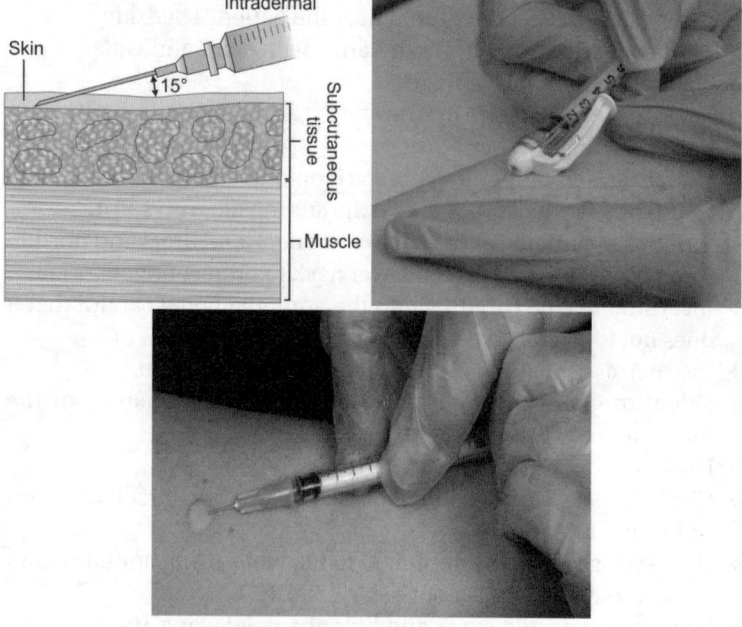

Fig. 36.2: Administering intradermal injection.

- Observe the site of injection for at least 10 minutes for any signs of reaction.
- Document the procedure.
- Discard the materials in appropriate places.
- Clean and replace articles.

CHAPTER 37

Subcutaneous Injection Administration

INTRODUCTION

Subcutaneous injections are commonly used for a variety of purposes, including the administration of insulin for people with diabetes, the delivery of certain vaccines, the administration of hormonal therapies, and the provision of other medications such as anticoagulants, growth factors, and immunosuppressant's. It is important to note that subcutaneous injections should be performed with proper sterile technique to minimize the risk of infection. Nurses should provide guidance on the appropriate technique and assist patients in learning how to self-administer subcutaneous injections if necessary.

DEFINITION

Subcutaneous injection administration refers to the process of delivering medication or other substances into the subcutaneous tissue, which is the layer of tissue located between the skin and the underlying muscle. This route of administration involves using a syringe and a fine-gauge needle to inject the substance into the subcutaneous tissue, allowing for slow and controlled absorption into the bloodstream.

PURPOSES

- To administer medications.
- To provide therapeutic treatment and pain management.
- To administer vaccine.
- For diagnostic procedures such as allergy testing.

ARTICLES REQUIRED

- Medication as prescribed
- Syringe
- Needle

- Alcohol swabs or cotton balls soaked in alcohol
- Clean gloves
- Small adhesive bandage

STEPS OF PROCEDURE

- Identify the patient.
- Review the medication order.
- Explain the procedure regarding medication administration, purpose and potential side effects.
- Assess the patient's arm for any contraindications, such as skin lesions or inflammation, and choose an appropriate injection site.
- Arrange all materials required near the patient bedside.
- Perform hand hygiene: Wash hands with soap and water or use alcohol-based hand sanitizer.
- Instruct the patient to sit in comfortable position.
- Inspect and select the site for injection: Abdomen, thigh, or upper arm.
- Prepare the medication as prescribed.
- Clean the injection site with an alcohol swab or cotton ball soaked in alcohol, using circular motion from the inside to the outside of the area. Allow it to air dry.
- Remove the needle cap or safety cap from the syringe and hold the syringe using the dominant hand.
- Using the nondominant hand, pinch the already clean area of skin between the thumb and forefinger to create a firm surface for injection **(Fig. 37.1)**.

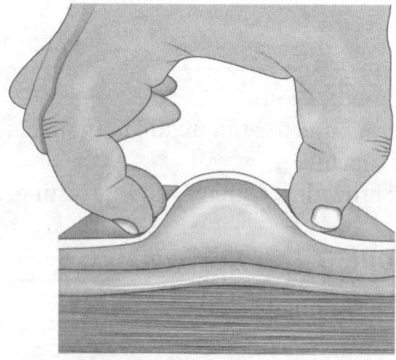

Fig. 37.1: Pinching the skin at the site of injection.

Subcutaneous Injection Administration

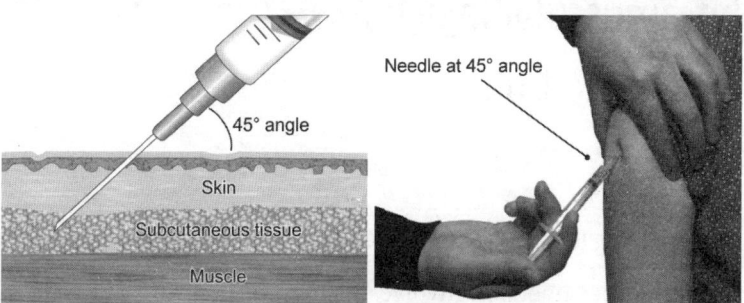

Fig. 37.2: Administration of medication subcutaneous route.

- Hold the syringe at a 45° angle and swiftly insert the needle into the subcutaneous tissue **(Fig. 37.2)**.
- After the needle is inserted, release the pinched skin.
- Pull back slightly on the plunger of the syringe to check for blood. If blood enters the syringe, remove the needle and start over with a new syringe and needle.
- If there is no blood, slowly and steadily depress the plunger to inject the medication.
- Once the medication is fully administered, withdraw the needle at the same angle it was inserted.
- Immediately dispose the used needle and syringe in a sharps container. Do not recap the needle.
- Gently apply pressure to the injection site with a cotton ball or swab and cover the site with a small adhesive bandage.
- Dispose of all used materials at appropriate places.
- Wash hands.
- Document the procedure.

CHAPTER 38

Intramuscular Injection Administration

INTRODUCTION

Intramuscular injection involves using a syringe and a needle to penetrate the skin and enter the muscle. The needle used for intramuscular injections is typically longer and thicker than the ones used for subcutaneous or intradermal injections. Before administering an intramuscular injection, the nurse should identify the appropriate injection site. Common sites for intramuscular injections include the deltoid muscle in the upper arm, the vastus muscle in the thigh, and the gluteus maximus muscles in the buttocks. The site for injection depends on the being administered and the age of the patient.

DEFINITION

Intramuscular injection administration refers to the process of delivering medication or substances directly into the muscle tissue using a syringe and needle. It involves penetrating the skin and inserting the needle into a specific muscle, typically at a 90° angle.

PURPOSES

- ❖ To deliver medication directly into the muscle tissue.
- ❖ To provide therapeutic treatment and pain management.
- ❖ To administer vaccine.

ARTICLES REQUIRED

- ❖ Medication as prescribed
- ❖ Syringe (1–5 mL)
- ❖ Needle (20–25 Gauges)
- ❖ Alcohol swabs or cotton balls soaked in alcohol
- ❖ Clean gloves
- ❖ Small adhesive bandages.

STEPS OF PROCEDURE

- ❖ Identify the patient.
- ❖ Review the medication order.
- ❖ Explain the procedure regarding medication administration, purpose and potential side effects.
- ❖ Arrange all materials required near the patient's bedside.
- ❖ Perform hand hygiene: Wash hands with soap and water or use alcohol-based hand sanitizer.
- ❖ Instruct the patient to sit in comfortable position.
- ❖ Prepare the medication as prescribed and withdraw the required amount of medication to be administered from the vial.
- ❖ Inspect and select the site for injection **(Fig. 38.1)**. If the buttock is used, upper and outer quadrant is preferred, position the patient in prone position or on his/her side. If the upper arm is selected, ask the patient to place his hand on the hip. In the case of a child the arm is steadied by holding it against the side of the body.
- ❖ Cleanse the injection site with an alcohol swab, using a circular motion from the center outward.
- ❖ Using nondominant hand, stretch the skin taut at the injection site.

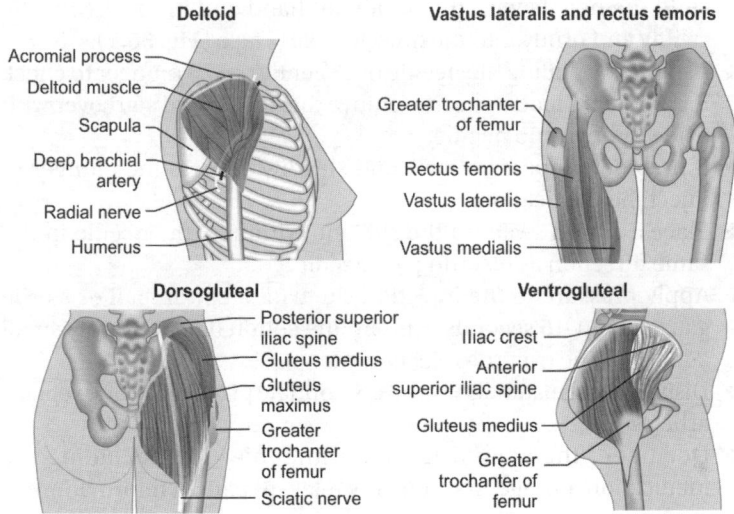

Fig. 38.1: Site for intramuscular injection.

Intramuscular Injection Administration

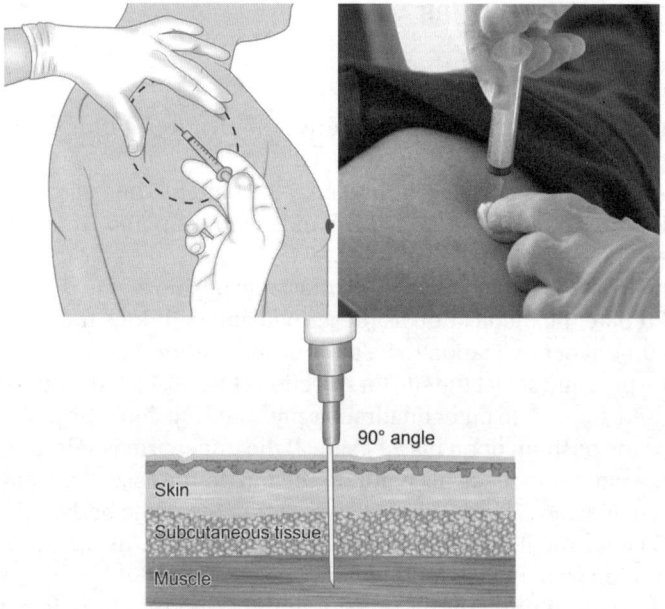

Fig. 38.2: Administration of intramuscular injection.

- Hold the needle with the dominant hand and insert the needle swiftly and firmly into the muscle at 90° angle **(Fig. 38.2)**.
- Aspirate by pulling the needle back gently on the plunger to check for blood. If blood appears, remove the needle and start over with a new syringe and needle.
- If no blood appears, slowly and steadily depress the plunger to inject the medication.
- Place a cotton swab on the site and withdraw the needle in the same direction as inserting the needle.
- Apply pressure to the injection site with a cotton ball or sterile gauze for 10–15 seconds. Discard the cotton ball and apply small adhesive tape over the injection site.
- Dispose of all materials used at appropriate place, clean and replace articles.
- Document the administration of the injection, including the medication, dosage, site, and any relevant patient information.

CHAPTER 39

Instillation

INTRODUCTION

The instillation of medication refers to the process of introducing or administering medication into a specific area of the body. It can be done through various routes depending on the desired effect and the type of medication being used. Irrigation refers to the process of flushing or cleaning a specific body part or area with a liquid solution. This technique is commonly used in medical settings or first aid situations to remove debris, foreign objects, or contaminants from the affected area. It is important to note that the specific method of instillation and irrigation, frequency of administration should be determined by a qualified healthcare professional based on the individual's condition and needs. Proper technique, cleanliness, and following the instructions provided by the healthcare professional or medication package insert are essential for safe and effective medication instillation.

DEFINITION

The instillation of medication refers to the process of delivering or introducing a medication into a specific area of the body. The medication can be instilled through various routes, such as oral, topical, ophthalmic, otic, nasal, inhalation, rectal, or parenteral, depending on the intended target area and the medication's formulation.

PURPOSES

- For therapeutic treatment.
- To provide symptomatic relief.
- For the purpose of diagnostic procedures.
- To provide preventive measures.

ARTICLES REQUIRED

- Medication as prescribed
- Droppers: Used for delivering eye drops, ear drops, or nasal drops.
- Cotton Balls or Swabs
- Clean gloves
- Tissues or paper towels
- Isotonic saline solution
- Alcohol or antiseptic solution

STEPS OF PROCEDURE

- Identify the patient.
- Review the medication order.
- Explain the procedure regarding medication administration, purpose and potential side effects.
- Arrange all materials required near the patient bedside.
- Prepare the medication.
- Perform hand hygiene: Wash hands with soap and water or use alcohol-based hand sanitizer.
- Instill the medication by using the appropriate technique for the specific route of administration:
  - **Eye drops:**
    - Turn the patient's head to the side of eye to be instilled.
    - Swab the eye with cotton soak in isotonic saline solution from inner canthus to outer canthus.
    - Gently pull down the lower eyelid to create a pocket and hold the dropper upside down with the tip directly over the eyelid pocket.
    - Instill the medication as prescribed into the lower eyelid pocket **(Fig. 39.1)**.
    - Instruct patient to close his/her eyes gently for at least 2 minutes.
    - Instruct patient not to touch or rub the eye after medication application.
  - **Ear drops:**
    - Position the patient in a side-lying position so that the affected ear is face upwards.
    - Straighten the patient ear canal by gently pulling the outer ear upwards and backwards for adults or downwards for children.

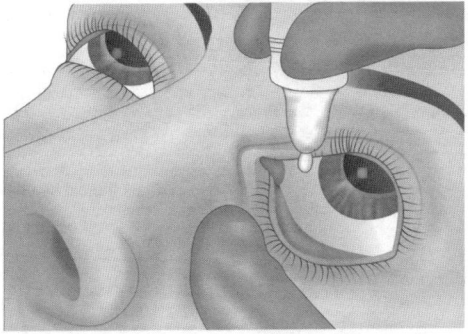

Fig. 39.1: Instillation of eye drops.

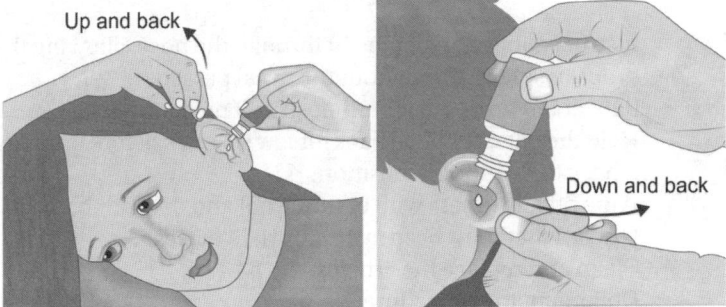

Fig. 39.2: Instillation of ear drops.

- Administer the prescribed number of drops into the ear canal **(Fig 39.2)**.
- Instruct patient to maintain the same position for at least 5 minutes.

- **Nose drops:**
    - Instruct the patient to blow out his nose gently to clean away the excess secretion.
    - Position the patient by having him sit with his head tilted backwards.
    - Hold the bottle of nose drops with the nozzle or dropper tip facing your nostril.
    - Ensure not to touch the dropper to any surfaces, including patient nose.
    - Instill the prescribed amount of nasal drops in the outer nostril **(Fig. 39.3)**.

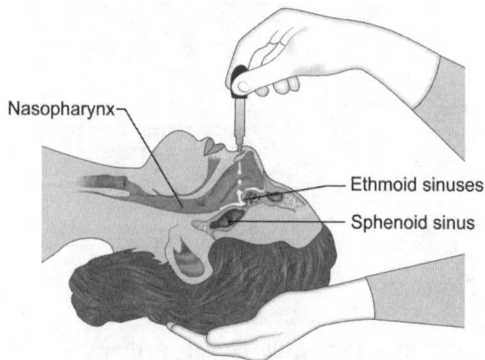

Fig. 39.3: Instillation of nasal drops.

- Instruct patient to breathe in through the nose, allowing the drops to spread throughout the nasal passage.
- Repeat the process for both nostrils if prescribed.
- Hold the patient's head back for few seconds before bringing it back to the upright position.
- Wipe off any excess with cotton wool and discard the swab.
- Discard materials used at appropriate places.
- Clean and replace the articles.
- Document the procedure.

CHAPTER 40

Irrigation

INTRODUCTION

Irrigation refers to a technique used to clean or flush a wound or body cavity using a steady flow of a liquid solution. Irrigation can be performed using sterile saline solution or other appropriate fluids. The solution is typically delivered through a syringe, a specialized irrigation device, or by gravity flow.

EYES

Irrigation of the eyes refers to the process of flushing the eyes with a sterile solution to clean out foreign substances, irritants, or chemicals that may have come into contact with the eyes.

PURPOSES

- To clean excess discharge from the eyes.
- To remove foreign bodies may be solid or chemicals.
- To reduce inflammation and congestion.
- To provide soothing effect to the eyes.

ARTICLES REQUIRED

- Small sterile undine or irrigation can with tube attached.
- Sterile solution, normal saline or sterile boric solution (4%).
- Bowl.
- Towel.
- Mackintosh.
- Sterile swabs.
- Forceps.
- Kidney tray.
- Eye pad, if necessary; and bandage.

STEPS OF PROCEDURE

- Explain the procedure to the patient.
- Perform hand washing with soap solution or alcohol hand rub.
- Warm solution to 100°F.
- Arrange all materials at bedside.
- Put mackintosh to avoid soiling of bed.
- Protect patient's clothing by fixing a towel.
- Ask the patient to hold a bowl to collect irrigated fluid or ask one assistant to help in holding.
- With the nondominant hand separate the eyelids using the thumb and forefinger gently.
- Hold the undine about 4 centimeters above the eye and allow the solution to flow **(Fig. 40.1)**.
- Direct the stream of the solution into the inner corner of the eye, allowing it to across the eye and out over the lower eyelid.
- Continue flushing the eye for at least 15 minutes and instruct the patient to blink or move the eye to ensure that the solution reaches all areas.
- Dry eyelids with dry gauze swab.
- Clean and wipe the face of the patient.
- Apply medication after irrigation if prescribed.
- Put a pad if necessary and bandage eye to fix the pad.
- Place patient in a comfortable position.
- Instruct him not to rub or disturb the pad, if applied.
- Document the procedure.

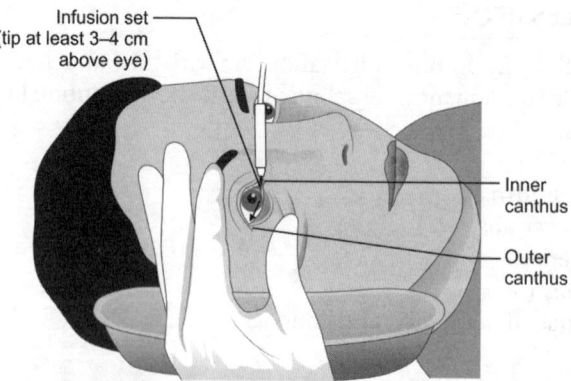

Fig. 40.1: Irrigation of the eye.

EARS

Irrigation of the ears, also known as ear irrigation or ear flushing, is a procedure used to remove excess earwax (cerumen) or foreign objects from the ear canal.

PURPOSES

- To remove wax or foreign body.
- To clean purulent materials.
- To relieve inflammation, congestion- and pain.

ARTICLES REQUIRED

- A small towel.
- Rubber bulb syringe or irrigation can with tip.
- Large kidney tray.
- Cotton.
- Irrigation fluid.

STEPS OF PROCEDURE

- Explain the procedure to the patient.
- Perform hand washing with soap solution or alcohol hand rub.
- Fill the rubber bulb syringe with irrigation fluid.
- Place patient in dorsal recumbent position with head near edge of the bed.
- First clean the ear with ear swab.
- Ask the patient to hold a bowl to collect irrigated fluid or ask an assistant to help in holding.
- Gently pull the outer ear upward and backward to straighten the ear canal.
- Insert the syringe into the ear canal, aiming slightly upward and away from the eardrum **(Fig. 40.2)**.
- Squeeze the bulb syringe to release a steady stream of the irrigation fluid into the ear canal. Avoid using excessive force to prevent damage to the eardrum.
- Allow the fluid to drain out of the ear into the kidney tray and repeat the process if necessary.
- When completely irrigated, clean the ear and insert one cotton wool pack.
- Document the procedure.

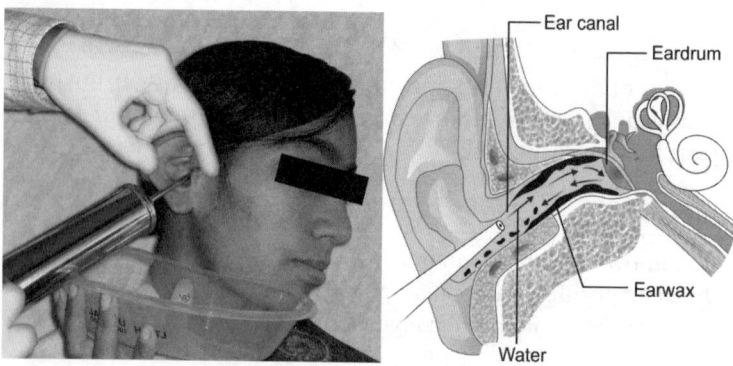

Fig. 40.2: Irrigation of ear.

NASAL

Nasal irrigation, also known as nasal rinsing or nasal lavage, is a practice that involves flushing out the nasal passages with a saline solution. It can help alleviate symptoms associated with nasal congestion, sinusitis, allergies, or colds.

PURPOSES

- To clean the nose.
- To relieve inflammation, congestion, swelling and pain.
- To check bleeding from nose.
- To remove foreign body.

ARTICLES REQUIRED

- Clean towel.
- Safety pins.
- Irrigation can fitted with rubber tip or nasal catheter.
- A bowl for return of wash out fluid.
- Sponges or small dressings.
- Irrigating fluid as ordered at 100–105°F (37.7 to 40.5°C).
- Irrigation stand.
- Mackintosh.
- Treatment towel.
- Torch.

Irrigation

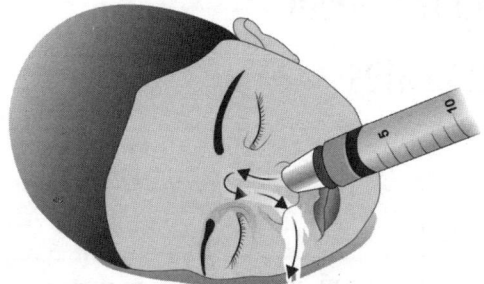

Fig. 40.3: Nasal irrigation.

STEPS OF PROCEDURE

- Explain the procedure to the patient.
- Perform hand washing with soap solution or alcohol hand rub.
- Instruct patient to lie on the side close to the edge of bed.
- Hang irrigation-can on stand at about 4 inches above the level of head of patient.
- Avoid soiling the bed and patient's clothing by putting a towel and fixing with safety pins.
- Expel air from tube by releasing solution to flow down and clamp.
- Instruct patient to tilt the head to the side, approximately at 45° angle. This allows the saline solution to flow in one nostril and out the other.
- Insert the tip of the nasal irrigation device into the top nostril gently.
- Slowly pour or squeeze the saline solution into the nostril, allowing it to flow through the nasal passage and out through the other nostril **(Fig. 40.3)**.
- Instruct patient to breathe through the mouth to prevent the solution from going down the throat.
- Repeat the same process with the other nostril.
- Observe any signs of bleeding or pain.
- After irrigating each nostril, wait for 30 minutes and instruct the patient to gently blow the nose to clear out any remaining solution, mucus, or debris.
- Discard materials used at appropriate places.
- Clean and air dry the nasal irrigation device before storing.
- Document the procedure.

CHAPTER 41

Assessing the Level of Consciousness

INTRODUCTION

Level of consciousness can be altered due to various reasons such as head injury, drug overdose, metabolic disorders etc. The Glasgow coma scale is used to assess the level of consciousness, which aids in the diagnosis of neurological function.

GLASGOW COMA SCALE

Glasgow coma scale (GCS) is used for assessing the level of consciousness in patient. GCS is a standardized scale/scoring system that uses three aspects of responsiveness such as eye-opening, motor response, verbal response.

PURPOSES

- To assess the impaired level of consciousness.
- To assess patient with head injury, hypoxia, neurological impairment, metabolic imbalances etc.
- For assessment of post-anesthesia patients.

ARTICLES REQUIRED

- Glasgow coma scale chart/performa **(Fig. 41.1)**.
- Pen.

STEPS OF PROCEDURE

- Identify the patient.
- Explain the procedure to the patient and family members.
- Place the patient in a comfortable position.
- Assess the responsiveness of the patient using Glasgow coma scale as follows:
  - **Eye opening (E)**
    - ***Eyes open spontaneously: 4 points***
      - *Assessment:* Initially observe if patient opens his/her eyes spontaneously.

Assessing the Level of Consciousness

Glasgow coma scale		
Response	Scale	Score
Eye opening response	Eyes open spontaneously	4 Points
	Eyes open to verbal command, speech, or shout	3 Points
	Eyes open to pain (not applied to face)	2 Points
	No eye opening	1 Point
Verbal response	Oriented	5 Points
	Confused conversation, but able to answer questions	4 Points
	Inappropriate responses, words discernible	3 Points
	Incomprehensible sounds or speech	2 Points
	No verbal response	1 Point
Motor response	Obeys commands for movement	6 Points
	Purposeful movement to painful stimulus	5 Points
	Withdraws from pain	4 Points
	Abnormal (spastic) flexion, decorticate posture	3 Points
	Extensor (rigid) response, decerebrate posture	2 Points
	No motor response	1 Point

Minor brain injury = 13–15 points; **moderate brain injury** = 9–12 points; **severe brain injury** = 3–8 points

Fig. 41.1: Glasgow coma scale.

- *Interpretation:* If patient open eyes spontaneously, assessment is complete with a score of 4, proceed to verbal response. If spontaneous eyes opening is not achieved move to the next step of eye opening.
- **Eyes open to sound: 3 points**
  - *Assessment:* Call patient by name and ask, "Are you ok?"
  - *Interpretation:* If patient open eyes in response to examiner voice, then score is 3. If no response, move to next step of eye opening.
- **Eyes open to pain: 2 points**
  Assessment: Can be done by using the following ways:
  - Apply pressure to one of the patient's fingertips **(Fig. 41.2 A)**
  - Apply pressure to the patient's supraorbital notch **(Fig. 41.2B)**.
  - Squeeze one of the patient's trapezius muscles (known as a trapezius squeeze) **(Fig. 41.2C)**.

Assessing the Level of Consciousness

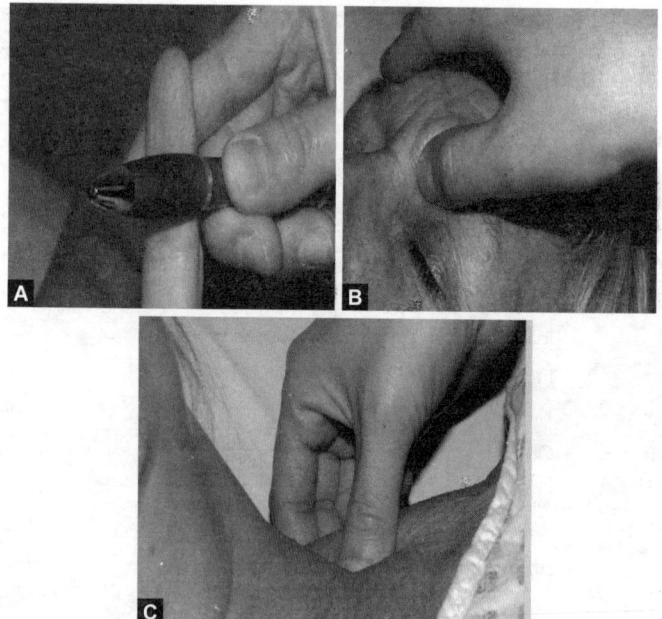

Figs. 41.2A to C: (A) Applying pressure on patient's fingertips; (B) Applying pressure on supraorbital notch; (C) Trapezius squeeze.

Interpretation: If a patient open eyes in response to pain, then score is 2. If no response, move to next step of eye opening.

- ***No response: 1 points***
  - *Assessment:* If patient does not open the eyes, then score is 1.
  - *Interpretation:* Eye response could not be assessed.
- ***Not testable: NT***

  If a patient cannot open the eyes due to certain conditions such as eye trauma, oedema, dressings etc. then it should be documented as NT.

- **Verbal response (V): 5 points**

  It involves engaging patients in conversation to assess the orientation level.

  Assessment: Ask the patient "Can you tell me your name?" or "Do you know what the date is today?"

  - ***Oriented: 5 points***
    - *Interpretation:* If patient gives appropriate answers, then score is 5.

Assessing the Level of Consciousness

- *Confused conversation: 4 points*
  - *Interpretation:* If patient response but answer is incomplete, then score is 4. Example: "I don't know what the date is" or "I am not able to recall the date".
- *Inappropriate words: 3 points*
  - *Interpretation:* If patient response with unrelated or inappropriate words, then score is 3.
- *Incomprehensible sounds: 2 points*
  - *Interpretation:* If patient makes incomprehensible sounds or speech with no meaning, then score is 3.
- *No verbal response: 1 point*
  - *Interpretation:* If patient does not response to the question asked, then score is 1.
- *Not testable: NT*
  - If patient response cannot be tested due to certain factors such as being intubated or other factors interfering with patient's inability to communicate, then it should be documented as NT.

- **Motor response (M): 6 points**
  - *Obeys command: 6 points*
    - *Assessment:* Ask the patient to perform a two-part request such as "Lift your right arm off the bed and make a fist".
    - *Interpretation:* If the patient is able to follow and obey commands appropriately, then score is 6.
  - *Localize to pain: 5 points*

    Assessment:
    - Squeeze one of the patient's trapezius muscles (known as a trapezius squeeze) **(Fig. 41.2C)**.
    - Apply pressure to the patient's supraorbital notch **(Fig. 41.2B)**.

    Interpretation: If a patient attempts to reach the site where painful stimulus is applied and brings his/her hand above the clavicle, then this is classed as localizing to pain. The score is 5.
  - *Withdraws to pain: 4 points*
    - *Assessment:* Follow the same assessment as **(Fig. 41.2B)** localize to pain.
    - *Interpretation:* If the patient try to withdraw away from the pain. Example: Patient tries to pull his/her arm away from the examiner when applying a painful stimulus to their fingertip. Then the score is 4.

- *Abnormal flexion response to pain (Decorticate posturing): 3 points*
  Interpretation: If patient response to painful stimulus involves adduction of the arm, internal rotation of the shoulder, flexion of the elbow, pronation of the forearm and wrist flexion (known as decorticate posturing) **(Fig. 41.3)**. Then score is 3.
  - **Decorticate posturing** indicates that there may be significant damage to areas including the cerebral hemispheres, the internal capsule, and the thalamus.
- *Abnormal extension response to pain (Decerebrate posturing): 2 points*
  Interpretation: If the patient head is extended, with the arms and legs extended and internally rotated, patient appears rigid with teeth clenched, and these signs can be present in one side or both sided of the body. This is also known as decerebrate posturing **(Fig. 41.3)**.
  - **Decerebrate posturing** indicates brain stem damage. It is exhibited by people with lesions or compression in the midbrain and lesions in the cerebellum.
  - **Progression** from decorticate posturing to decerebrate posturing is often indicative of uncal (transtentorial) or tonsillar brain herniation (often referred to as coning).
- **No response: 1 point**
  - *Interpretation:* If there is complete absence of motor response to painful stimulus, then score is 1.

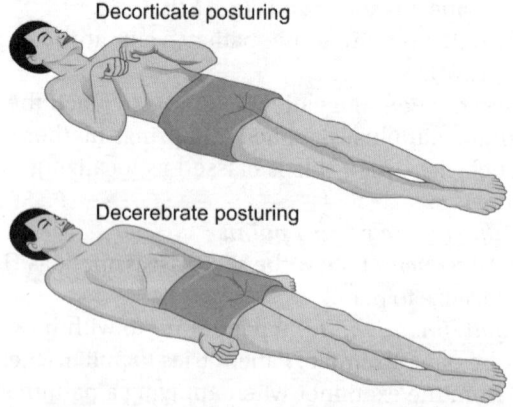

Fig. 41.3: Decorticate and decerebrate posturing.

Assessing the Level of Consciousness

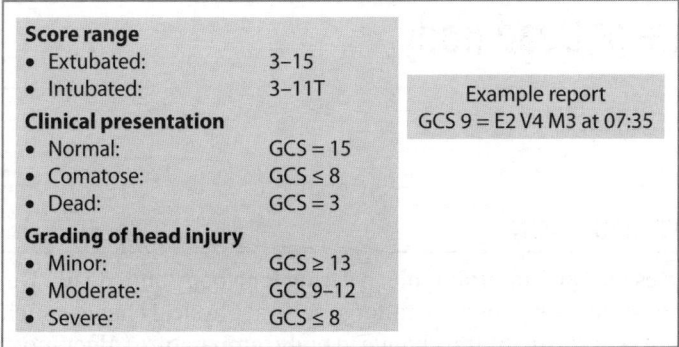

Fig. 41.4: Inference of GCS score with example.

- **Not testable: NT**
  If a patient is not able to perform any motor response due to certain condition such as paralysis, then it should be documented as NT.
- ❖ After the assessment of eye-opening, verbal response, motor response is completed, add all the scores together.
- ❖ Document the patient GCS score at the bottom of the sheet using the assessment performa with inference of score **(Fig. 41.4)**
- ❖ The documented score must show the score for each individual behavior tested, GCS 15 [E4, V5, M6].

Care of Dead Body

CHAPTER 42

INTRODUCTION

Nurses play an important role in caring for a body after death. Death either sudden or expected undergo several physical changes such as loss of skin elasticity and change in body temperature (Algor mortis), purple discoloration of the skin (livor mortis), and a stiffening of the body (rigor mortis). The nurses' responsibilities after dead continues as physical care of the body as well as care of family members.

DEFINITION

Care given to the body 30–45 minutes after death following the declaration of death by the physician.

PURPOSES

- To release the dead body to relatives with dignity and respect.
- To maintain normal body alignment before rigor mortis sets in.
- To reduce mental distress of the family.
- To protect the body from postmortem discharge.
- To facilitate transportation to mortuary/residence.

ARTICLES REQUIRED

- Tray lined with towel.
- Clean sheet.
- Long artery clamp.
- Bandage.
- Clean gloves, mask, and gown.
- Absorbent and nonabsorbent cotton.
- Hospital gown or patient's clothes.
- Mackintosh.
- Mortuary cards in transparent plastic cover.
- Valuables envelope.

- Shroud/body bag/sheet.
- Articles for cleaning or bathing the body.

STEPS OF PROCEDURE

- Confirm physician order regarding covering the body with clean sheet after death.
- Assess the presence of family members and encourage them to ask questions.
- Identify the family religious and culture belief.
- Identify the cause of death and assess if certain precautions must be taken during the procedure.
- Place all articles near the bedside.
- Wash hands.
- Wear gloves, a mask and gown.
- Place the body in a supine position with arms at the side or across the abdomen.
- Elevate the head of the bed using a pillow.
- Close the eyelids by placing fingers over it for a few seconds.
- Place a rolled towel under the chin to close the mouth.
- All bottles, sacks, or receptacles such as urinary catheters, nasogastric tubes, IV lines, or drainage tubes must be removed.
- Replace soiled dressings with new gauze dressings.
- Wash the body parts and put on a clean gown.
- Wrap a jaw bandage (four-tailed bandage).
- Body orifices such as the nostrils, mouth, vagina, and rectum should be plugged with absorbent cotton first, followed by nonabsorbent cotton.
- Unless specifically requested, take all jewelry off.
- Close eyes by placing wet cotton balls on eyelids.
- Fold hands in prayer posture and bind the thumbs together.
- Place the legs straight, feet kept together, and toes should be tied **(Fig. 42.1)**.
- Fill the mortuary card, place it inside a plastic bag with the big foot tied together.
- Place an absorbent pad under the patient's buttocks.
- Comb and brush the patient's hair. Take off any elastic bands, hairpins, or clips.
- List, identify and label all valuables that are still present in the patient's room.

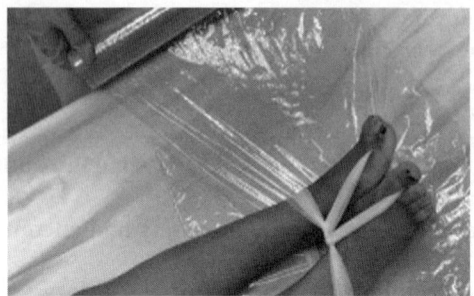

Fig. 42.1: Tying of the toes and feet.

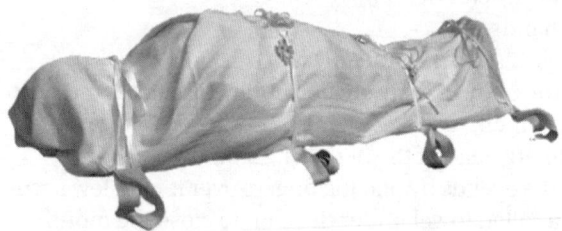

Fig. 42.2: Draping of dead body with a shroud.

- Place patient's personal belongings in a labelled bag and return to family members.
- Fill out identifying tags, then affix one to the patient's big ankle.
- If the family asks to see the body, cover it with a sheet or thin blanket, leaving only the head and upper shoulders visible.
- Place the body in a body bag or drape it with a shroud after removing all linens and the patient's gown **(Fig. 42.2)**.
- Attach the completed label to outside of the body bag or shroud.
- Use special label in case of death due to infectious disease.
- Arrange for transportation of the body to the morgue or mortuary.
- Close the other patients' rooms and make plans to transport the body.
- Transfer the body to a stretcher with care, maintaining the body aligned. Cover with a new clean sheet.
- Following the procedure, remove any remaining items and linen from the patient's room.
- Wash hands.

- Record the date, time when physician was informed, the name of the physician who announced the death, time of death, the disposition of valuables and belongings, the care provided to the family, the consent form signed by the family, the disposition of the body, and the information given to family members.
- Document any wounds, bruise, marks and specific observation made during the procedure.

CHAPTER 43

Poisoning

INTRODUCTION

Poisoning is an injury or death caused by the touching, ingestion, inhalation and injection of hazardous substance or chemicals to the body. Certain compounds are hazardous when consumed only in large quantities or concentrations while some can cause poisonous effects even in small quantities. Poisons have varying effects, ranging from minor illness to severe disease, coma, and death. Poison management differs depending on the material.

DEFINITION

A poison may be defined as any substance when taken in sufficient quantity produce ill health, disease or death. The damage caused by poison can be either temporary or permanent.

CLASSIFICATION OF POISON WITH FIRST AID MANAGEMENT (TABLE 43.1)

Table 43.1: Classification of poison.

Poison	Common source	First aid treatment
Acids (strong)	• Dispensaries • Laboratories • Garages • Industries	• Do not make the casualty induce vomiting • Give plenty of water to dilute the acid and if possible, 2 tablespoons of chalk, milk of magnesia, plaster or whitewash, to a pint of water
Alkalis (strong)	• Dispensaries • Laboratories • Some industries or in the home (ammonia)	• Do not make the casualty induce vomiting • Give plenty of water to dilute the alkali, add if possible 2 tablespoons of vinegar, orange, lemon or lime juice to a pint of water

Contd...

Contd...

Poison	Common source	First aid treatment
Disinfectants (e.g. carbolic acid, Lysol, Izal and Cresol)	• Hospitals • Dispensaries or in the home	• Do not make the casualty induce vomiting • Give 2 tablespoons of Epsom salts in a pint of water or in a teacup full of medicinal paraffin
Other poisons		
Arsenic	In some weed-killers, rat poisons and sheep dips	• Make the casualty induce vomiting • Give the soothing drinks
Aspirin		• Make the casualty induce vomiting • Give water to which add 2 teaspoons of bicarbonate of soda to the tumbler may be added • Give strong tea or coffee
Carbon monoxide from gas stoves or exhaust fumes		• Apply artificial respiration • Give oxygen, if available can be obtained in some garages and chemists

GENERAL GUIDELINES FOR MANAGEMENT OF POISONS

- ❖ Call for help (emergency helpline).
- ❖ Assess the area for remaining poisons bottle, box, container, vomited manner.
- ❖ Take history of poisoning—time, type, quantity, etc. from attendants or relatives.
- ❖ If the patient is unconscious, place him/her in recovery position and start artificial respiration.
- ❖ If the patient is conscious, induce vomiting.
- ❖ If poison is identified, administer antidote for the poison.
- ❖ Give an adequate amount of water to the patient so that the poison consumed is diluted.
- ❖ Provide symptomatic treatment.

TYPES OF ANTIDOTE

- ❖ **Chemical antidote:** Acids for alkalis, alkalis for acids, vinegar for caustic soda, potassium permanganate in solution of 10–15 grain in pint of water.

Poisoning

- ❖ **Mechanical antidote:** Finely powdered charcoal, egg albumin, fats and oils, bulky food for glass powder.
- ❖ **Physiological antidote:** Which produces opposite effect in body to the poison, atropine, physostigmine, etc.

Some toxic substances with their antidotes are presented in **Table 43.2**.

Table 43.2: Toxic substances with antidotes.

Sl. No.	Antidote	Toxic exposure
1.	Acetylcysteine IV	Acetaminophen
2.	Activated charcoal PO	Oral poisons bound to charcoal
3.	Atropine sulfate	Organophosphorus bradycardia
4.	Calcium chloride	Calcium channel blockers, hypermagnesemia hyperkalemia
5.	Calcium gluconate	Hydrofluoric acid burns
6.	Calcium gluconate gel	Hydrofluoric burns
7.	Hydroxocobalamin (Cyanokit®)	Cyanide
8.	Sodium nitrite	Cyanide
9.	Sodium thiosulphate	Cyanide
10.	Flumazenil	Over-sedation with benzodiazepines
11.	Glucagon	For beta blockers/calcium channel blockers
12.	Dextrose	Calcium channel blockers cardiotoxicity reversal
13.	Lipid emulsion (Intralipid 20%)	Severe, systemic local anesthetic toxicity
14.	Methylthioninium chloride (methylene blue)	Methemoglobinemia
15.	Naloxone (Narcan®)	Opioids
16.	Procyclidine injection	For extra-pyramidal symptoms
17.	Sodium bicarbonate	Tricyclic antidepressants
18.	Thiamine (Vit. B1)	Ethanol
19.	Sugammadex	Neuromuscular blockade drug
20.	Prothrombin complex concentrate	Reversal of acquired coagulation factor deficiency
21.	Antisnake antivenin	Snake venoms

Contd...

Contd...

Sl. No.	Antidote	Toxic exposure
22.	Antiscorpion antivenin	Scorpion venoms
23.	Bromocriptine mesylate (Parlodel®)	Drugs causing Neuroleptic Malignant syndrome
24.	Calcium folinate	Methotrexate/Methanol
25.	Cyproheptadine	Drugs causing Serotonin syndrome
26.	L-Carnitine	Valproic acid
27.	Dantrolene	Drugs causing Neuroleptic Malignant syndrome
28.	Desferrioxamine (Desferal®)	Iron
29.	Digoxin specific antibody fragments fab	Digoxin
30.	Fomepizole	Ethylene glycol
31.	Idarucizumab	Dabigatran
32.	PEG solution (polyethylene glycol)	Whole bowel irrigation
33.	Octreotide acetate (sandostatin)	For sulfonylureas, hypoglycemia
34.	Pralidoxime	Organophosphate insecticides
35.	Phentolamine	Digital ischemia, resistant hypertension
36.	Phytomenadione IV (Vitamin K1)	Warfarin
37.	Phytomenadione PO (Vitamin K1)	Warfarin
38.	Protamine sulphate	Heparin and low molecular weight heparins
39.	Pyridoxine (Vit. B6)	For isoniazid seizures
40.	Calcium disodium EDTA	Heavy metals particularly lead, zinc
41.	Physostigmine	Atropine poisoning
42.	Potassium iodide	Radioactive iodine
43.	Succimer (dimercaptosuccinic acid)	Chelating agent for lead and mercury

Universal Antidote

When the poison nature and source of poison are unknown, a universal antidote is applied. The antidote listed below must be blended with a glass of water. One tablespoon should be administered once or twice.

- Powdered charcoal—2 parts.
- Tannic acid (strong tea)—1 part.
- Magnesium oxide (milk of magnesium)—1 part.

FIRST AID MEASURES

Unabsorbed Poisons

- If inhaled poison is a gas **(Fig. 43.1)**, transfer the patient away from the source of exposure and into fresh air. Check breathing and perform CPR if necessary.
- If poison is from bites, apply a tourniquet above bite site for 15-20 minutes and loosen for 20-30 seconds **(Fig. 43.2)**.
- If poison is swallowed to stomach, do gastric lavage by stomach wash tube as per described procedure.

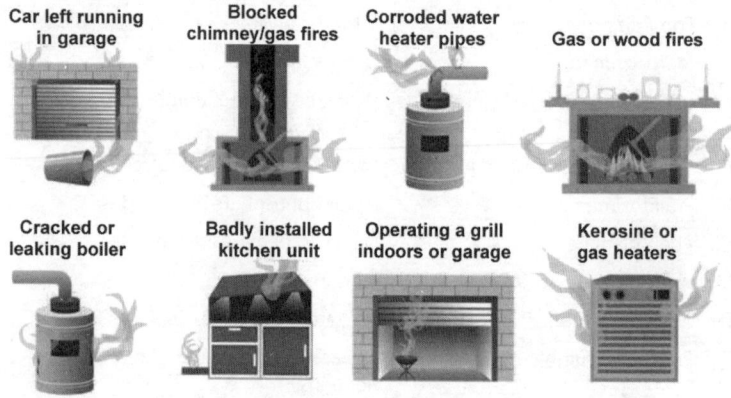

Fig. 43.1: Gas poisons.

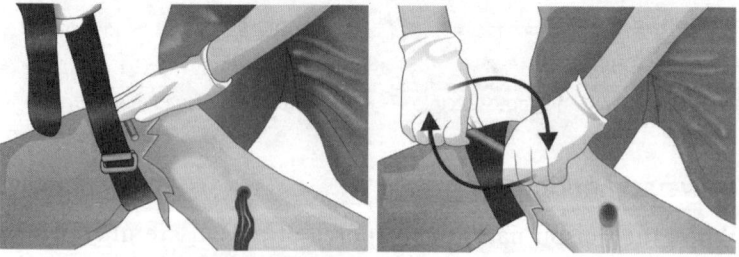

Fig. 43.2: Applying tourniquet above area of bite.

- Never introduce stomach tubes in corrosive poisoning except carbolic acid.
- If the patient is conscious and stomach wash facility is not available try to induce vomiting to remove stomach contents.
- The vomited matter should be preserved for medicolegal examination.
- Vomiting procedures are as follows (vomiting should not be attempted in corrosive acid poisoning):
  - Copious draughts of warm water.
  - A tablespoonful of grounded mustard seeds or 2 tablespoonful of common salt.
  - Half drachm of zinc sulphate in a glass of warm water repeated at 15 minutes interval.
  - 20/30 grains of ipecacuanha powder or 2-6 drachm of ipecacuanha wine.
  - 15-30 grains of ammonium carbonate dissolved in water.
  - Apomorphine hydrochloride 3-6 mg hypodermally.
  - Mechanical tickling of fauces or inserting fingers in mouth.

Absorbed Poisons

- This is done by common practice of giving IV fluids to eliminate excretion by kidney.
- Peritoneal dialysis can be done in acute cases of snakebite.
- Diuresis can be promoted by diuretics infusions/injections.
- Elevate the foot-end of patient by putting 9" block till BP reached 106/60 mm Hg.
- Provide warmth to the patient by covering with blankets or hot water bottles.
- If the temperature is high, lower body temperature by sponging.
- Relieve pain by analgesics usually morphine or pethidine in consultation with doctor.
- Give IV fluids to restore fluid balance and promote kidney excretion of poison.
- Record BP, TPR regularly.
- Maintain intake and output chart and other general condition of patient.
- In conscious patient, give artificial respiration, clean air way, administer oxygen.

COMMON POISONS WITH MANAGEMENT

Corrosive Acids (Fig. 43.3A)

Some examples of corrosive acids includes sulfuric acid, hydrochloric acid, nitric acid, acetic acid, hydrogen peroxide, etc.

Signs and Symptoms

- Intense burning pain from mouth down to stomach.
- Vomiting and retching.
- Intense thirst.
- Excoriation of lips and angles of mouth.
- Hoarse voice, fall of BP, mind remains clear till death.

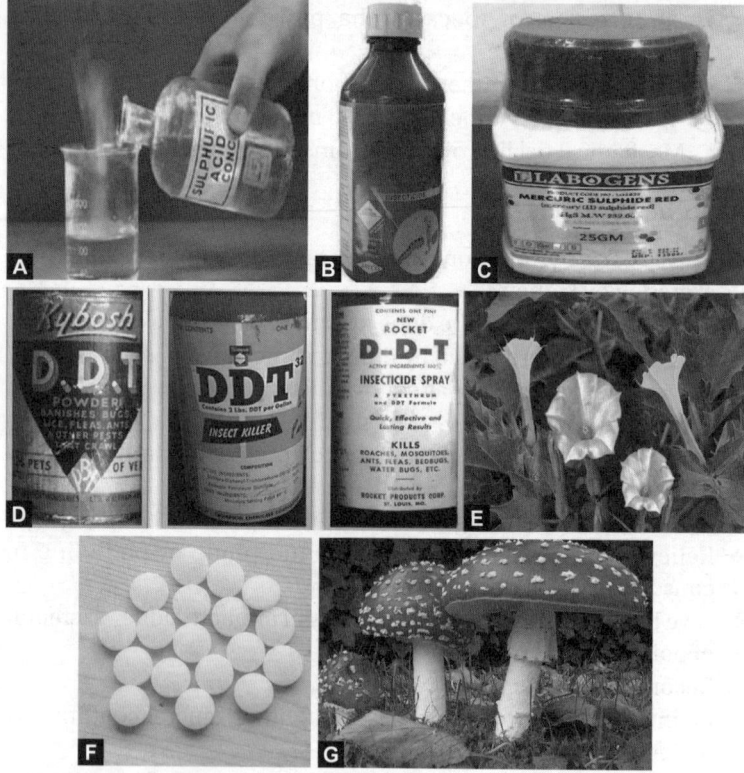

Figs. 43.3A to G: Various types of poisonous substances: (A) Corrosive acids sulfuric acid; (B) Organophosphorus insecticides; (C) Mercuric sulfide; (D) DDT; (E) Dhatura plant; (F) Camphor; (G) Fly agaric mushroom.

Management

- Do not introduce stomach wash tube.
- Neutralize acid by a pint of water or milk with 4 tablespoonful of calcium or magnesium oxide or aluminum hydroxide.
- Alternately vegetable oil, soap solution, lime water or egg white are used to reduce the effect.
- Morphine for relieving pain.
- IV fluid drip.

Washing Soda (Sodium Carbonate)

Symptoms

- The taste is acrid and soapy.
- The vomited matter does not cause gas formation when comes in contact with earth or floor like in acids.
- Purging is frequent with severe pain and strain.
- Vomiting and pain chest.

Management

- Neutralize alkali by vegetable acid like acetic acid (vinegar), citric acid (orange or lemon juice).
- Administer egg white, olive oil, milk for soothing effect.
- Morphine for pain.
- IV fluid to combat dehydration and anuria.

Organophosphorus Compounds (Fig. 43.3B)

It includes Malathion, Parathion, Chlorthion, Tik-20 Endrex, and other agriculture insecticides.

Symptoms

- Headache, nausea, vomiting.
- Giddiness, tightness over chest, dimness of vision.
- Constricted pupils.
- Profuse frothing.
- Later on convulsion, twitching, mental confusion may develop.
- Diarrhea, tenesmus, delirium.

Management

- Atropine sulphate: 1-2 mg every 10–30 minutes till pupil dilate, IV or IM.

- Stomach wash by 2% potassium permanganate solution.
- Oxygen inhalation, artificial respiration.
- IV fluid.

Iodine

Signs and Symptoms

- Burning pain in stomach, mouth and throat.
- Intense thirst.
- Salivation, vomiting, purging.
- Dark coloration of vomited matter and stool.
- Odour of iodine in vomitus and stool.
- Scanty urine.
- Collapsing state with weak pulse.

Management

- Administer emetics to cause vomiting.
- Wash out stomach with water containing soluble starch or albumin.
- Give barley water.
- Symptomatic treatment of dehydration and shock by IV fluid, steroids.

Mercury Poisoning (Fig. 43.3C)

Mercury poisoning, also known as mercury toxicity, occurs when there is an excessive accumulation of mercury in the body. Mercury is a heavy metal that can exist in different forms, including elemental (liquid) mercury, inorganic mercury compounds, and organic mercury compounds like methylmercury.

Symptoms

- Acrid, metallic taste.
- Feeling of constriction and choking.
- Hoarse voice.
- Nausea and retching.
- Later on diarrhea.
- Scanty urine.

Management

- Give emetics for vomiting.
- Wash stomach with warm water.

- ❖ Administer egg white and milk.
- ❖ 3 to 4 tablespoonful of charcoal suspended in about, a pint of water should be administered immediately which absorbs mercuric salts.

Opium

Symptoms

- ❖ Initial stage of mental excitement, freedom from anxiety.
- ❖ Restlessness, hallucination, flushing of face.
- ❖ The stage of stupor—nausea—vomiting, giddiness, lethargic condition, drowsiness.
- ❖ Uncontrollable desired to sleep.
- ❖ Pupils are contracted.
- ❖ Deep coma.

Management

- ❖ Perform gastric lavage with potassium permanganate.
- ❖ Administer magnesium-sulphate.
- ❖ Never allow the patient to sleep, pinch him, slap him.
- ❖ Administer oxygen, if necessary.
- ❖ Antidote like nalorphine hydrochloride or lethidrone IM can be given.
- ❖ IV fluid.

Alcohol (Liquor)

Symptoms

- ❖ Sense of well-being, self-confidence, flushing of face.
- ❖ Carefree behavior, argumentativeness.
- ❖ Gradual loss of self-control.
- ❖ Sense of confusion, in coordination of gait, slurred voice, blurred vision.
- ❖ Unconsciousness.
- ❖ Dilated pupils

Management

- ❖ Administer emetics.
- ❖ Cover body and maintain body temperature.
- ❖ Give strong coffee.
- ❖ Give soda-bicarb by mouth.
- ❖ Symptomatic treatment of shock, fall of BP.

DDT (Dichloro-diphenyl-trichloroethane) (Fig. 43.3D)

Symptoms
- Nausea, vomiting, cough.
- Excitability, vertigo.
- Weakness, muscular tremors, convulsions.
- Paralysis of legs.
- Unconsciousness and collapse.

Management
- Perform gastric lavage.
- Atropine inj. Hypodermally.
- Calcium gluconate IV.
- Paraldehyde or luminol for convulsions.
- Artificial respiration and oxygen.

Phenobarbitone Luminol (Gardenol)

Symptoms
In therapeutic dose it produces sleeping effect. In overdose or suicidal or homicidal case it produces poisonous effect.
- Loss of memory.
- Instability and muscular weakness.
- Insensibility and unconsciousness.
- Slow respiration.

Management
- There is no specific antidote for phenobarbitone Luminal (Gardenol).
- Assess airway, breathing and circulation.
- Administration of activated charcoal via nasogastric tube.
- Force administration of alkaline diuresis and hemodialysis for severe cases.

Kerosene Poisoning

Symptoms
- Burning pain in stomach, throat and chest.
- Cough, thirst, nausea, vomiting.
- Colics, diarrhea.
- Giddiness, heaviness in head.

- Drowsiness, stupor, coma.
- Pupils are first constricted but later dilated in coma.
- Convulsion may occur.

Management

- Gastric lavage keeping head low to avoid aspiration to lungs, by warm water with soda bicarbonate.
- Purgatives and stimulants.
- Artificial respiration.
- Penicillin injection.
- Steroids are usually given parenterally.
- IV fluid.
- High carbohydrate diet and B complex to protect liver. Do not give oils or fats.

Dhatura (Fig. 43.3E)

Symptoms

- Vomiting, bitter taste.
- Dryness of mouth, throat, burning pain in stomach.
- Difficulty in swallowing.
- Giddiness.
- Staggering gait.
- In coordination of muscles.
- Photophobia.
- Dilated pupils.
- Loss of accommodation, scanty urine.
- Delirium and drawing of imaginary threads.

Management

- Gastric lavage with potassium permanganate.
- Physostigmine Hypodermically.
- Phenobarbitone to control delirium.
- Caffeine or strong coffee.
- Artificial respiration.

Bhang (Cannabis indica) Ganja, Charas

Symptoms

- Stage of well-being in form of hallucination, euphoria, laughter.
- Talkativeness, increased appetite.

- ❖ Purpose full muscular movements.
- ❖ Disorientation of time, space.
- ❖ Giddiness, drowsiness.
- ❖ Suicidal tendency.
- ❖ Dilated pupils.
- ❖ Death usually does not occur.

Management

- ❖ Stomach wash or emetics.
- ❖ Saline purgatives.
- ❖ Oxygen.
- ❖ Artificial respiration.
- ❖ Symptomatic treatment.

Camphor (Kapur) (Fig. 43.3F)

Symptoms

- ❖ Burning pain in mouth, throat and stomach.
- ❖ Thirst, nausea and vomiting.
- ❖ Excitement and confusion.
- ❖ Flushed face, cyanosed lips.
- ❖ Dilated pupils.
- ❖ Vertigo, smell of camphor in urine.

Management

- ❖ Wash stomach with normal saline.
- ❖ Warm up body.
- ❖ Saline purgatives.
- ❖ Inhalation of ether.
- ❖ Respiratory stimulants.
- ❖ Paraldehyde if compilations.
- ❖ Do not give fats or oils.

Mushrooms (Fig. 43.3G)

Symptoms

- ❖ Constriction in throat, burning pain in stomach.
- ❖ Nausea, painful retching and vomiting.
- ❖ Diarrhea with blood.
- ❖ Urine may contain blood or albumin.

- ❖ Convulsions.
- ❖ Giddiness, mental excitement, delirium, constricted pupils, double vision.

Management

- ❖ Wash out stomach with potassium permanganate.
- ❖ Castor oil or magnesium sulphate purgatives.
- ❖ Atropine hypodermically.
- ❖ Pethidine for pain.
- ❖ Antibiotics.
- ❖ Oxygen or artificial respiration if required.

CHAPTER 44

Care of Newborn

INTRODUCTION

The care of newborns is a critical aspect of ensuring their health and well-being during the early stages of life. Newborns require special attention and care to adapt to their new environment and meet their nutritional needs.

CARE OF NEWBORN AT BIRTH

A healthy infant born at term between 38–42 weeks, should have average birth weight, cries immediately following birth, establishes independent rhythmic respiration and quickly adapts to the changed environment **(Fig. 44.1)**.

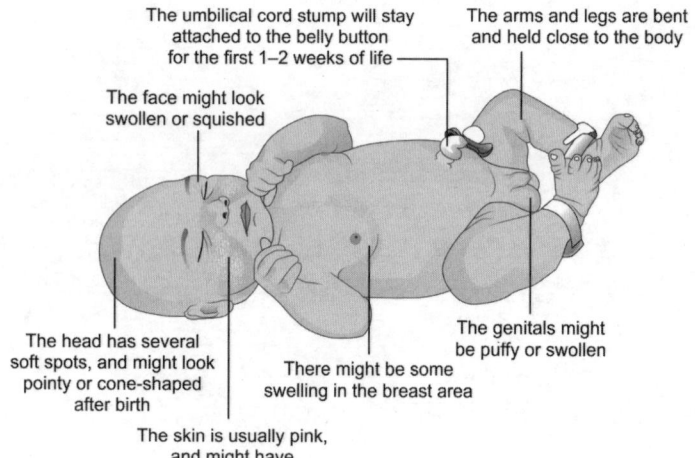

Fig. 44.1: Healthy newborn.

Care of Newborn

IMMEDIATE BASIC CARE TO THE NEWBORN

Maintenance of Body Temperature

- The baby needs to be covered with a warm and dry cloth, especially if the temperature of labor room is < 25°C.
- A baby who is small (<2.5 kg at birth or born before 37 weeks gestation) and sick needs additional thermal protection and warmth to maintain normal body temperature. These babies become hypothermic very quickly, and rewarming the baby can take a long time.

Methods of Maintaining Temperature in Newborn

See **Table 44.1**.

Table 44.1: Methods of maintaining body temperature in newborn.

Method	Guidelines for selection and use	Advantages	Disadvantages
Skin-to-skin contact	a. Appropriate for all stable babies b. Appropriate for re-warming a baby with moderate hypothermia (32°C to 36.4°C) c. Not appropriate for babies with life threatening problems (sepsis, severe breathing difficulty)	a. Mother can closely monitor baby. b. Another person can provide skin-to-skin contact if the mother is unavailable c. Babies usually maintain normal body temperature	
Kangaroo mother care (KMC)	Appropriate for low-birth-weight babies	a. Mother can closely monitor baby b. Babies usually maintain normal body temperature	a. Mother may not always be available.

Contd...

Contd...

Method	Guidelines for selection and use	Advantages	Disadvantages
Radiant warmer	a. Appropriate for sick babies and babies weighing 1.5 kg or more b. Used to keep baby warm during initial assessment, treatment, and procedures and to re-warm a cold baby	a. Allows observation of baby b. Many procedures can be performed while baby is under warmer	a. Baby can become hyperthermic if temperature is not monitored b. Baby can become dehydrated
Incubator	a. Appropriate for continuous care of babies weighing <1.5 kg who are not eligible for kangaroo mother care b. Appropriate for babies who have life threatening problems (sepsis, severe breathing difficulty)	a. Maintains constant temperature b. Allows observation of baby c. Oxygen can be easily provided	a. Baby can become hyperthermic or hypothermic if temperature is not monitored b. Baby can become dehydrated

Immunization (Fig. 44.2)

BCG and first dose of OPV and hepatitis B vaccine (HBV) are given at birth. Within 1 hour of birth, intramuscular vitamin K should also be administered.

Breastfeeding (Fig. 44.3)

* Early skin-to-skin contact and breastfeeding initiation are key to successful breastfeeding.
* Skin-to-skin contact enhances the transition of the newborn, boosts the production of maternal milk, and makes breastfeeding more effective.

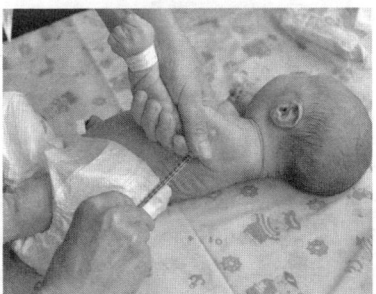

Fig. 44.2: Immunization.

- In the first 48 hours, effective sucking and latching should be established.
- Educate the mother about the benefits of early and exclusive breastfeeding.

Skin Care and Baby Bath

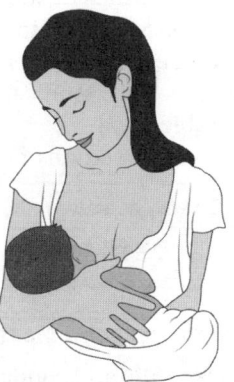

Fig. 44.3: Breastfeeding.

Skin care: Full-term newborn's skin is covered by vernix caseosa which protects the epidermis in the uterus from water damage due to its high lipid content and hydrophobic properties. It is recommended to keep it in contact with the skin for at least 6 hours after birth. Use clean, soft cotton clothes to dress the baby.

Bathing: Until the umbilical stump falls, bathing should be done with a sponge to keep the cord dry and is not required frequently. Soaps usually contain surfactants to remove dirt, and this can damage subcutaneous lipid and cause irritation. After 1 month, oil massage can be given. There after skin can be exposed to sunlight for added advantage of Vitamin D.

Care of Umbilical Cord

The umbilical cord is susceptible to bacterial colonization and can serve as a port of entry for bacteria into the systemic circulation. Dry cord care is the preferred method as per the World Health Organization (WHO). The umbilical cord should be kept exposed to the air, and if covered, it should be loosely covered with a clean garment. The umbilical stump usually falls off naturally in 10 to 14 days.

NEWBORN ASSESSMENT

Initial Assessment

The most essential assessment is the 'first cry'. Good cry helps in establishment of satisfactory breathing. The respiration, heart rate and skin color are the basic criteria's which should be evaluated immediately to determine the need for resuscitation.

The physiological status including temperature, degree of consciousness, general level of activity, gross congenital anomalies, presence of birth injury, meconium staining and evidence of shock also need to be ascertained immediately and promptly after birth.

Another significant assessment of the neonate is 'Apgar scoring' **(Table 44.2)**.

Interpretation of Apgar score

Severely depressed	0–3
Moderately depressed	4–6
Excellent condition	7–10

Anthropometric Measurements

Assess the anthropometric measurements.
- **Weight (Fig. 44.4):** The average weight of a normal full-term newborn infant is about 2.9 kg with a variation of 2.5–3.9 kg or

Table. 44.2: Apgar score.

Score	0 points	1 point	2 point
Appearance (Skin color)	Cyanotic/Pale all over	Peripheral cyanosis only	Pink
Pulse (Heart rate)	0	<100	100–140
Grimace (Reflex irritability)	No response to stimulation	Grimace or weak cry when stimulated	Cry when stimulated
Activity (Tone)	Floppy	Some flexion	Well flexed and resisting extension
Respiration	Apneic	Slow, irregular breathing	Strong cry

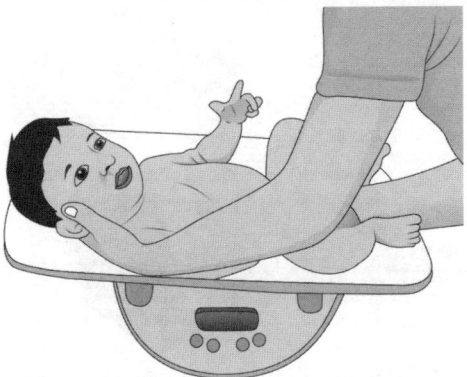

Fig. 44.4: Measuring weight of newborn.

more. It varies country-to-country and in different socioeconomical status.
- **Length (Fig. 44.5):** At birth the average crown heel length of the term newborn is 50 cm with the range of 48–53 cm. The length is a more reliable criterion of gestational age than the weight.
- **Head circumference (Fig. 44.6):** The head circumference is usually varying from 33 to 37 cm, with the average of 35 cm.
- **Chest circumference (Fig. 44.7):** The chest circumference is about 3 cm < head circumference. The chest is rounded rather than flattened anteroposteriorly.

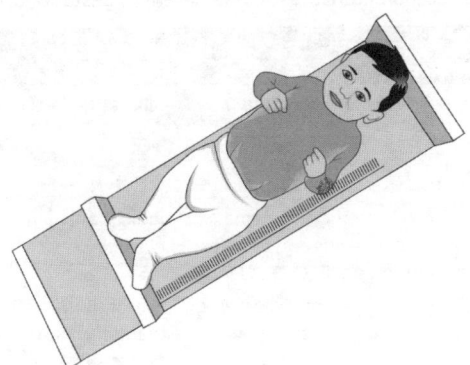

Fig. 44.5: Measuring length of newborn.

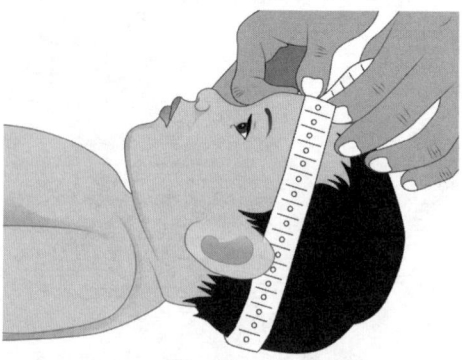

Fig. 44.6: Measuring the head circumference of newborn.

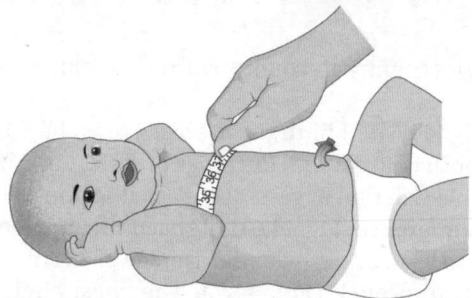

Fig. 44.7: Measuring the chest circumference of newborn.

Assessment of Gestational Age at Birth (Table 44.3)

Table. 44.3: Physical characteristics for assessment of gestational age at birth.

Physical characteristics	Preterm	Term
Hair texture and hair distribution on scalp	Wool, fuzzy and very fine	Silky and black coarse
Skin texture	Shiny oily plethoric, edema with visible veins and venules on abdomen and excess lanugo	Pink, scanty lanugo. Good elasticity
Breast	Breast tissue <5 mm diameter. Nipples are absent	Breast tissue >10 mm diameter. Nipples raised above skin level
Ear cartilage	Pinna feels soft with no cartilage and no recoil	Pinna is firm with definite cartilage and instant recoil.

Contd...

Contd...

Physical characteristics	Preterm	Term
Plantar creases	Absent or faint red marks over sole	Deep creases
Genitalia-Male	Small scrotum with few rugae and light pigmentation. Undescended testis	At least one testis descends in scrotum. Prominent rugae and deep pigmentation
Genitalia-Female	Labia majora widely separated with labia minora and clitoris	Labia majora completely cover the labia minora and clitoris

Premature Baby

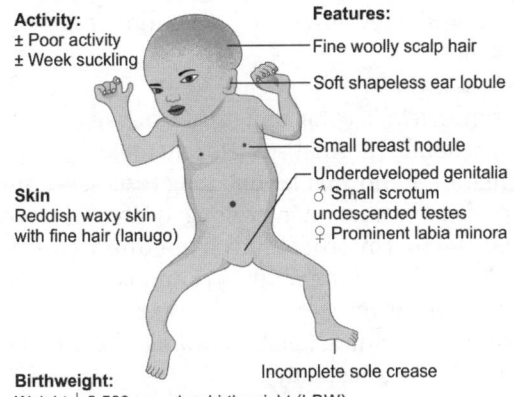

Activity:
± Poor activity
± Week suckling

Features:
- Fine woolly scalp hair
- Soft shapeless ear lobule
- Small breast nodule
- Underdeveloped genitalia
  ♂ Small scrotum undescended testes
  ♀ Prominent labia minora

Skin
Reddish waxy skin with fine hair (lanugo)

Incomplete sole crease

Birthweight:
Weight ↓ 2,500 gm = low birthweight (LBW)
Weight ↓ 1,500 gm = very low birthweight (VLBW)
Weight ↓ 1,000 gm = extremely low birthweight (ELBW)

Normal Newborn

LOC and activity:
Conscious
Active
Good sukling

Appearance:
Pink in color

Vital signs:
H.R.: ± 120/minute
R.R.: ± 40/minute
Temp.: ± 37°C

Measurements:
Weight: ± 3 kg
Length: ± 50 cm
Head c.: ± 35 cm

Regional:
Normal

Systemic:
Normal

No prematurity
No congenital anomalies
No birth trauma

Head-to-Toe Examination

- ❖ **General appearance**
  - *Body structure:* Well developed healthy newborn (normal baby) or poorly developed (low birth weight baby).
  - *Skin:* Pink (normal baby), red (low birth weight baby), blue (cyanosed/asphyxiated baby) or yellow (jaundiced baby) or any cracks, spots or birthmarks.
  - *Cry:* Listen whether cry is loud and strong (normal baby), weak or whiny (low birth weight baby) or absent (asphyxiated baby).
  - *Activity:* Whether baby is active (normal baby), less active or in active (low birth weight/asphyxiated).
- ❖ **Body size and shape:** Observe for achondroplasia.
- ❖ **Head and face**
  - *Inspect the head for:*
    - Presence of hair, color, and texture of hair.
    - *Shape:* Round (normal), oval (slight molding or a small caput formation in normal labor), long (excessive molding or a large caput formation in prolonged labor) or asymmetrical.
    - *Size:* Small (microcephaly), medium (normal), large (hydrocephaly or prematurity) or unusual (anencephaly).
  - *Palpate the head for*
    - *Sutures:* Overriding (slight molding or excessive molding) and wide (hydrocephaly).
    - *Fontanelle:* Front and back whether normal or tense (hydrocephaly).
  - Measure the head circumference.
  - Look for color, shape, size, and symmetry of face.
- ❖ **Eyes**
  - Inspect the eyes for symmetry, alignment, and any discharge.
  - Assess the pupillary reflex by shining a light and observing the constriction of the pupils.
  - Check for the red reflex by using an ophthalmoscope to ensure the absence of any abnormalities in the retina.
- ❖ **Ear**
  - Inspect the external ears for shape, position, and any abnormalities.
  - Observe for any signs of discharge, swelling, or abnormalities in the ear canal.

- ❖ **Nose**
  - Observe the nose for symmetry, patency, and any nasal discharge.
  - Gently palpate the nasal bridge to check for any abnormalities or tenderness.
- ❖ **Mouth**
  - Inspect the mouth for cleft lip and cleft palate, frothy mucus (esophageal atresia), tongue tie, and false teeth.
  - Check for a suck reflex by gently stimulating the newborn's lips.
  - Inspect the neck. Normally it is so short that head seems to rest on shoulders.
- ❖ **Neck**
  - Assess the range of motion of the neck by gently moving it from side to side.
  - Check for any masses, swelling, or abnormalities in the neck area.
- ❖ **Chest**
  - Observe the chest for symmetry, noting any retractions or abnormal movements.
  - Auscultate the lung sounds using a stethoscope to assess for any abnormal breath sounds or murmurs.
  - Palpate the chest to check for any tenderness or abnormalities.
  - Measure the chest circumference.
- ❖ **Abdomen**
  - Observe the abdomen for symmetry, noting any distension or visible organs.
  - Auscultate the bowel sounds using a stethoscope to assess their presence and character.
  - Palpate the abdomen for tenderness and masses.
- ❖ **Genitalia:**
  - Observe the genitalia to determine the sex of the newborn and assess for any abnormalities or swelling.
  - Check for the presence of testes in male newborns.
  - Note the appearance of the labia and clitoris in female newborns.
- ❖ **Extremities**
  - Inspect the arms and legs for symmetry, noting any deformities or abnormalities.

- Assess the range of motion in the joints by gently moving the limbs.
- Palpate the pulses in the extremities to ensure adequate circulation.

❖ **Spine and back**
- Observe the spine for alignment and any visible abnormalities or defects.
- Inspect the buttocks and anal area for any abnormalities, such as skin tags or imperforate anus.

❖ **Reflexes:** *See* **Table 44.4** for newborn reflexes.

Table 44.4: Reflexes in newborn.

Reflex	Stimulus	Response	Age when reflex disappear
Moro reflex (startle reflex)	Sudden loud noise or a change in head position	The newborn throws their arms and legs out, then pulls them back in, often accompanied by crying	3–4 months
Rooting reflex	Light touch or stroke on the cheek or around the mouth	The newborn turns their head toward the stimulus and opens their mouth, seeking to suck or feed	3–4 months when awake and 7–8 months when asleep
Sucking reflex	Sensation of the lips or mouth being touched	The newborn begins to suck rhythmically	Begins to diminish at 6 months

Contd...

Contd...

Reflex	Stimulus	Response	Age when reflex disappear
Swallowing reflex	Accompanies the sucking reflex	Food, reaching the posterior of the mouth is swallowed	Does not disappear
Gag reflex	When more food is taken into the mouth that can be successfully swallowed	Immediate return of undigested food	Does not disappear
Tonic neck reflex (fencing reflex)	Turned head to one side while lying on the back	The arm on the side the newborn is facing extends, while the opposite arm bends at the elbow	6 months
Babinski reflex	Stroke along the outer edge of the sole of the foot, from the heel toward the toes	The toes fan out, and the big toe moves upward	12 months
Stepping or dancing reflex	Holding the newborn upright and allowing their feet to touch a flat surface	The newborn lifts one foot after another, mimicking a stepping motion	3-4 weeks

Contd...

Contd...

Reflex	Stimulus	Response	Age when reflex disappear
Palmar reflex	Place a finger in the newborn's open palm	The newborn closes their hand around the finger, tightens the grip if the examiner attempts to withdraw the finger	6 weeks–3 months
Sneezing and coughing reflex	Foreign substance entering the upper and lower airways	Clearing of upper air passages by sneezing and lower air passage by coughing	Does not disappear
Blinking	Exposure of eyes to bright light	Protection of eyes by rapid eyelid closure	Does not disappear
Doll's eye	Turn the newborn's head slowly to right or left side	Normally eyes do not move	When fixation develops

CHAPTER 45

Assisting in Diagnostic Procedures

Assisting in the diagnostic procedures is one of the prime responsibilities of the nurse. The results of these diagnostic procedures help the physician in making a diagnosis and in providing proper treatment. This chapter will deal with different diagnostic and therapeutic procedures.

RESPIRATORY SYSTEM

CHEST X-RAY

Chest radiograph or chest X-ray is the imaging study to visualize respiratory structures and organs using X-rays **(Fig. 45.1)**. Normally the pulmonary tissues are radiolucent (transparent to X-rays) therefore, densities produced by fluid, tumors, foreign bodies, and other pathologic conditions can be detected by X-ray examination. It may reveal an extensive pathologic process in the lungs in the absence of symptoms.

Commonly two views are taken in the routine chest X-rays (i.e., posterior-anterior (PA) and lateral view) **(Fig. 45.2)**.

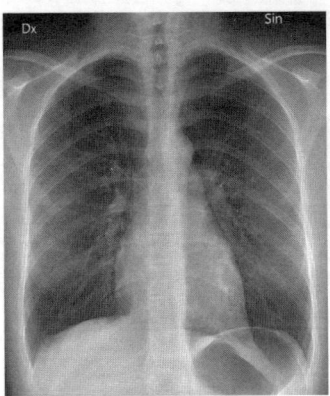

Fig. 45.1: Imaging in Chest X-ray.

Assisting in Diagnostic Procedures

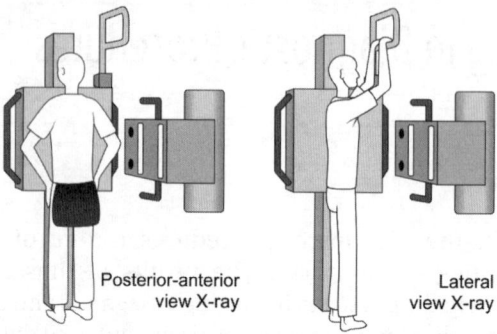

Fig. 45.2: Posterior-anterior (PA) and lateral view.

 Nursing Responsibilities

- Identify the patient and check for the physician's order.
- Explain the procedure to the patient that this is the noninvasive procedure, causes no discomfort.
- Ask the patient to remove all the clothing, jewelry, metals, etc. and make the patient wear hospital gown.
- Instruct the patient that the technician will ask to take a deep breath and hold on during the procedure.

CT SCAN

CT scan is an imaging method in which the lungs are scanned in the successive layers by a narrow-beam X-ray **(Fig. 45.3)**. A cross-sectional view of chest is produced by these images. It

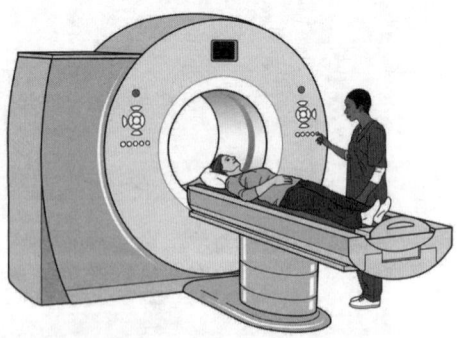

Fig. 45.3: CT scan procedure.

is used to define pulmonary nodules and tumors adjacent to pleural surfaces that are not visible in the chest X-rays. Contrast enhanced CT scan is used to detect mediastinal abnormalities and hilar adenopathy.

Nursing Responsibilities

- Informed consent.
- Explain the procedure to the patient.
- Look for history of allergies from iodinated dye or shellfish if contrast enhanced CT is indicated.
- If patient is undergoing contrast enhanced CT, check for NPO status for 4 hours.
- Ask the patient to remove all the clothing, jewelry, metals, etc.
- Provide comfortable loose-fitting clothes to the patient.
- Instruct the patient that the technician will ask to take a deep breath and hold on during the procedure.
- Instruct the patient to resume the usual diet after the procedure.
- In case of contrast enhanced CT scan, encourage patient to increase the fluid intake in order to promote the excretion of contrast.

MRI

MRI is like CT scan but in MRI magnetic fields and radiofrequency signals are used instead of a narrow-beam X-ray **(Fig. 45.4)**. It yields much more detailed diagnostic image than CT because it visualizes soft tissues. It is used to stage cancer and to evaluate inflammatory activity in interstitial lung disease and acute pulmonary embolism.

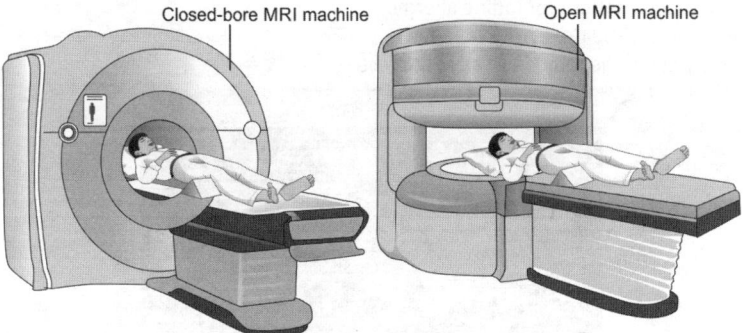

Fig. 45.4: MRI procedure.

Nursing Responsibilities

- Informed consent.
- Explain the procedure to the patient.
- Inform the patient that test may take 30–90 minutes.
- Explain about the jackhammers, clanking, banging, whirring, thumping and industrial noises from the MRI machine.
- Ask whether the patient has any surgically implanted joints, pins, clips, valves, pumps, or pacemakers containing metal that could be attracted to strong MRI magnet. If he does, he won't be able to have the test.
- Note and report all allergies.
- Provide patient with comfort measures as needed.
- Tell the patient to resume his normal diet and activities unless otherwise indicated.
- Monitor vital signs.
- Monitor the patient for orthostatic hypotension.

LUNG SCAN

Ventilation (V) and perfusion (Q) lung scan is a nuclear test that uses the perfusion scan to delineate the blood flow distribution and the ventilation scan to measure airflow distribution in the lungs **(Fig. 45.5)**. The primary utilization of the V/Q scan is to help diagnose lung clots called pulmonary embolisms.

 ### Nursing Responsibilities

- Informed consent.
- Explain the procedure to the patient.
- Check patient for iodine allergy.
- Follow the prescriptions.
- Encourage force fluid after the test.

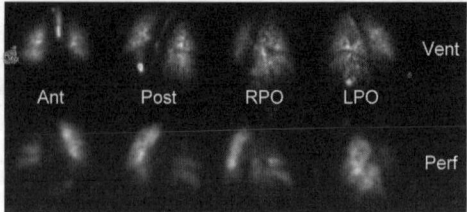

Fig. 45.5: Imaging the lung scan.

POSITRON EMISSION TOMOGRAPHY (PET) SCAN

PET scan is an advanced radioactive study which is used to evaluate the lung nodules for malignancy **(Fig. 45.6)**. It also detects and displays the metabolic changes in the tissues, differentiate viable from dead or dying tissue, show regional blood flow, and determine the distribution and fate of medications in the body. PET is more accurate in detecting malignancies than CT scan.

In PET scan, radioisotope that releases positron is inhaled by or injected into the individual. As short-lived radioisotope decays, it releases gamma rays that are recorded by the computerized scanner.

Nursing Responsibilities

- Obtain consent from the patient.
- Explain the procedure to the patient.
- Tell the patient to refrain from strenuous exercised for 24–48 hours prior investigation.
- Ask the patient to adhere to low carbohydrate and no sugar diet before test.
- Maintain NPO status for 4–6 hours before test.
- Remove jewelry before test and wear hospital gown.
- Ask patient to void before taking isotope injection.
- After the procedure, patient can resume usual activities.
- Encourage the patient to increase the fluid intake in order to promote the excretion of contrast.

PULMONARY ANGIOGRAPHY

It is used to investigate thromboembolic disease of the lungs, such as pulmonary emboli, and congenital abnormalities of the pulmonary vascular tree **(Fig. 45.7)**.

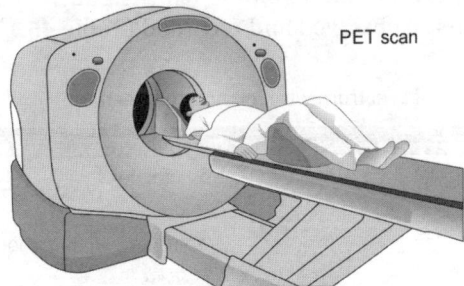

Fig. 45.6: PET scan procedure.

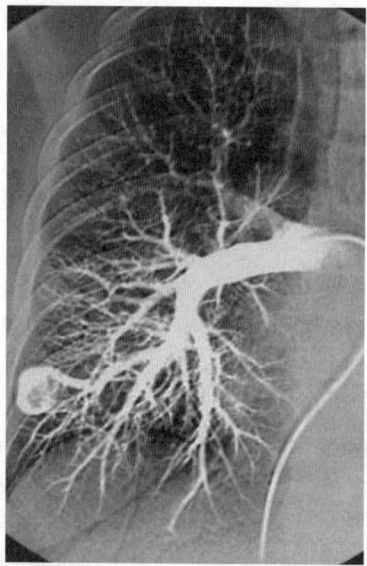

Fig. 45.7: Imaging in pulmonary angiography.

In this procedure, a radiopaque material is injected via a catheter into a systemic vein, or the pulmonary artery and the distribution of this material is recorded on film.

The nursing responsibilities are similar to lung scan.

SPUTUM EXAMINATION

Sputum examination is performed to identify the pathogen and to determine the presence of malignant cells. Expectoration is the usual method for collecting a sputum specimen.

In sputum examination volume, consistency, color, and odor of the sputum are observed and recorded **(Table 45.1)**. It includes

Table 45.1: Color of spectrum with relation to infection.

Colour of sputum	Infection
Clear/colorless	Noninfectious
Green	*Pseudomonas*
Creamy yellow	Staphylococcal pneumonia
Rusty	*Klebsiella*
Pink frothy	Pulmonary edema

culture and sensitivity, gram staining, AFB, smear, t-Cytology and quantitative test.

Nursing Responsibilities

- Instruct the patient to clear the nose and throat and rinse the mouth to decrease contamination of the sputum.
- Ask the patient to collect the sputum that has come from deep in the lungs.
- Collect the first sputum raised in the morning.
- Provide a wide mouthed container and instruct to expectorate directly into it.
- Encourage to have more fluid in case patient has tenacious sputum.
- Collect the specimens before meals to avoid possible emesis from coughing after eating instruct patient rinse mouth with water before collecting sputum to decrease contamination.
- Send the specimens to the laboratory as soon as it is collected.

In some patient's nasogastric tube may be passed into the stomach and a specimen of stomach contents is greatly withdrawn and placed in a covered container. This is done in case there is no coughed sputum available specially in tuberculosis patients.

MANTOUX TEST

The Mantoux method is used to determine whether a person has been infected with the tubercle bacillus. It is a standardized, intradermal injection procedure that should be performed by trained personnels **(Fig. 45.8)**.

Tubercle bacillus extract (tuberculin), purified protein derivative (PPD), is injected into the intradermal layer of the inner aspect of the forearm, approximately 4 inches below the elbow. Only 0.1 mL of PPD is injected, creating an elevation in the skin or wheal 6 to 10 mm in diameter. The site, antigen name, strength, lot number, date, and time of the test are recorded. The test result is read 48 to 72 hours after injection.

The largest diameter of induration should be measured and recorded in millimeters. Any erythema at the site should be noted. 10 mm or more is highly significant for past or present infection. 5 to 9 mm is doubtful reaction except in persons with HIV infections and 0 to 4 mm indicate little or no sensitivity.

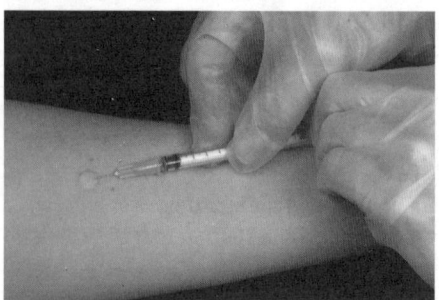

Fig. 45.8: Mantoux test procedure.

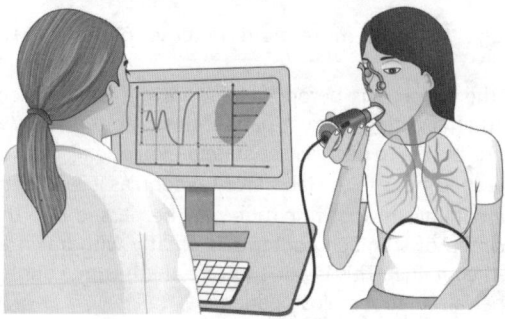

Fig. 45.9: Pulmonary function test.

PULMONARY FUNCTION TEST

Pulmonary function tests (PFTs) are performed in patients with chronic respiratory disorders **(Fig. 45.9)**. This procedure is used to assess the respiratory function and determine the extent of dysfunction.

Pulmonary function test measures the lung volumes, ventilatory function, and the mechanics of breathing, diffusion, and gas exchange **(Figs. 45.10 and 45.11)**.

 Nursing Responsibilities

- Check for the physician's order for the test.
- Explain the procedure to the patient.
- Patient while wearing a nose clip breath through a mouthpiece connected through the apparatus. The spirometer is connected to the recording device that documents air volume in liters. The residual volume is calculated, as it cannot be measured.

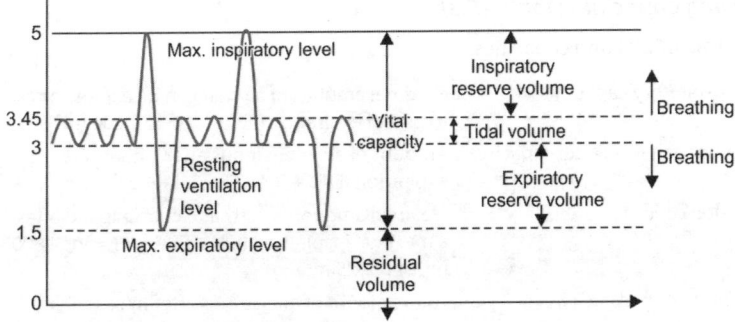

Fig. 45.10: Overview of lung volumes and capacities.

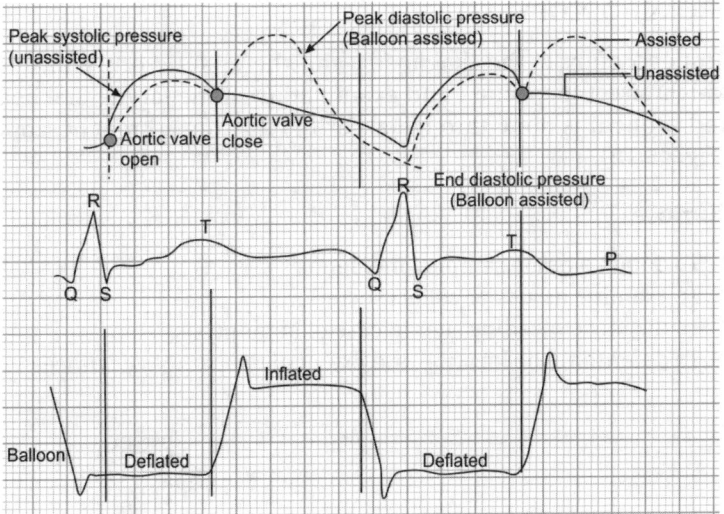

Fig. 45.11: Spirogram of lung volumes and capacities.

Lung Volume (Table 45.2)

Table 45.2: Lung volume.

Tidal volume	Volume of air inspired or expired during a normal breath at rest (VT 500 mL).
Inspiratory reserve volume	Maximum volume that can be inspired from the end of normal inspiration (IRV 3,100 mL).
Expiratory reserve volume	Maximal volume that can be exhaled by forced expiration after a normal expiration (ERV 1,200 mL).
Residual volume	Volume of air left in the lungs after maximal expiration (RV 1,200 mL)

Lung Capacities (Table 45.3)

Table 45.3: Lung capacities.

Inspiratory capacity	Maximal amount of air that can be expired after a normal expiration (IRV + VT = IC 3,600 mL)
Functional residual capacity	Amount of air left in lungs after a normal expiration (ERV + RV = FRC 2,400)
Vital capacity	Maximal amount of air that can be expired after a maximal inspiration (IRV + ERV + VT = VC 4,800 mL or 65–75 mL/kg)
Total lung capacity	Total amount of air in lungs after maximal inspiration (VT + IRV + ERV + RV = TLC 6,000 mL)

BRONCHOSCOPY

Bronchoscopy is the diagnostic and therapeutic procedure in which direct inspection and examination of the larynx, trachea, and bronchi is done through a flexible fiberoptic bronchoscope (**Fig. 45.12**).

Purpose

- To obtain a tissue sample for diagnosis
- To examine tissues or collect secretions.
- To diagnose bleeding sites in case of hemoptysis.
- To determine the location and extent of the pathologic process.

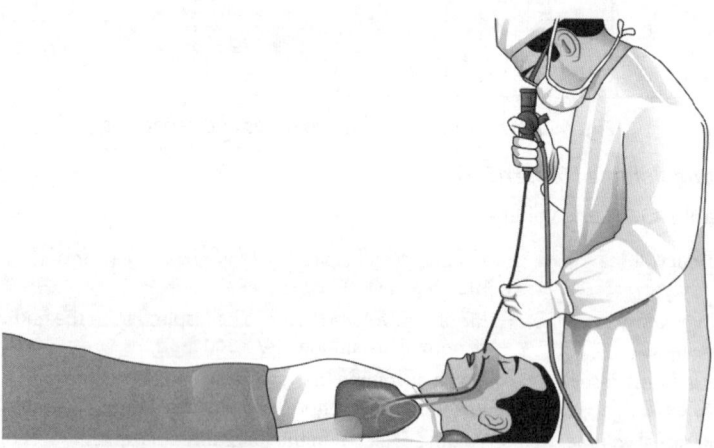

Fig. 45.12: Bronchoscopy.

Nursing Responsibilities

- Written and informed consent.
- Explain the procedure to the patient.
- Instruct the patient to maintain NPO status for 6 to 8 hours prior to the procedure.
- Remove dentures, document any loose teeth.
- Premedicate as prescribed
- After the procedure, withhold fluid and food until gag reflex returns.
- Encourage deep breathing, coughing, and moving to clear the airway after the procedure.

THORACOSCOPY

Thoracoscopy is a diagnostic procedure in which the pleural cavity is examined with an endoscope **(Fig. 45.13)**. It is usually indicated in pleural effusions, pleural disease, and tumor staging.

Procedure

- Small incisions are made into the pleural cavity in an intercoastal space depending upon the clinical and diagnostic findings.
- After any fluid present in the pleural cavity is aspirated, the fiberoptic mediastinoscope is inserted into the pleural cavity, and its surface is inspected through the instrument.
- After the procedure, a chest tube may be inserted, and the pleural cavity is drained by negative-pressure water-seal drainage.

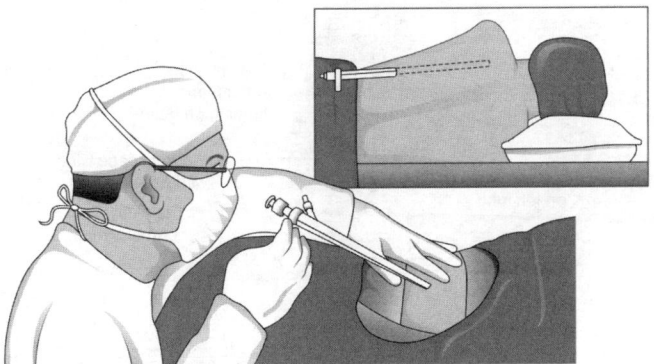

Fig. 45.13: Thoracoscopy.

Nursing Responsibilities

- Written and informed consent.
- Explain the procedure to the patient.
- Instruct the patient to maintain NPO status for 6 to 8 hours prior to the procedure.
- Follow-up care in the hospital involves monitoring the patient for shortness of breath (which might indicate a pneumothorax) and minor activity restrictions, which vary depending on the intensity of the procedure. If a chest tube was inserted during the procedure, monitoring of the chest drainage system and chest tube insertion site is essential.

THORACENTESIS

Thoracentesis is the aspiration of fluid or air from the pleural space which is performed for diagnostic or therapeutic reasons **(Fig. 45.14)**.

Nursing Responsibilities

- Arrange the required articles for the procedure.
- Explain the procedure to the patient, emphasizing the importance of not moving, breathing quietly, and not coughing during the procedure to avoid damage to the pleura.
- Position the patient: Patient should sit on the bed maintaining a position with head resting upon folded arms on the overbed table or patient turned to the unaffected side with head of bed elevated 30 degrees.

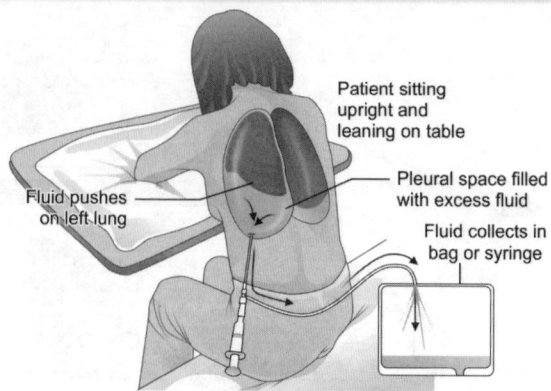

Fig. 45.14: Thoracentesis.

Assisting in Diagnostic Procedures

- Reassure and provide physical comfort.
- The physician inserts the aspiration needle and remove the fluid for diagnostic purposes and connect to the drainage system. No >1,500 mL of pleural fluid should be removed within a 30-minutes period because of the risk of intravascular fluid shift.
- Apply sterile occlusive dressing applying pressure after the needle is withdrawn.
- Make the patient comfortable, position on the unaffected side with insertion site up.
- Observe the vitals and any signs of complications.
- Document the procedure and its findings.

CARDIOVASCULAR SYSTEM

ECG

Electrocardiogram (ECG) is a graphical recording of electrical activity of the heart detected by surface electrodes and measured using a galvanometer **(Fig. 45.15)**.

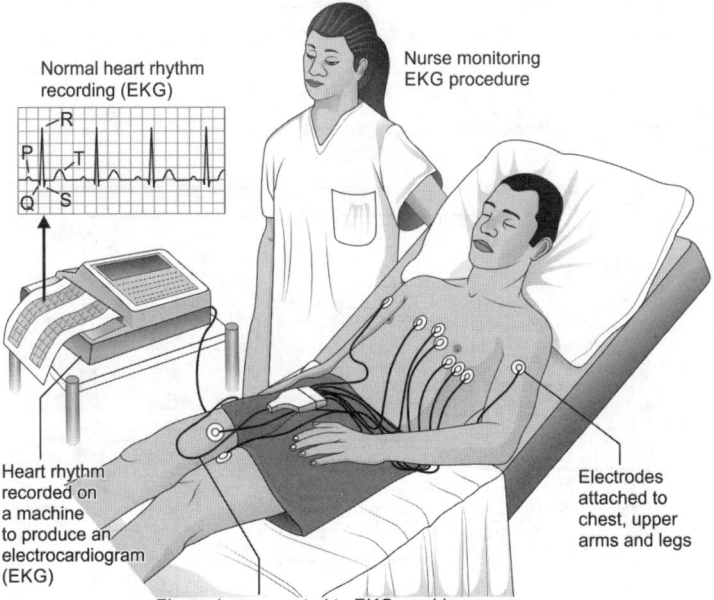

Fig. 45.15: ECG procedure.

Components of ECG

See **Table 45.4 and Figure 45.16**.

Nursing Responsibilities

Preprocedure
- Explain the purpose of the test.
- Advise to wear loose clothing with front buttoning tops.

Table 45.4: Components of ECG.

Wave/Segment	Duration (in secs)	Description
P wave	0.12	Atrial depolarization
PR segment	0.05–0.12	Conduction delay through AV node; used as baseline to evaluate ST segment elevation or depression
PR interval	0.12–0.2	Atrial depolarization+ conduction delay through AV node
QRS complex	0.06–1	Ventricular depolarization
ST segment	0.08	Isoelectric; ventricles still depolarized
QT interval	0.3–0.4	Ventricular depolarization+ ventricular repolarization; mechanical contraction of ventricles
T wave	0.10–0.25	Ventricular repolarization

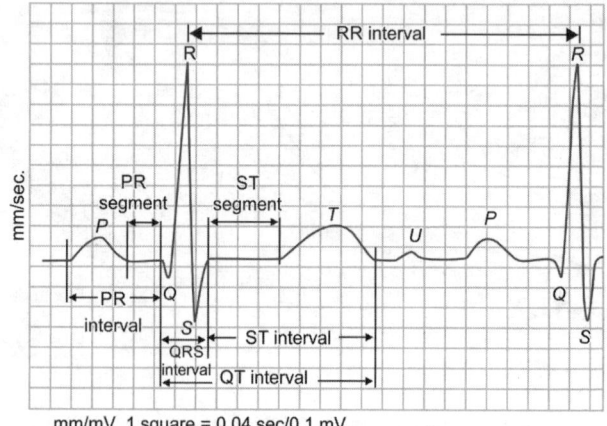

Fig. 45.16: Normal ECG waveform.

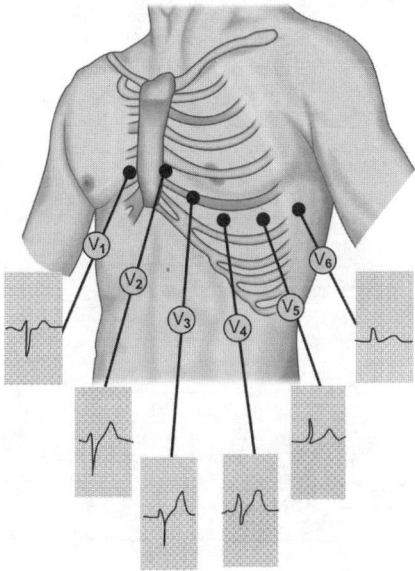

Fig. 45.17: Placement of electrodes.

During the Procedure
- Shave the site and apply electrodes **(Fig. 45.17)**.
- The electrode cable is accurately attached to the monitor.
- The monitor and case are positioned as the patient will wear it, then the leads are attached to the electrodes. A fully charged or new battery is installed into the recorder, the tape is inserted, and the recorder is turned on.
- The electrode attachment circuit is tested by connecting the recorder to a standard ECG machine.

Postprocedure
Remove all electrodes and clean electrode sites.

EXERCISE STRESS TESTING

This procedure evaluates the action of heart during physical stress and tests the cardiac reaction to increased demand for oxygen.

Types

- Treadmill **(Fig. 45.18)**
- Bicycle ergometer **(Fig. 45.19)**

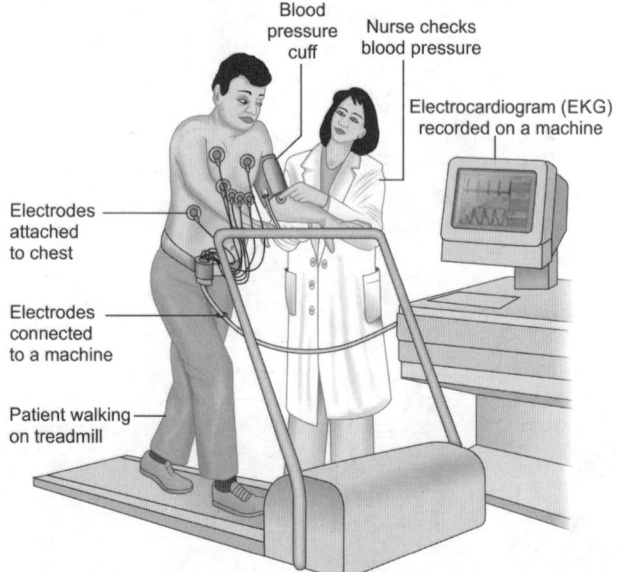

Fig. 45.18: Treadmill test.

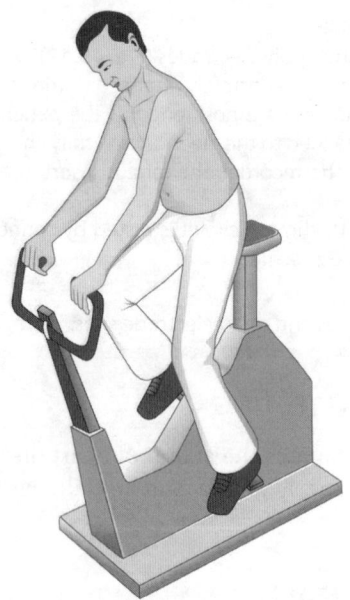

Fig. 45.19: Bicycle ergometer test.

Nursing Responsibilities

Preprocedure
- Written and informed consent.
- Explain about the test.
- Instruct the patient for not to eat, smoke or drink alcoholic or caffeine beverages for 3 hours before the test as it may cause fatigue, slight breathlessness, and sweating.
- If scheduled for multi-stage treadmill test, explain that the speed and incline of the treadmill increase at predetermined intervals, and he will be informed of each adjustment.
- If for a bicycle ergometer test, explain that the resistance he experiences in pedaling increases gradually.

During Test
Encourage patient for informing any discomfort. Monitor pulse, BP, and ECG.

Post Test
- Assist patient to a chair and continue monitoring heart rate and B.P. for 10–15 minutes, until ECG returns to the base line.
- Remove electrodes and clear sites.
- Inform the patient to take a rest for 30–60 minutes.

ECHOCARDIOGRAPHY

Echocardiography is a noninvasive ultrasound procedure that is used to measure the ejection fraction and examine the size, shape, and motion of cardiac structures **(Fig. 45.20)**.

In this procedure, high-frequency sound waves are transmitted into the heart through the chest wall and recording of the return signals. The ultrasound is generated by a handheld transducer applied to the front of the chest. The transducer picks up the echoes, converts them to electrical impulses, and transmits them for display on an oscilloscope and recording on a videotape.

An ECG is recorded simultaneously to assist with interpreting the echocardiogram.

Nursing Responsibilities

Before the procedure, the nurse informs the patient about the test, explaining that it is noninvasive, painless. It is performed while a transducer

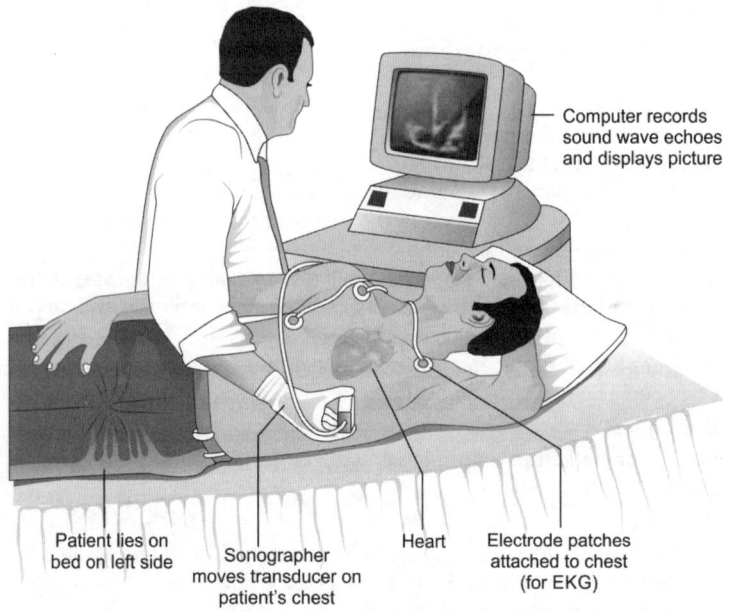

Fig. 45.20: Echocardiography.

that emits sound waves is moved over the surface of the chest wall. Gel applied to the skin helps transmit the sound waves.

At intervals, the patient may ask to turn onto the left side or hold a breath. This procedure takes about 30 to 45 minutes.

CARDIAC CATHETERIZATION

Cardiac catheterization is an invasive diagnostic procedure in which radiopaque arterial and venous catheters are introduced into selected blood vessels of the right and left sides of the heart **(Fig. 45.21)**. Catheter advancement is guided by fluoroscopy. Most commonly, the catheters are inserted percutaneously through the blood vessels, or via a cutdown procedure if the patient has poor vascular access. Pressures and oxygen saturation levels in the four heart chambers are measured.

Cardiac catheterization is usually performed with angiography, a technique in which a contrast agent is injected into the vascular system to outline the heart and blood vessels.

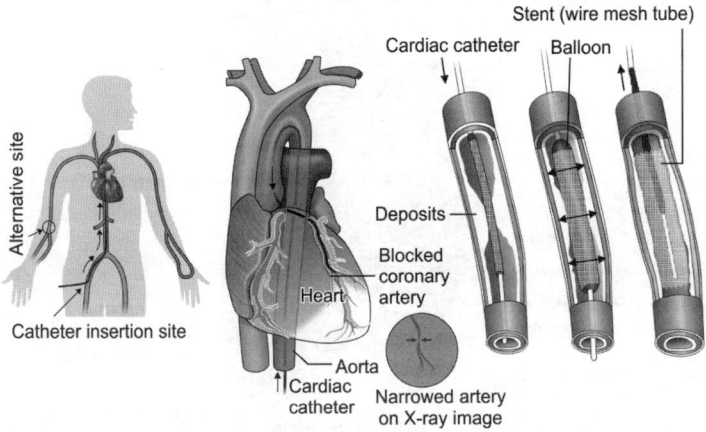

Fig. 45.21: Cardiac catheterization.

Right Heart Catheterization

A sterile, radio-opaque catheter of 100–125 cm is introduced through the antecubital vein or femoral vein into the vena cava, then through the right atrium and ventricle into the pulmonary artery (pulmonary artery wedge pressure monitoring). The ECG is constantly monitored during the procedure. The pressure within the atrium, ventricles and the pulmonary artery are measured. Contrast is injected into the right side of the heart and the X-ray pictures are taken to depict the right side of the heart and the pulmonary vessels.

Left Sided Cardiac Catheterization

The catheter is passed retrograde from brachial or femoral artery into the aorta into the left side of the heart. Once the catheter is positioned, the left side of the heart can be studied by means of pressure readings, blood studies, contrast injection and X-ray films. Coronary and aorto-arteriography are done in conjunction with left sided cardiac catheterization.

Pressure and Oxygen Concentration in Great Vessels and Chambers of Heart

See **Figures 45.22 and 45.23**

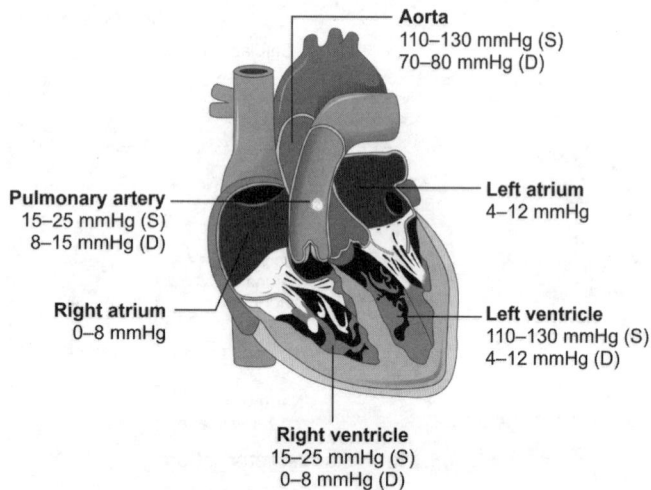

Fig. 45.22: Pressure in great vessels and chambers of heart.

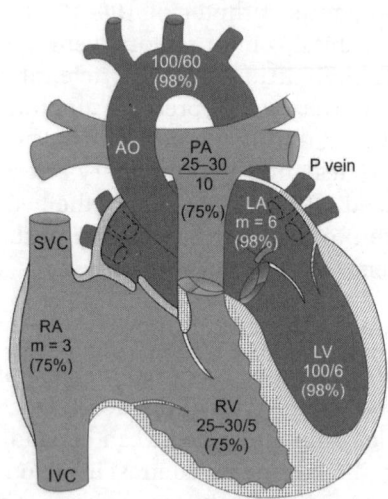

Fig. 45.23: Oxygen concentration of great vessels and chambers of heart.

Parameters of Heart and its Associated Conditions

See **Table 45.5.**

Table 45.5: Parameters of heart and its associated conditions.

Parameters	Associated conditions
↑ Pressure in chambers	Stenosed valves
↑ Ventricular end diastolic pressure	Ventricular failure
↑ Oxygen content of blood in the right side of heart	Septal defects
↑ Pulmonary artery pressure	Septal defects, chronic lung diseases
↑ Pulmonary wedge pressure	Congestive heart failure, mitral stenosis
↑ Left ventricular pressure	Aortic stenosis
↑ Left ventricular end diastolic pressure	Aortic insufficiency, mitral insufficiency, constrictive pericarditis, congestive heart failure
↓ Aortic pressure	Aortic insufficiency

Nursing Responsibilities

Before the Procedure
- Explain the procedure to the patient.
- Written and informed consent.
- NPO status for 6–8 hours.
- Prophylactic antibiotics.
- Check for allergies.
- Premedication as prescribed.
- Record the vital signs.
- Mark the site of the peripheral pulses.
- Arrange articles for immediate resuscitation in case of any emergency.
- Local preparation as for a surgical procedure.
- Arrange for continuous cardiac monitoring during the entire procedure.
- Watch for the early signs of complications such as cardiac dysrhythmias, pulmonary embolism, myocardial infarction, pneumothorax, anaphylactic shock, pericardial tamponade etc.

After the Procedure
- Complete bed rest for 12–24 hours.
- Application of pressure on the site to prevent bleeding or hematoma formation, 5 minutes in venous puncture and 10–15 minutes in case of arterial puncture.
- Continuous cardiac monitoring until the vital signs are stabilized.
- Assess for skin color and peripheral pulses.
- Keep the affected extremity straight to prevent clot formation in the vessel.

ELECTROPHYSIOLOGIC TESTING (EPS)

Electrophysiologic studies is an invasive method of recording intracardiac electrical activity **(Fig. 45.24)**. It is used in diagnosis and management of serious dysrhythmias.

Procedure

An electrophysiologic catheter has four electrodes at the distal tip to record or stimulate. it is introduced into the heart under fluoroscopy via the femoral, basilic, or subclavian vein. The selection of catheter sites depends on the purpose of examination (e.g., it can be placed at bundle of His, right atrium, coronary sinus, or right ventricle).

The procedure is designed to initiate dysrhythmias so that the origin may be isolated. Antiarrhythmic drugs may be administered during the study to evaluate their effect. When irritable focus has been identified, an ablation may be performed using radiofrequency, direct current, ethyl alcohol or cryosurgery. Radio-frequency ablation is more popular because its effect may be localized, with less damage to surrounding tissue.

The nursing responsibilities of electrophysiologic studies are similar to cardiac catheterization.

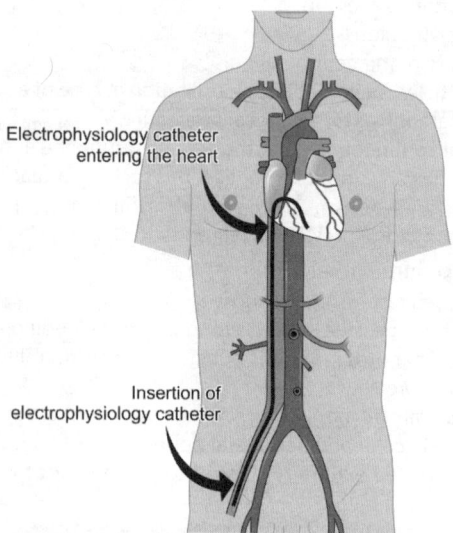

Fig. 45.24: Electrophysiology study.

GASTROINTESTINAL (GI) SYSTEM

UPPER GI ENDOSCOPY

Endoscopy of the upper GI tract allows direct visualization of the esophageal, gastric, and duodenal mucosa through a lighted endoscope (gastroscope) **(Fig. 45.25)**.

Nursing Responsibilities

- **Patient preparation:** Nurses should ensure that the patient is well-informed and prepared for the procedure. This may include providing preprocedure instructions, explaining the procedure, answering any questions that the patient may have and maintaining the NPO status.
- **Monitoring vital signs:** Nurses should closely monitor the patient's vital signs throughout the procedure and be prepared to act if there are any significant changes.
- **Administration of medications:** Nurses may be responsible for administering medications and sedation during the procedure, as directed by the physician or endoscopist. They should be familiar with the effects and side effects of these drugs and be prepared to intervene if necessary.
- **Maintaining sterile technique:** Nurses should ensure that sterile techniques are followed throughout the procedure to prevent infection.
- **Documentation:** Nurses should accurately document the patient's medical history, procedure-related information, and any complications that may arise during the procedure.

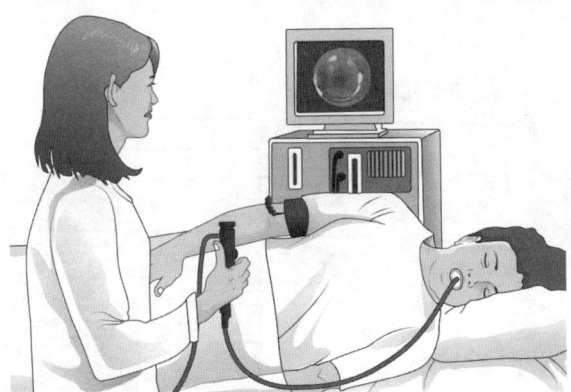

Fig. 45.25: Upper GI endoscopy procedure.

- **Patient education:** Nurses should provide the patient with instructions on postprocedure care, including any necessary dietary restrictions or medications.

Note

- Give a mouth wash to the patient after the treatment, if desired.
- Maintain NPO status for at least 1 to 2 hours postprocedure as the throat is anesthetized.
- Observe the patient for signs of bleeding from the stomach, or any other symptom.

LOWER GI ENDOSCOPY

Lower GI endoscopy is the direct visualization of the bowel through a proctoscope, sigmoidoscope, or colonoscope. It is often termed as colon endoscopy **(Fig. 45.26)**. This procedure is used when a client has a history of constipation, diarrhea, lower GI bleeding, or a strong family history of rectal or colon cancer.

Colonic endoscopy is useful in diagnosing cancer, strictures, polyps, and ulcerative or inflammatory bowel lesions. Colon endoscopy is contraindicated in patient with inflammatory bowel disease. Toxic megacolon, or strictures.

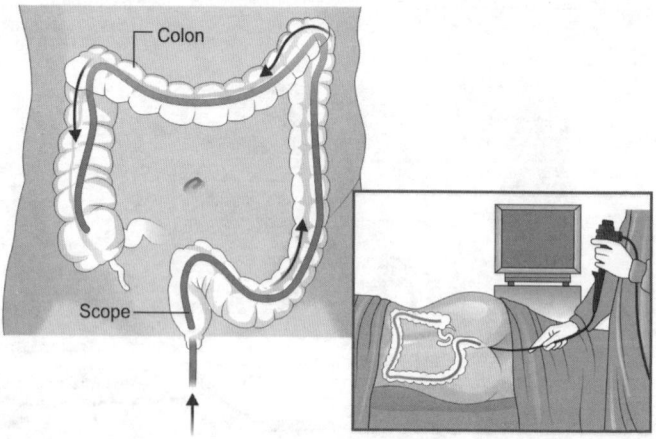

Fig. 45.26: Lower GI endoscopy procedure.

Nursing Responsibilities

- **Patient preparation:** Nurses should ensure that the patient understands the procedure and is adequately prepared for it. This may involve providing instructions on bowel preparation and fasting requirements.
- **Monitoring vital signs:** Nurses should monitor the patient's vital signs, including blood pressure, heart rate, and oxygen saturation, throughout the procedure.
- **Administration of medications:** Nurses may be responsible for administering medications, including sedatives and pain relievers, as directed by the physician or endoscopist.
- **Assisting with the procedure:** Nurses may assist the physician or endoscopist during the procedure by positioning the patient, providing suction, and adjusting the endoscope.
- **Maintaining sterile technique:** Nurses should ensure that sterile technique is maintained throughout the procedure to prevent infection.
- **Documenting the procedure:** Nurses should accurately document the procedure, including the findings and any complications that may arise.
- **Providing postprocedure care:** Nurses should provide the patient with instructions on postprocedure care, including any necessary dietary restrictions or medications.

BARIUM SWALLOW AND MEAL

Barium swallow and meal refers to providing the barium sulphate emulsion through the mouth followed by an X-ray examination.

Barium swallow: When the investigations are done in relation to the esophagus (**Figs. 45.27 and 45.28**).

Barium meal: When the investigations are done in relation to the stomach or the intestines.

Barium sulphate is a radio-opaque substance which given in the form of an emulsion. Generally, 10 ozs. of barium sulphate is dissolved in 12 ozs. of plain water. As the barium sulphate passes through it forms a coating on the lumen of the organ that to be examined.

Nursing Responsibilities

- Assess the patient's medical history and previous experiences with barium swallow and meal procedures.
- Explain the procedure to the patient and answer any questions they may have.

- Ensure the NPO status of the patient before the procedure.
- Check that the patient has removed any metal objects such as jewelry, dentures, or eyeglasses, as these can interfere with the imaging.

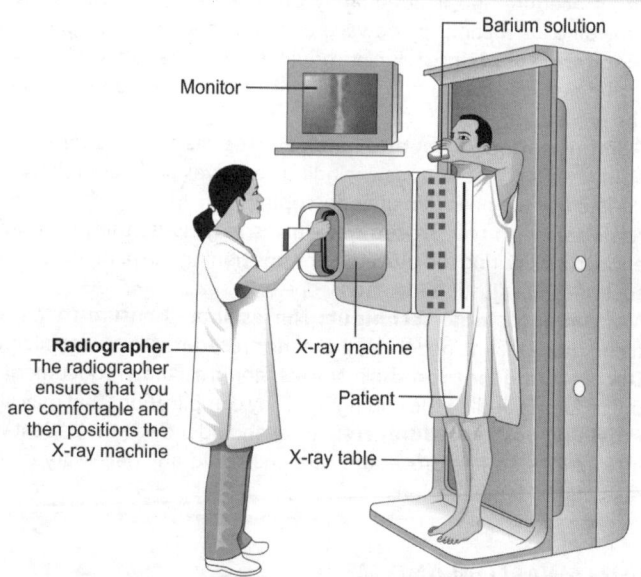

Fig. 45.27: Barium swallow procedure.

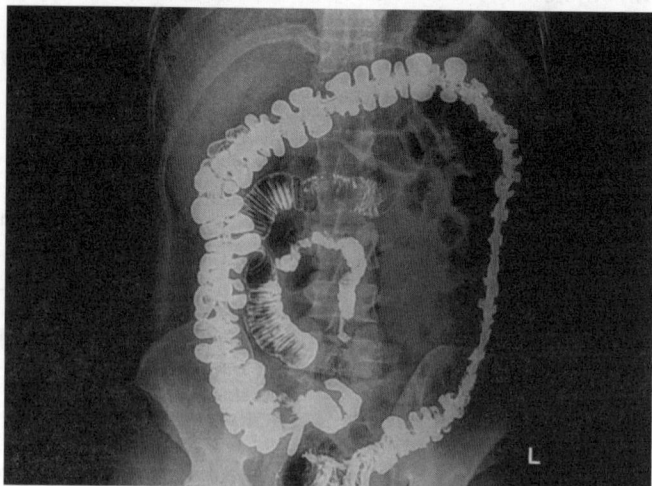

Fig. 45.28: Imaging in barium studies.

- Assist the radiologist or physician in positioning the patient correctly for the procedure.
- Monitor the patient's vital signs throughout the procedure.
- Observe the patient for any adverse reactions or side effects, such as nausea, vomiting, or allergic reaction.
- Make sure that the patient stays hydrated after the procedure and monitor for any signs of dehydration or other complications.
- Document the procedure and any relevant information in the patient's medical records.

BARIUM ENEMA

Barium enema is performed to visualize the position, movements, and filling of the colon **(Fig. 45.29)**. It can aid in the detection of tumors, diverticuli, stenosis, obstructions, inflammation, ulcerative colitis, and polyps.

In this investigation, a radiopaque contrast (i.e., barium is instilled via rectal catheter and radiographs are taken), with or without fluoroscopy **(Fig. 45.30)**.

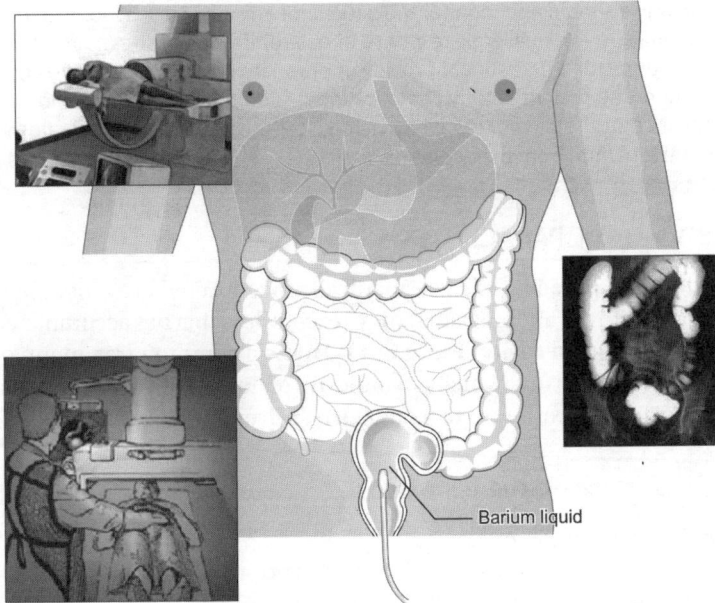

Fig. 45.29: Barium enema procedure.

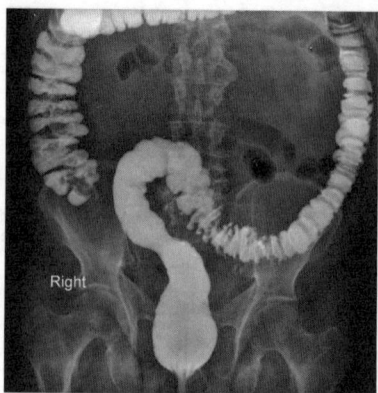

Fig. 45.30: Imaging in barium enema.

Nursing Responsibilities

During a barium meal, the nurse plays an important role in preparing the patient for the procedure, explaining the procedure to the patient, and ensuring that the patient is comfortable and calm during the procedure. The nurse should also monitor the patient for any adverse reactions to the barium, such as an allergic response or gastrointestinal distress. After the procedure, the nurse should provide appropriate postprocedure care and monitor the patient for any complications. Additionally, the nurse should ensure that the patient is well-hydrated after the procedure to help flush out the barium from their system.

ABDOMINAL PARACENTESIS

Abdominal paracentesis is a medical procedure where a needle is inserted into the abdomen to remove excess fluid that has accumulated in the peritoneal cavity **(Fig. 45.31)**. This is a common treatment for patients with ascites, which is a build-up of fluid in the abdomen that can occur for a variety of reasons, such as liver failure or cancer.

Nursing Responsibilities

Before the Procedure
- The nurse should ensure that the patient's consent has been obtained.
- Explain the procedure to the patient.

Assisting in Diagnostic Procedures

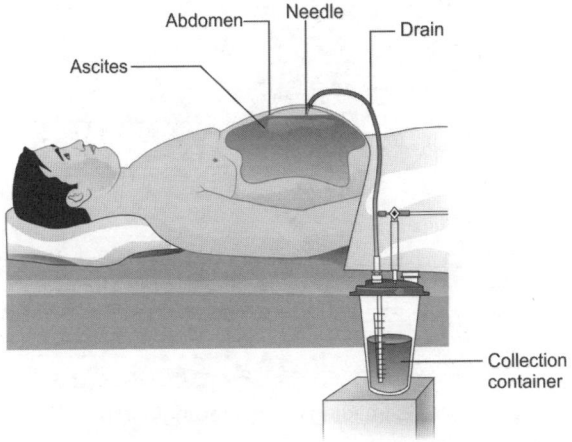

Fig. 45.31: Abdominal paracentesis procedure.

- Assess the patient's vital signs and check the abdomen for any signs of tenderness or distension.

During the Procedure
- Assist the physician or other healthcare provider by positioning the patient correctly and providing any necessary equipment or supplies.
- Monitor the patient's vital signs and keep the patient calm and comfortable.

After the Procedure
- Monitor the patient closely for any signs of complications, such as bleeding, infection, or changes in vital signs.
- Document the procedure and the patient's response to it and provide any necessary follow-up care or instructions.

NEUROLOGICAL SYSTEM

CEREBRAL ANGIOGRAPHY

It is an X-ray study of the cerebral circulation with a contrast agent injected into a selected artery. This procedure is used in investigating vascular disease or anomalies, to determine vessel patency, and identify the presence of collateral circulation **(Fig. 45.32)**.

It is performed by inserting a catheter via femoral artery in the groin and up to the desired vessel. Alternatively, direct puncture of the carotid artery or retrograde injection of a contrast agent into the

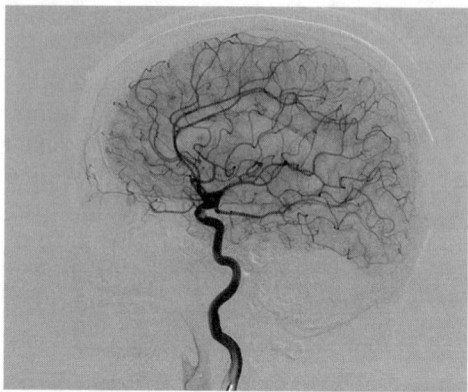

Fig. 45.32: Imaging in cerebral angiography.

brachial artery may be performed. X-ray images are obtained as the contrast agent flows through the vessels; the carotid and vertebral arterial systems are visualized, as well as venous drainage.

 Nursing Responsibilities

Before the Procedure
- The patient's blood urea nitrogen (BUN) and creatinine should be checked.
- The patient should be well hydrated, and clear liquids are usually permitted up to the time of the test.
- The patient is instructed to void immediately before the test, and locations of the appropriate peripheral pulses are marked with a felt-tip pen.

During the Procedure
- The patient is instructed to remain immobile during the angiogram process and is told to expect a brief feeling of warmth in the face, behind the eyes, or in the jaw, teeth, tongue, and lips, and a metallic taste when the contrast agent is injected.
- After the groin is shaved and prepared, a local anesthetic agent is administered to minimize pain at the insertion site and to reduce arterial spasm.
- A catheter is introduced into the femoral artery, flushed with heparinized saline, and filled with contrast agent. t
- Fluoroscopy is used to guide the catheter to the appropriate vessels.
- Neurologic assessment is conducted during and immediately following cerebral angiography to observe for embolism or arterial dissection that may occur during the test.

After the Procedure
- Observe the injection site for bleeding or hematoma formation.
- Assess the color and temperature of the involved extremity to detect possible embolism.

MYELOGRAPHY

It is an X-ray of the spinal subarachnoid space taken after the injection of a contrast agent into the spinal subarachnoid space through a lumbar puncture **(Fig. 45.33)**.

The water-based contrast agent disperses upward through the CSF to outline the spinal subarachnoid space and show any distortion of the spinal cord which can be caused by tumors, cysts, herniated vertebral disks, or other lesions. It is not performed commonly because of the sensitivity of CT and MRI scanning.

Nursing Responsibilities
- Written and informed consent.
- Explain the procedure to the patient.
- Prepare the skin for lumber puncture and assist the physician during the procedure.
- Seal the wound with Tr. Benzoin and apply sterile dress.

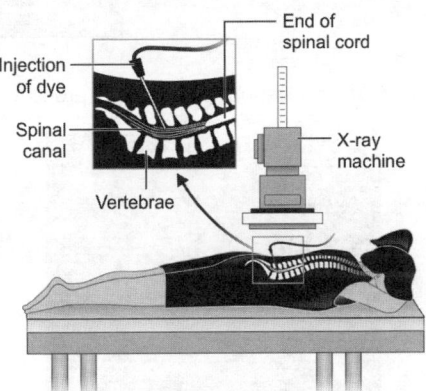

A myelogram requires the injection of dye into the spinal canal under X-ray guidance. The dye is usually injected in the lower back region (lumbar) and in some cases, in the neck (cervical) area.

Fig. 45.33: Myelography procedure.

- Make the patient comfortable on the bed.
- Document the procedure, time, date, and reaction of patient.
- Monitor vital signs.
- Evaluate the patient for signs of meningeal irritation.

RENAL SYSTEM

INTRAVENOUS PYELOGRAPHY

Intravenous pyelography (IVP) **(Figs. 45.34 and 45.35)** is a diagnostic imaging test that uses a contrast dye to visualize the urinary tract

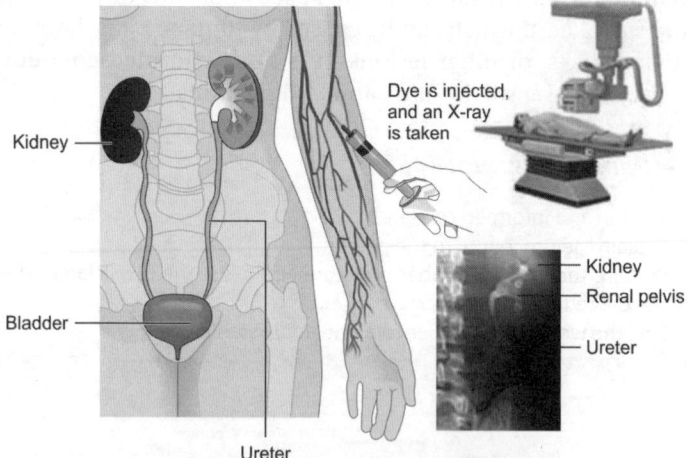

Fig. 45.34: Intravenous pyelography procedure.

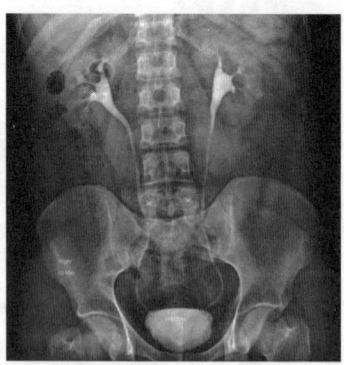

Fig. 45.35: Imaging in IVP.

system. It is used as the initial assessment of many suspected urologic conditions, especially lesions in the kidneys and ureters. It also provides an approximate estimate of renal function.

Nursing Responsibilities

Before the Procedure
- Written and informed consent.
- Explain the procedure to the patient.
- Assess the patient's medical history, allergies, and current medications to ensure that the contrast dye will not cause an adverse reaction.

During the Procedure
- Monitor the vital signs and keep the patient comfortable.
- Maintain the hydration status of the patient.

After the Procedure
- Observe the patient for any adverse reactions to the contrast dye, such as an allergic reaction or kidney damage.
- Encourage the patient to drink plenty of fluids to help flush the contrast dye out of their system.

CHAPTER 46

Family Planning-Contraception

INTRODUCTION

National programme for family planning was launched in 1952. The program has expanded to all areas of India and has penetrated the primary health centers and sub centers in rural areas, urban family welfare centers and postpartum centers in the urban areas. Family planning emerged as one of the interventions to reduce maternal and infant mortalities and morbidities, it is confirmed that area where there is easy availability of contraceptives have lower maternal and infant mortalities.

DEFINITION

Family Planning

According to World Health Organization (WHO), family planning is defined as "the ability of individuals and couples to anticipate and attain their desired number of children and the spacing and timing of their births".

Contraception

Contraception means the method used by male or female partner to prevent conception or pregnancy.

CONTRACEPTIVE METHODS (FERTILITY REGULATING METHODS) (FLOWCHART 46.1)

Spacing Methods

Barrier Methods

- ❖ **Physical methods**
  - ♦ **Diaphragm:** Diaphragm is also known as a "Dutch cap", invented by a German physician in 1882. The diaphragm is a shallow cup made up of synthetic rubber, silicon or plastic material that acts as a barrier for entry of sperm into the uterus.

Flowchart 46.1: Contraceptive methods.

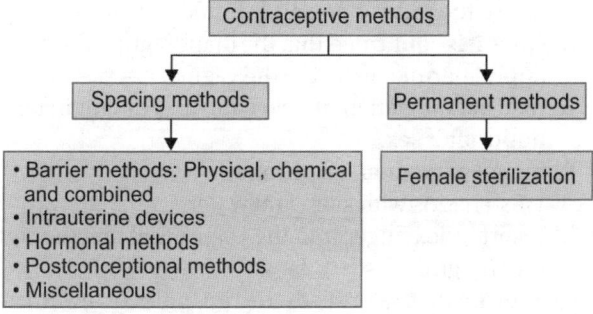

The vaginal diaphragm is inserted before sexual intercourse and comes in different size ranging in diameter from 5–10 cm (2–4 inches), it is 92–96% effective if used correctly with spermicide (foam, cream, gel, or suppository) but it doesn't prevent from transmission of STD's.

- **Insertion of vaginal diaphragm (Fig. 46.1)**
  - Wash hands with soap and water.
  - Apply spermicide inside the rim of the diaphragm.
  - Ask patient to lie on her back, squatting or standing with one leg propped on a chair or counter.
  - Using one hand part the inner labia to access the vaginal opening, holding the diaphragm with the other hand.
  - Insert the diaphragm gently by compressing the sides so that it fits into the vaginal opening. Push the diaphragm as far back as it will go.
  - After insertion of diaphragm into the vagina, use index (pointer) finger to nudge the rim so that it covers the

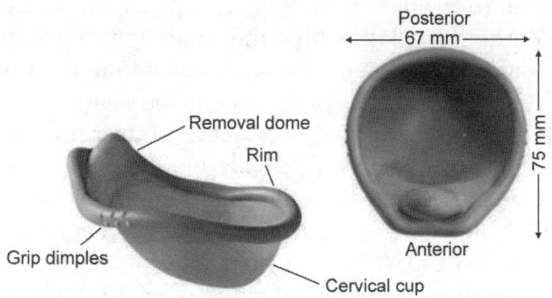

Fig. 46.1: Vaginal diaphragm.

cervix. A properly positioned diaphragm should fit snugly above the pubic bone and should not cause irritation.
- Once it is confirmed that the diaphragm is fitted properly, apply spermicide inside the vagina.
- Instruct the patient to leave the diaphragm in place for 6 hours after sex.

- **Removal of vaginal diaphragm**
  - Wash hands with soap and water.
  - Insert index finger into the vagina and feel the rim of the diaphragm.
  - Slide finger underneath the rim, pull downward and out.
  - Wash the diaphragm using soap and water and air dry it.
  - Replace the diaphragm in its container and store in a cool and dry place.

- **Condoms:** These are also called sheaths or French leather. Condoms is the most widely used barrier methods of contraception, made out of thin rubber. "NIRODH" is the trade name used in India for condom. This is worn over penis before intercourse as it prevents the semen from depositing into the vagina and prevent the transmission of sexually transmitted diseases (STD). There are two varieties—disposable and washable.
  - **Application of male condom (Fig 46.2)**
    - Open the condom package carefully.
    - Ensure that the condom is not damaged.
    - Before intercourse, fit the condom on the erect penis.
    - Expelled the air from the condom by pinching the teat end.
    - Using one hand hold the condom over the tip of the penis, unroll it down to the base of the penis with the other hand.
    - After ejaculation hold the condom firmly and carefully around the penis and withdraw it from the vagina. This prevents spillage of semen into the vagina.
    - **Advantage of male condom:** It is easy to use, reliable, light compact, easily disposable and no side effects.
    - **Disadvantages of male condom:** Failure rate is 2–12 per cent mainly due to rupture of condom and carelessness. It may slip by incorrect use. Some people feel that it does not provide natural feeling during intercourse being barrier between vaginal mucosa and penis.

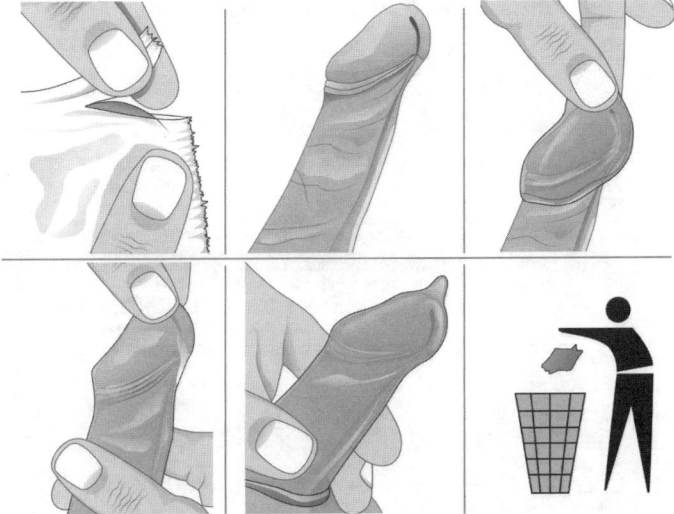

Fig. 46.2: Insertion of male condom.

- **Application of female condom:** Female condom is a pouch which lines the vagina with a ring and is made up of polyurethane. It has internal ring and external ring. The internal ring covers the cervix and the external ring remains outside the vagina. *See* **Figure 46.3** for steps of insertion of female condom.
- **Vaginal sponge (Fig. 46.4):** In the USA vaginal sponge is commercially available under the trade name TODAY.
  - Sponges used for birth control purposes are small polyurethane foam measuring 5 cm × 2.5 cm saturated with spermicide nonoxynol-9.
  - Vaginal sponge can be inserted into the vagina 24 hours before intercourse.
  - During insertion of vaginal sponge ensure that it covers the cervix by pushing it as far back as possible into the vagina.
  - Instruct the patient to leave the vaginal sponge in place for 6–8 hours after intercourse.
- **Chemical methods (Fig. 46.5):** Chemical agents are certainly helpful but not reliable on their own. They can form a very important second line of defense. Hence, they should only be used in conjunction with other contraceptive methods. Certain chemicals when introduced into the vaginal passage rapidly kill or

How to insert and remove a female condom

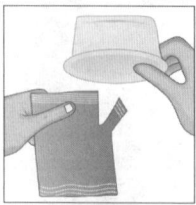

Carefully open and remove condom from package to prevent tearing

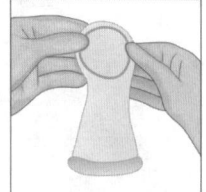

The thick, inner ring with closed end is used for placing in the vagina and holds condom in place. The thin, outer ring remains outside of body, covering vaginal opening

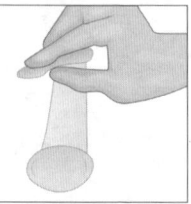

Find a comfortable position. While holding outside of condom at closed end, squeeze sides of inner ring together with your thumb and forefinger and insert into vagina.
It is similar to inserting a tampon

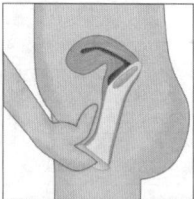

Using your finger, push inner ring as far up as it will go - until it rests against cervix. The condom will expand naturally and you may not feel it

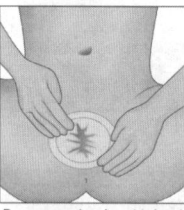

Be sure condom is not twisted. The thin, outer ring should remain outside vagina

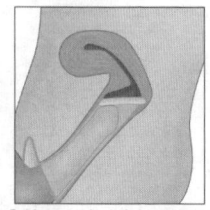

Guide partner's penis into opening of condom. Stop intercourse if you feel penis slip between condom and walls of vagina or if outer ring is pushed into vagina

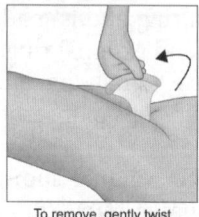

To remove, gently twist outer ring and pull condom out of vagina

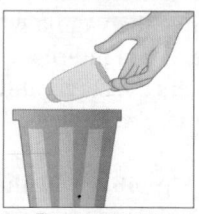

Throw away condom is trash after using it one time. Do not reuse

Fig. 46.3: Insertion and removal of female condom.

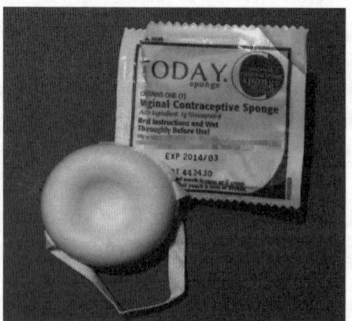

Fig. 46.4: Vaginal sponge.

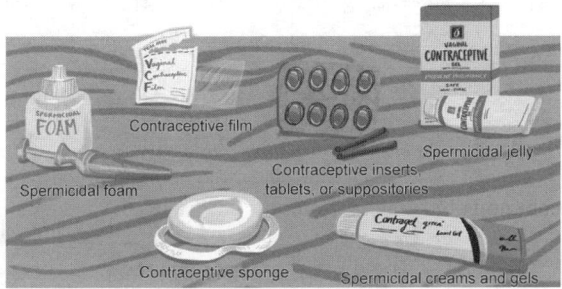

Fig. 46.5: Various types of chemical methods of contraceptives.

paralyze sperms. Sperms are also easily destroyed by the weakest chemicals—in fact plain water can immobilize them in a matter of seconds. The most commonly used modern spermicides are "surface-active agents" which attach themselves to spermatozoa and inhibit oxygen uptake and kill sperms.

- Chemical foams comprises of four categories:
  - *Foams:* Foam tablets, foam aerosols.
  - *Creams, jellies and pastes*: Squeezed from a tube.
  - *Suppositories:* Inserted manually.
  - *Soluble films–C:* Film inserted manually.

Intrauterine Contraceptive Device (IUCD)

These are small plastic devices which are introduced into uterine cavity by means of a special applicator. Still by mechanical intervention and metallic touch of copper, the uterine environment is changed to prevent implantation of ovum thus serving as a contraceptive device. IUCD's are devices made up of polyethylene or other polymers, and there are two basic types:
1. **Nonmedicated:** First generation IUDs. Lippes loop is most commonly used.
2. **Medicated:** Release metal ions (copper) also called second generation IUDs or hormones (progestogens) also called third generation IUDs.

Lippes Loop (First-Generation)

Lippes loop is made up of flexible plastic called polyethylene in the shape of double "S". It is available in four different size and color A, B, C, D, where A being the smallest and D the largest **(Figs. 46.6A to D)**. A plastic tail or thread is attached to the lower end of the loop

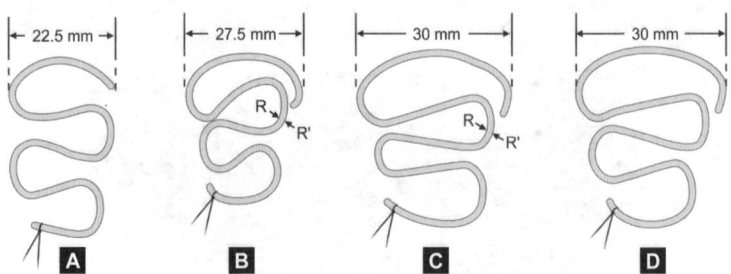

Figs. 46.6A to D: Types of Lippes loop.

to facilitate removal and identification of correct placement of the loop. The larger size has greater antifertility effect, size C and D are recommended for multiparous women.

Insertion of Lippes Loop

For sterilization purposes a loop should not be boiled or autoclaved. It is sterilized chemically by keeping in 1/1,000 Savlon solution or 1/2,500 aqueous solution of iodine for 20 minutes. It should be kept in the solution only for the duration required for sterilization.

- The patient is put on table/bed in supine position with thighs flexed and knees bend and separated.
- The cervix is prepared by swabbing with an antiseptic lotion. Dilatation of the cervix is not necessary.
- The loop is threaded into the applicator by means of forceps. It straightens when it is threaded into the tube of the plastic applicator.
- A Sim's speculum is introduced and cervix is visualized.
- The anterior lip of cervix can be held by means of an ovum forceps or vulsellum.
- The applicator is then introduced into the cervical canal after which the plunger of the applicator pushes the loop gently into the uterine cavity where it resumes its characteristic shape.

Copper Releasing IUD (Second-Generation)

There are different types of second-generation IUDs. The numbers included in the names of the devices refer to the surface area (in sq.mm) of the copper on the device. The newer devices are more effective in preventing pregnancies as compare to the older ones. The newer multiload devices have an affective life of at least 5 years. Cooper releasing intrauterine device includes **(Fig. 46.7)**:

Family Planning-Contraception

Earlier devices	Newer devices

• Cooper -7
• Copper T-200
	• Variants of the T device
	  ➢ CuT 220C
	  ➢ CuT380A or Ag
	• Nova T
	• Multiload devices
	  ➢ ML Cu 250
	  ➢ ML Cu 375

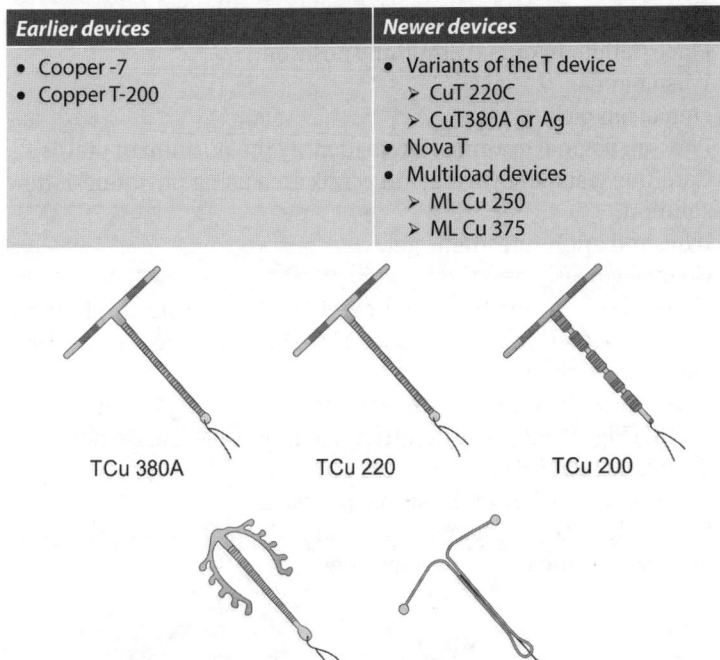

Fig. 46.7: Types of copper releasing IUD.

Insertion of Copper T 380A

Articles required

- Clean gloves
- Sterile gloves
- Cervical tenaculum
- Cotton balls soaked in antiseptic solution or povidone-iodine
- Long suture scissors
- Ring forceps
- Sterile and nonsterile examination gloves
- Sterile IUD package with IUD
- Sterile tray for the procedure
- Sterile vaginal speculum
- Uterine sound

Steps of procedure

- Identify the patient.
- Confirm negative pregnancy test.

- ❖ Obtained informed consent.
- ❖ Place patient in dorsal lithotomy position.
- ❖ Wash hands.
- ❖ Don clean gloves.
- ❖ Perform vaginal examination to identify the position of uterus.
- ❖ Carefully clean the vagina and cervix area using povidone-iodine solution.
- ❖ If desired apply anesthetic gel.
- ❖ Change gloves.
- ❖ Grasp the anterior lip of the cervix with a sterile single tooth tenaculum and apply gentle traction to straighten the cervical canal and uterine chamber.
- ❖ Determine the depth of the uterine cavity using sterile uterine sound **(Fig. 46.8A)**. The depth should be 6 cm–9 cm. Do not insert if depth is below 6 cm.
- ❖ Remove the IUD from the sterile package.
- ❖ Ensure that the blue flange is aligned with the IUD arms and set at the distance the uterus was sounded.

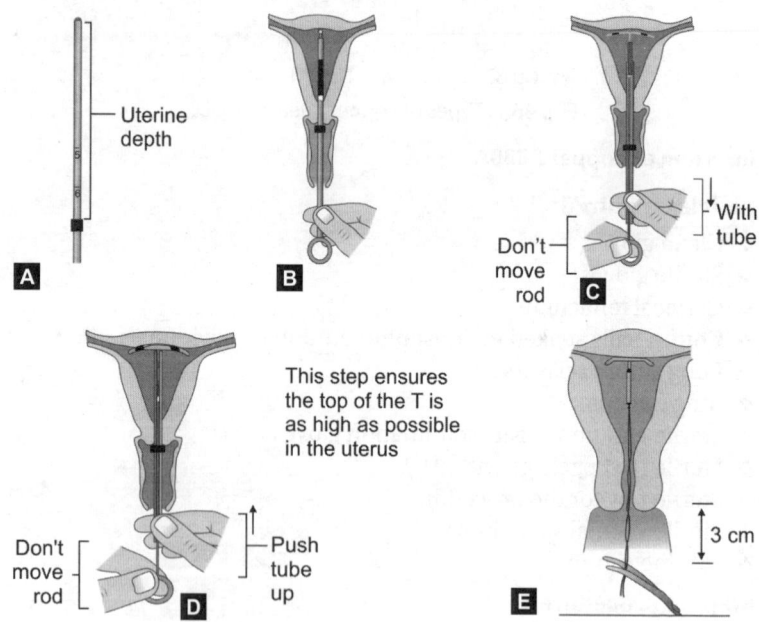

Figs. 46.8A to E: Insertion of copper releasing IUD.

- Gently place the loaded inserter tube through the cervical canal **(Fig. 46.8B)**. Ensure that the blue depth gauge is in horizontal position.
- Continue the insertion of the IUD into the uterus until the flange is against the cervical OS.
- With one hand hold the tenaculum and white rod, with the other hand withdraw the inserter tube until it touches the thumb grip of the white rod **(Fig. 46.8C)**.
- After this, the arms of the TCu 380A will be released high in the uterine fundus **(Fig. 46.8D)**.
- Gently push the inserter tube upward, towards the top of the uterus until a slight resistance is felt. This means that the arms of the T are as high as possible in the uterus.
- Hold the inserter tube and remove the white rod.
- Then, gently and slowly withdraw the inserter tube from the cervical canal.
- The thread will emerge from the cervical OS, cut the thread to a length of 3 cm **(Fig. 46.8E)**.
- Remove the tenaculum. If the cervix is bleeding from the tenaculum site, press a swab to the site, using clean forceps, until the bleeding stop.
- Gently and slowly remove the speculum and put all of the instruments used in 0.5% chlorine solution for 10 minutes for decontamination.
- Record the procedure and note length of the thread in the vagina.

Insertion of Hormone Releasing IUD (Third-Generation IUD)

Third-generation IUD release hormones that makes the uterus unsuitable for survival of sperms and implantation of embryo. Some of the second-generation IUD includes Progestasert, LNG-20 etc.

Articles required

Same as copper releasing hormone.

Steps of procedure

- Arrange all materials required.
- Identify the patient.
- Wash hands.
- Don clean gloves and perform bimanual vaginal examination.
- Carefully clean the vagina and cervix area using povidone-iodine solution.

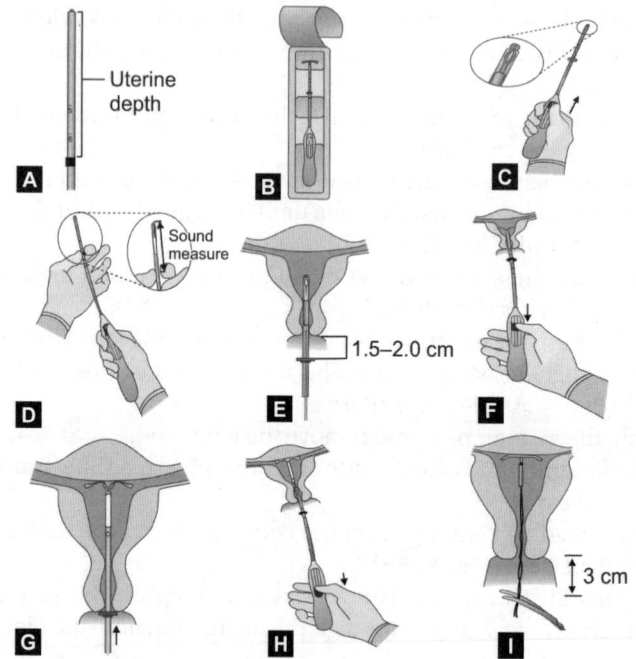

Figs. 46.9A to I: Insertion of levonorgestrel intrauterine device.

- If desired apply anesthetic gel.
- Determine the depth of the uterine cavity using sterile uterine sound **(Fig. 46.9A)**. The depth should be 6 cm–9 cm. Do not insert if depth is below 6 cm.
- Open the sterile IUD package **(Fig. 46.9B)** and put on sterile gloves.
- Move the slider in forward position by giving forward pressure with the thumb or forefinger on the slider **(Fig. 46.9C)**.
- Set the flange's upper edge to the uterine depth (in centimeters) measured during sounding **(Fig. 46.9D)**.
- The loaded insertion tube should be advanced through the cervical canal until the upper edge of the flange is 1.5–2.0 cm from the cervical OS **(Fig. 46.9E)**.
- To release the LNG IUD arms, move the slider down to the mark. Allow 10 seconds for the horizontal arms to fully open **(Fig. 46.9F)**.

Family Planning-Contraception

- Gently move the inserter towards the uterine fundus until the flange hits the cervix **(Fig. 46.9G)**.
- Holding the inserter firmly in position, move the slider all the way down to release the LNG-IUD. Then withdraw the inserter from the uterus **(Fig. 46.9H)**.
- The thread will emerge from the cervical OS, cut the thread to a length of 3 cm **(Fig. 46.9I)**.
- Record the procedure and note length of the thread in the vagina.

Hormonal Contraceptives

Hormonal contraceptives contains estrogen and progesterone, or progesterone only and act on the endocrine system. Hormonal contraceptive works by blocking the release of eggs from the ovaries and prevent sperm from reaching the eggs.

Classification

- **Oral pills**
  - **Combined pills:** Combine pill contain 30–35 mcg of synthetic estrogen and 0.5 to 1.0 mg of progestogen. Combined pill must be taken for 21 consecutive days staring from the 5th day of the menstrual cycle, followed by a break of 7 days during which period menstruation occurs. The first day of the next cycle occurs when then the next bleeding starts. In India it is available under the brand name MALA-N and MALA-D **(Fig. 46.10A)**.
  - **Progesterone only pill (POP) (Fig. 46.10B):** This pill contains only progesterone and it is called as "minipill" or "micropill". The pill is taken in small doses throughout the cycle. Norethisterone and levonorgestrel are commonly used.
  - **Postcoital pill (Fig. 46.10C):** This pill is also called as "morning after" pill. The pill should be taken within 72 hours after unprotected sexual intercourse.
  - **Once-a-month (long-acting) pill (Fig. 46.10D):** Quinestrol, a long acting estrogen is given in combination with a short-acting progestogen. This is not recommended as the pregnancy rate is high.
  - **Male pill (Fig. 46.10E):** Male pill is made up of gossypol which is a derivatives of cotton-seed oil. It works by producing azoospermia or severe oligospermia. The side effects of this pill

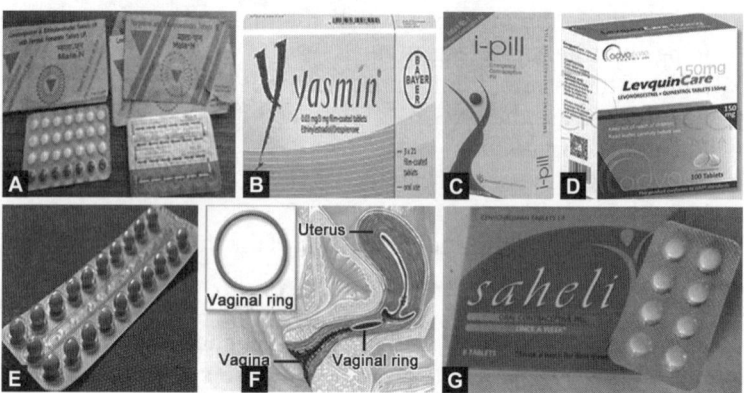

Figs. 46.10A to G: Different types of hormonal contraceptives.

is that it can cause permanent azoospermia after taking it for 6 months.

- ❖ **Depot (slow release) formulations**
  - ♦ **Injectables:** Injectables contraceptives are of two types:
    - Progesterone only injectables
    - Once a month combined injectables
  - ♦ **Subcutaneous implants:** This capsule contains progesterone. The capsule is implanted in subcutaneous tissue which slowly releases progesterone to produce contraceptive effect.
  - ♦ **Vaginal rings (Fig. 46.10F):** This is an approach of releasing progesterone to bloodstream at low level by inserting vaginal rings. The ring is introduced in vagina which slowly releases hormones. This is slowly absorbed by vaginal mucosa. The device can be inserted by the woman herself.
  - ♦ **Centchroman nonhormonal pill (Chhaya) (Fig. 46.10G):** This pill is commonly known as weekly pill. The pill is taken biweekly for the first three months and from fourth month onwards it is taken once weekly. It is available in the market as "Saheli" tablet.

Postconceptional Methods

Postconceptional methods includes:

- ❖ **Menstrual regulation:** In this, aspiration of uterine contents is done 6 to 14 days of a missed period before any other pregnancy can determine whether a woman is pregnant or not **(Fig. 46.11)**

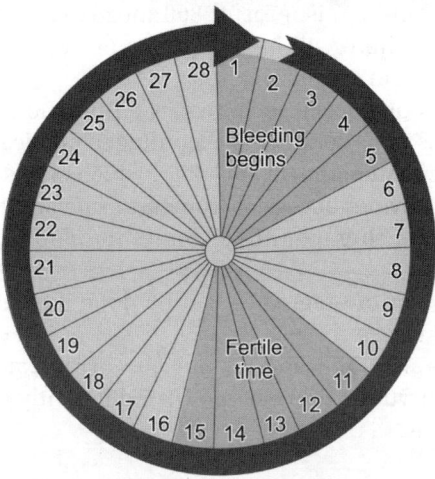

Fig. 46.11: Menstrual cycle regulation.

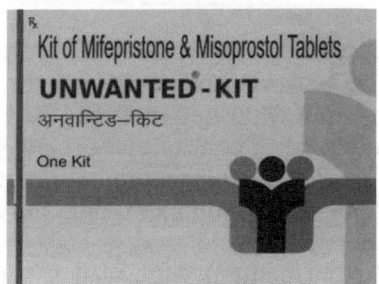

Fig. 46.12: MTP kit.

- **Menstrual induction:** This is done by intrauterine application of 1–5 mg solution (or 2.5–5 mg pellet) of prostaglandin F2 to disturb the normal progesterone-prostaglandin balance. The bleeding starts a few minutes after the application and continues for 7–8 days.
- **Oral abortifacient:** Oral abortifacient meaning "Oral pills which will cause a miscarriage". In this, two medications are used namely mifepristone and misoprostol. Commercially, it is available as MTP kit **(Fig. 46.12)** and has 95% success rate for terminating pregnancies.
  - Mifepristone 200 mg is taken orally on day 1. Mifepristone works by blocking the production of progesterone preventing the pregnancy from growing.

- After 48 hours, misoprostol 800 mcg is to be administered vaginally. There will be symptoms of heavy bleeding with cramping pain within 24 hours.
- **Abortion:** Abortion is also known as termination of pregnancy. Abortion has to be conducted according to Medical Termination of Pregnancy (Amendment) Bill, 2021 which includes:
  - The act provides access of women to safe and legal abortion services on therapeutic, eugenic, humanitarian or social grounds.
  - Termination of pregnancy can be done if gestational age is below 24 weeks.
  - The act is also applicable for survivors of rape, victims of incest and other vulnerable women (like differently abled women, minors) etc.

Miscellaneous

- **Abstinence:** Abstinence means avoiding sexual intercourse by both partners.
- **Coitus interruptus:** This is a method of interruption in coitus or intercourse. The penis is withdrawn before discharge of semen so that semen is not deposited in vagina. The method wholly depends on timing and control by husband as semen often leaks prior to discharge. This method also puts psychological strain on both partners leading to frustration and incomplete satisfaction.
- **Safe period (rhythm method):** The ovulation (coming out of ovum from ovary) occurs 14 days prior to menses. In a regular cycle of 28 days, ovulation will occur on 14th day. By giving a margin of 5 days on either side that is from 9th to 19th is considered as unsafe period when conception can occur, if intercourse is done. So the rest of the days of the month are considered safe period comparatively as there will be no ovum to fertilize.
- **Natural family planning methods:** In this three methods are used namely:
  1. Basal body temperature method (BBT)
  2. Cervical mucus method
  3. Symptothermal method
- **Birth control vaccine:** Immunization of women with vaccine prepared from beta sub-unit of human chorionic gonadotropin (hCG).

Permanent Methods

Vasectomy Male

It is commonly carried out through one incision or two. In vasectomy it is customary to remove a piece of the vas deferens at least 1 cm long after clamping. The current trend is to make vasectomy a reversible operation as far as possible, but there is no assurance of its success.

Following vasectomy, sperm production and hormone output from the testicular interstitial cells continue normally, but the sperms are destroyed intraluminally by phagocytosis. This is a normal process in the male genital tract. The rate of destruction is greatly increased after vasectomy.

Reversible Method

- **Vas clips:** Tantalum clips are applied without removing a segment of the vas deferens.
- **Intravasal thread:** Nonabsorbable suture material such as surgical black nylon are threaded into the vas for plugging the passage of the semen. For reversing the operation the vas is exposed and the thread is removed.
- **Vie plug:** Occlusion of the vas lumen with a variety of materials such as silicone gel, silicone rubber, etc. are under testing.
- **Vas valve:** A 'T' shaped micro-valve which could produce azoospermia in the 'off position and allow sperms through in the 'on' position is being tested.

Female Sterilization (Tubectomy)

Normally when a woman gets her first menstrual period, it indicates that the ovary has started producing the ova and these ova after maturing by about the 14th day, reach the ampulla of the uterine tube and wait for fertilization by the spermatozoa of the male. If somehow the ova do not reach the tubes to meet the spermatozoa, pregnancy cannot take place.

- In case of tubectomy, the operation takes place a few days after delivery.
- As per the abdominal route, the tube is ligated about an inch apart and the intervening segment of the tube is excised. The length of tube is 4 inches and breadth are 3 mm.
- The cut ends of the tubes are buried separately, to avoid the remote possibility of reunion of the divided ends of the tube and recanalization.

- The pre-eminance of the abdominal tubectomy has been recently challenged by the vaginal tubectomy operation.
- **Advantages:** Scar is not visible and early ambulation after a shorter hospital stay is possible.

The other types of instruments used are the laparoscope, inserted through the abdomen, the kaleidoscope, inserted through the vagina and the hysteroscope which is inserted through the uterine cavity.

Laparoscopic Application of Clip or Ring

This is a good technique followed for female sterilization.
- The method consists of blocking the fallopian tubes by applying an inert silicone clip or ring.
- The procedure is with an instrument called laparoscope.
- The instrument has a long body with lighting arrangement. It is introduced through a small incision below the umbilicus.
- Air is introduced for distension of abdominal organs and proper visibility.
- Then tubes are seen and one after and other the clip or ring is fixed to block the tubes and thus to stop entrance of ovum to uterine cavity.
- The procedure is carried by trained gynecologist under local or general anesthesia. It takes about 5-10 minutes. The patient need not to be kept hospitalized.

CHAPTER 47

Antenatal Care

INTRODUCTION

Antenatal care includes all management and supervision given to women during pregnancy to monitor the health of the mother and fetus. It is the initial step that provides care, prepare a birth plan and identify facility for delivery and referral in case of complications. There are certain complications that can arise during pregnancy such as pre-eclampsia, anemia etc., routine checkup during antenatal period helps in the identification of complication and early management.

DEFINITION

Antenatal care refers to the medical care and routine checkups that women receive during their pregnancy.

PURPOSES

- To maintain the health of mother during pregnancy.
- To identify high risk cases and complications.
- To prevent complications of pregnancy.
- To reduce maternal and infant mortality and morbidity rate.
- To educate the mother regarding family planning, hygiene, childcare, health and nutrition.
- To prepare the mother for delivery physically and mentally.

ARTICLES REQUIRED

- Fetoscope/stethoscope/Doppler machine.
- Measuring tape.
- BP apparatus, thermometer.
- Weighing machine.
- Bedside screen.

GENERAL ASSESSMENT

- ❖ Identify the patient.
- ❖ Collect history: Medical, surgical, obstetric and family.
- ❖ Assess vital signs.
- ❖ Assess height, weight, gestational age using Naegele's rule.
- ❖ Complete blood investigations and urine examination.
- ❖ Assess for general appearance.
- ❖ Conduct head to toe examination.

Abdominal Examination

Examination of the abdomen during pregnancy to monitor fetal growth and well-being. Abdominal examination includes:
- ❖ Measurement of fundal height.
- ❖ Determination of fetal lie and presentation by fundal palpation, lateral palpation and pelvic grips.
- ❖ Auscultation of FHS.
- ❖ Inspection of scars and any abnormal findings.

Steps of Procedure

- ❖ Explain the procedure to the patient.
- ❖ Ask the patient to empty her bladder.
- ❖ Put the bedside screen to maintain privacy.
- ❖ Wash hands.
- ❖ Instruct patient to lie on her back with upper part of the body supported by pillows, with hips and knees partially flexed.
- ❖ Expose her abdomen from below the breasts to the symphysis pubis.
- ❖ Stand on the right side of the patient to conduct systematic examination.
- ❖ Ensure that the hands are warm before conducting abdominal examination.
- ❖ Inspect the abdomen to identify any scars, diastasis recti, hernia, linea nigra, striae gravidarum, contour of the abdomen, state of umbilicus, skin condition.

Fundal Height Measurement

- ❖ Using the ulnar side of the palm determine the fundal height (**Fig. 47.1**).

Antenatal Care

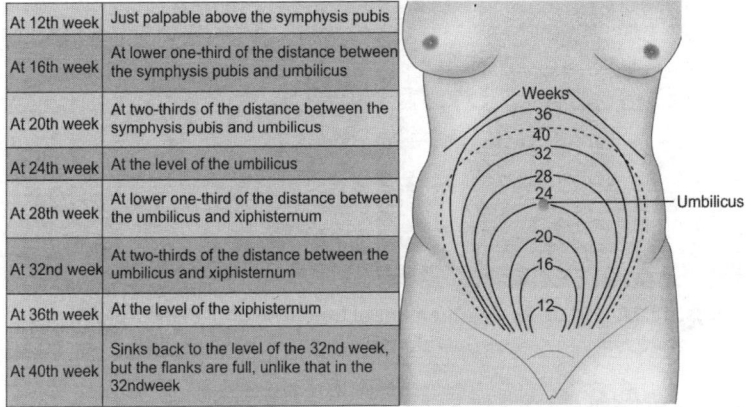

At 12th week	Just palpable above the symphysis pubis
At 16th week	At lower one-third of the distance between the symphysis pubis and umbilicus
At 20th week	At two-thirds of the distance between the symphysis pubis and umbilicus
At 24th week	At the level of the umbilicus
At 28th week	At lower one-third of the distance between the umbilicus and xiphisternum
At 32nd week	At two-thirds of the distance between the umbilicus and xiphisternum
At 36th week	At the level of the xiphisternum
At 40th week	Sinks back to the level of the 32nd week, but the flanks are full, unlike that in the 32nd week

Fig. 47.1: Fundal height at different gestational age.

- Measure the height of the fundus using a measuring tape from the superior border of the symphysis pubis extending across the contour of the abdomen to the top of the fundus along the midline **(Fig. 47.2A)**.
- Encircle the abdomen with a tape at the level of the umbilicus to measure abdominal girth **(Fig. 47.2B)**.
  - If measurement is 2 inches less than the weeks of gestation it is normal, but if it exceeds 100 cm/39 and half inches it is abnormal at any week of gestation.
  - The following conditions can be suspected if the height of the uterus is more or less than that indicated by the period of amenorrhea:

Height of the uterus more than that indicated by the period of amenorrhea	Height of the uterus less than that indicated by the period of amenorrhea
• Wrong date of LMP • Full bladder • Multiple pregnancy/large baby • Polyhydramnios • Hydrocephalus • Hydatidiform mole	• Wrong date of LMP • IUGR • Missed abortion intrauterine death (IUD) • Transverse lie

Fetal Lie and Presentation/Leopold's Maneuvers

- Instruct the woman to bend her knees slightly and perform relaxation breathing. This helps in relaxation of abdominal muscles.

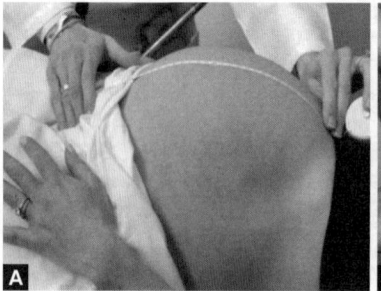
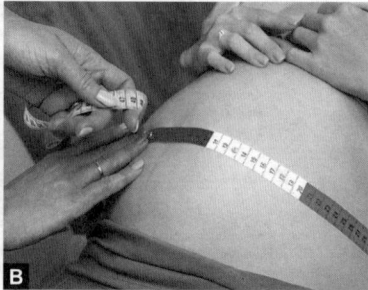

Figs. 47.2A and B: (A) Measurement of fundal height. (B) Measurement of abdominal girth.

- Use the palmer side of the fingers and apply smooth deep pressure as firm as necessary to perform abdominal palpation.
- Perform four pelvic grips (Leopold's maneuvers) as shown in **Box 47.1**.

Box 47.1: Abdominal palpation or Leopold's maneuvers.

A. First maneuvers/Fundal palpation:
- The palpation is done by facing the women's face.
- Place your hands on the fundus's sides and wrap your fingers over the top of the uterus.
- Palpate for size, shape, consistency, and mobility of the fetal part in the fundus.
  - *Head of the fetus:* A round, hard, movable part that is felt between the fingers of both hands.
  - *Breech presentation:* Irregular, bulkier, less firm and not well defined movable part.

First maneuver/Fundal palpation or fundal grip.

This maneuver helps determine the lie and presentation of the fetus

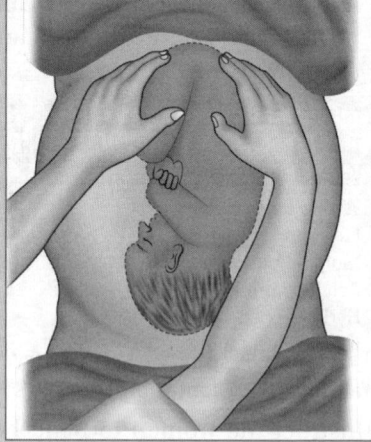

Contd...

Contd...

B. Second maneuver (lateral palpation):

- Place hands on both sides of the abdomen midway between the symphysis pubis and fundus.
- Apply pressure to the uterus with one hand, pushing the fetus to the opposite side and stabilizing it there.
- Using smooth pressure and rotatory movements, palpate the other side of the abdomen with the examining fingers from the midline to the lateral side and from the fundus.
- Repeat the same steps for examination of opposite side of the abdomen.
  - *Fetal back:* Smooth, firm convex, resistant mass extending from breech to neck.
  - *Fetal small parts:* Small irregular mass that moves when pressed or kick.

Second maneuver/lateral palpation/lateral grip

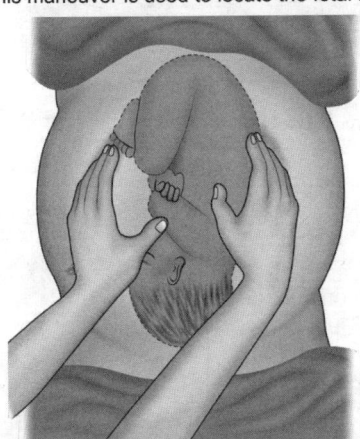

This maneuver is used to locate the fetal back

C. Third maneuver (Pawlik's grip)

- Using the thumb and middle finger grasp the area of the lower abdomen just above the symphysis pubis.
  - *Fetal head above the brim:* head will be easily movable.
  - *Engaged head:* Not easily movable.

Contd...

Contd...

Third maneuver/First pelvic grip or superficial pelvic grip

The third maneuver must be performed gently. It helps to determine whether the head or the breech is present at the pelvic brim. If the head cannot be moved, it indicates that the head is engaged.
In the case of a transverse lie, the third grip will be empty

D. Fourth maneuver (pelvic palpation)

- Instruct the patient to bent the knees.
- Position yourself facing the women's feet.
- Place both hands on the side of the abdomen just below the umbilicus and fingers towards the symphysis pubis.
- Deeply press your fingertips into the lower abdomen and move them towards the pelvic inlet.
    - *Engaged head:* Hands will diverge away from the presenting part.
    - *Head not engage:* Hands converge around the presenting part.

Fourth maneuver/second pelvic grip/ deep pelvic grip

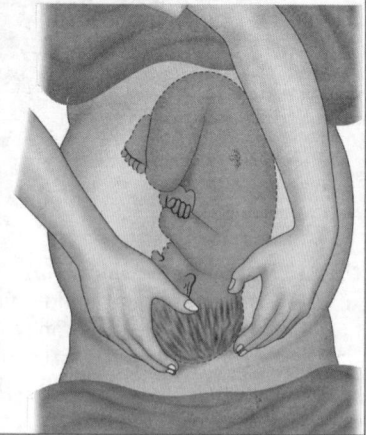

This maneuver in experienced hands, will be able to tell us about the degree of flexion of the head

Location of FHS Using Fetoscope

- ❖ Place the fetoscope or stethoscope on the convex area of the fetus nearest to the anterior uterine wall.
  - *Vertex and breech presentation:* FHS are heard over fetal back.
  - *Face presentation:* FHS are heard over the chest.
- ❖ Listen to the fetal heart sounds **(Fig. 47.3)** according to the fetal position given below **(Fig. 47.4)**:
  - *ROA:* Right occiput anterior.
  - *LOA:* Left occiput anterior.

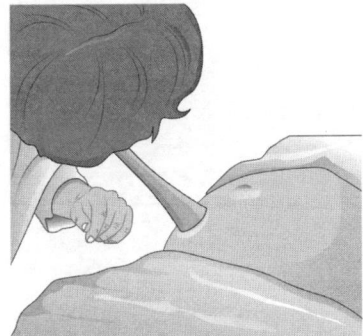

Fig. 47.3: Listening to FHS using fetoscope.

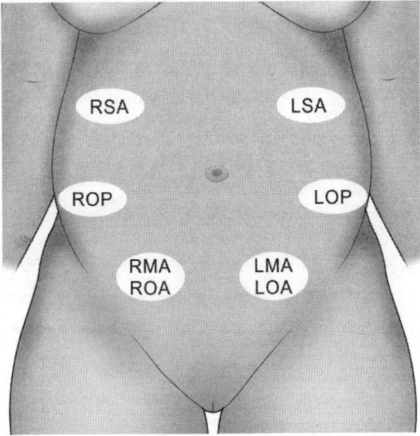

Fig. 47.4: Fetal position for listening to fetal heart sound.

- *RSP:* Right sacrum posterior.
- *LSP:* Left sacrum posterior.
- *RSA:* Right sacrum anterior.
- *LSA:* Left sacrum anterior.

❖ Cover the patient and make the patient comfortable.
❖ Inform the patient regarding the findings.
❖ Replace articles and wash hands.
❖ Records the findings.

CHAPTER 48

Postnatal Care

INTRODUCTION

The postnatal period is pivotal for the mother and new-born babies since maternal and infant deaths are prevalent within the first month after birth. Providing essential care to the mother and new-born baby within 24 hours of birth, regardless of the type of delivery, lays the groundwork for long-term health and well-being for both the woman and her infant. As a result, it is critical for health team members to create excellent postpartum care in order to improve the health of both the mother and the newborn.

DEFINITION

According to World Health Organization (WHO) postnatal care is defined as "a care given to the mother and her newborn baby immediately after the birth of the placenta and for the first six weeks of life".

POSTNATAL ASSESSMENT AND EXAMINATION

It is the systematic assessment and examination of women for the first three postnatal days up to 28 days during postpartum period.

PURPOSES

- To promote the physical wellbeing of mother and baby.
- To identify any physiological changes during postpartum period.
- To assess the involution of various organs.
- To detect any complications during postpartum period.
- To provide health teaching regarding postnatal to the mother.

ARTICLES REQUIRED

- Gloves
- Gown
- Mask
- TPR Tray
- Weighing machine
- Measuring tape
- Articles for perineal examination
- Bedside screen
- Flashlight

STEPS OF PROCEDURE

- Explain the procedure to the patient.
- Instruct patient to empty the bladder 30 minutes prior to examination.
- Open bedside screen to maintain privacy.
- Instruct patient to assume comfortable position.
- Wash hands.
- Assess vital signs, height and weight.
- Conduct head to toe examination.
- Conduct postnatal assessment using the "BUBBLE HE" acronym **(Table 48.1)**.
    - B: Breast
    - U: Uterus
    - B: Bowel
    - B: Bladder
    - L: Lochia
    - E: Episiotomy
    - H: Homan's sign
    - E: Emotions
- Instruct patient to maintain comfortable position.
- Replace all articles.
- Inform the date and time of next visit.
- Teach regarding postnatal exercise.
- Encourage family planning counselling.
- Educate regarding breast feeding and perineal care.
- Record the findings.

Table 48.1: Postnatal assessment using the "BUBBLE HE" acronym.

BREAST	• Inspect the color, shape, contour and abnormal discharge • Palpate the breast gently for any nodule, tenderness, firmness and fullness **(Fig. 48.1)** • Gently remove the milk to check the presence of colostrum • Check for the presence of cracked, inverted, erected, bleeding and bruised nipple **(Fig. 48.1)** 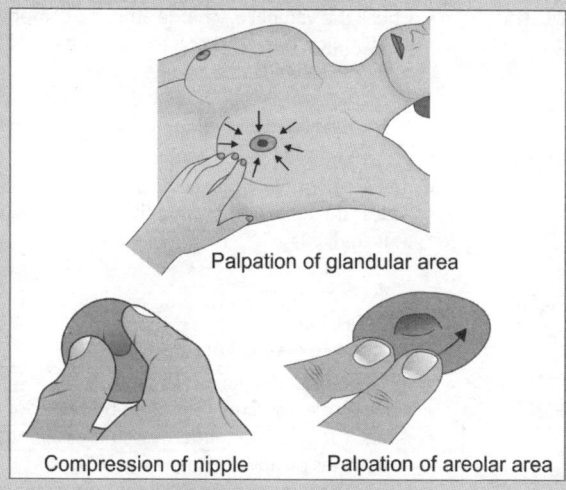 **Fig. 48.1:** Breast examination.
UTERUS	• Place hands on the lower abdomen and massage the uterus before palpation **(Fig. 48.2)** • Check for any discharge of blood during massage • Palpate the uterus for position, consistency and tonicity • Assess for pain and tenderness during palpation 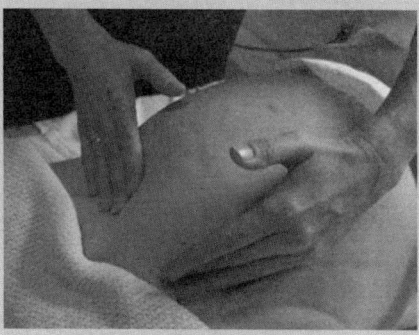 **Fig. 48.2:** Palpation of uterus.

Contd...

Contd...

BLADDER	• Inspect and palpate the bladder • Assess for retention of urine, pain or burning sensation while voiding • Assess for bruising and swelling around the urinary meatus
BOWEL	• Ask for presence of abnormal bowel movements • Auscultate for bowel sounds

LOCHIA	• Check the vaginal discharge amount, composition, color, consistency, odor and presence of clots.
	  ➢ *Lochia rubra (Red):* 1–4 days
	  ➢ *Lochia serosa (Pinkish brown):* 5–9 days
	  ➢ *Lochia alba (Pale white):* Pale/yellowish white

EPISIOTOMY	• Place patient in sim's position
	• Use flashlight when necessary
	• Assess the episiotomy using the acronym "REEDA"
	  ➢ R: Redness
	  ➢ E: Edema
	  ➢ E: Ecchymosis
	  ➢ D: Discharge
	  ➢ A: Approximation of suture line

HOMAN'S SIGN	• Instruct patient to lie on her back • Ask her to extend the leg flat on bed and dorsiflex her foot • Assess for pain and tenderness in the calf muscles. If present, it indicates positive Homan's sign **(Fig. 48.3)** • Assess for signs of superficial thrombophlebitis • Assess for presence of red, and painful edema 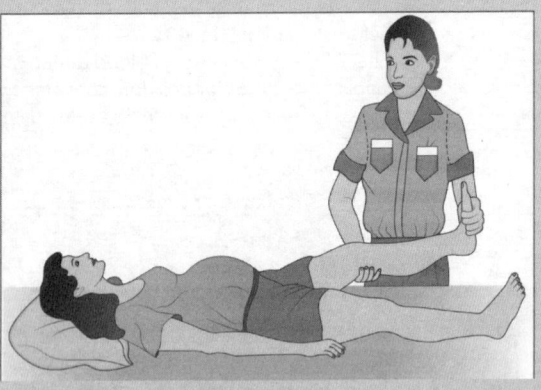 **Fig. 48.3:** Assessment of Homan's sign.
EMOTIONS	• Assess for presence of insomnia, anxiety, irritability, mood swings, and apathy • Assess for presence of postpartum blues or baby blues or postpartum depression

CHAPTER 49

Perioperative Care

INTRODUCTION

Surgery is a crucial treatment option for any acute or chronic illness, the success of the surgery largely depends on the care provided since the planning of the surgery to the period of rehabilitation. Perioperative care includes all strategies used by medical professional to care for patient during preoperative, intraoperative and postoperative phases of surgery. The care given to patients are physical, psychological, safety and security.

DEFINITION

Perioperative care, also known as perioperative medicine, is the practice of providing patient-centered, interdisciplinary, and integrated medical care to patients from the time of planning surgery till the time of full recovery.

PHASES OF PERIOPERATIVE CARE

- ❖ **Preoperative care:** Begins with the decision to perform surgery till patient arrives in the operating room.
- ❖ **Intraoperative care:** Begins when patient is transferred to the operating room and ends when patient is transfer to the post anesthesia care unit (PACU).
- ❖ **Postoperative care:** Begins with admission from the recovery area till discharge from the rehabilitation unit.

PREOPERATIVE CARE (FIG. 49.1)

Role of Nurse in Preoperative Care

- ❖ To ensure that the patient understands the nature of the surgery to be perform.
- ❖ To make patient understand about postoperative complications.
- ❖ To assess areas of anxiety and provide remedy.

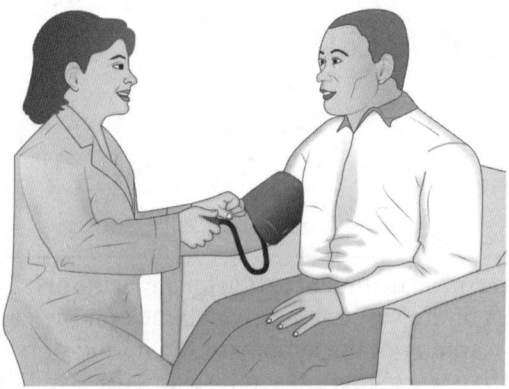

Fig. 49.1: Preoperative care.

- To identify, physical condition of the patients so that complications can be prevented.
- To ensure that the patient is in optimum physical condition before surgery.
- To ensure that surgical safety checklist is use for patient safety **(Fig. 49.2)**.

Patient Preparation

- To avoid infection, the patient is given a proper bath.
- Shaving of the part is also a common preoperative procedure.
- Nothing should be given to the patient to keep stomach empty. It takes 6 hours for solid food to come out of stomach.
- Ensure that the patient is wearing proper identification slip.
- Record the patients pulse, BP, respiration and temperature.
- Before giving preoperative medication ensure his personal belongings are kept safely.
- Check that the operation site and side is marked properly.
- Shift the patient carefully.
- Carry his complete record of findings and investigations to the OT.

INTRAOPERATIVE CARE (FIG. 49.3)

It is the physical and psychological care given in anesthesia room till transferred to recovery room. Nursing care includes:
- Make patient understand regarding the outcome of surgery, to minimize anxiety.

Perioperative Care

Surgical safety checklist
World Health Organization — Patient safety: A world alliance for safer healthcare

Before induction of anesthesia (with at least nurse and anesthetist)	Before skin incision (with nurse, anesthetist and surgeon)	Before patient leaves operating room (with nurse, anesthetist and surgeon)
Has the patient confirmed his/her identity, site, procedure, and consent? ☐ Yes **Is the site marked?** ☐ Yes ☐ Not applicable **Is the anesthesia machine and medication check complete?** ☐ Yes **Is the pulse oximeter on the patient and functioning?** ☐ Yes **Does the patient have a: Know allergy?** ☐ No ☐ Yes **Difficult airway or aspiration risk?** ☐ No ☐ Yes, and equipment/ assistance available **Risk of >500 mL blood loss (7 mL/kg in children)?** ☐ No ☐ Yes, and two IVs/central access and fluids planned	☐ **Confirm all team members have introduced themselves by name and role** ☐ **Confirm the patient's name, procedure, and where the incision will be made** **Has antibiotic prophylaxis been given within the last 60 minutes?** ☐ Yes ☐ Not applicable **Anticipated critical events** **To surgeon:** ☐ What are the critical or nonroutine steps? ☐ How long will the case take? ☐ What is the anticipated blood loss? **To Anesthetist:** ☐ Are there any patient-specific concerns? **To nursing team:** ☐ Has sterility (including indicator results) been confirmed? ☐ Are there equipment issues or any concerns? **Is essential imaging displayed?** ☐ Yes ☐ Not applicable	**Nurse verbally confirms:** ☐ The name of the procedure ☐ Completion of instrument, sponge and needle counts ☐ Specimen labeling (read specimen labels aloud, including patient name) ☐ Whether there are any equipment problems to be addressed **To surgeon, anesthetist and nurse:** ☐ What are the key concerns for recovery and management of this patient?

Fig. 49.2: Surgical safety checklist.

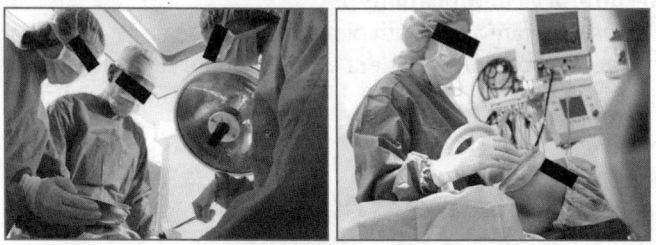

Fig. 49.3: Intraoperative care.

- To ensure correct part has been operated of which consent was taken.
- Minimize postoperative problems by keeping the patient in proper position.
- Maintain asepsis.

- Have proper staff to shift the patient.
- Ensure that all limbs are supported on table.
- Ensure all equipment, oxygen cylinder, etc. is in order.
- The surgeon is to be informed that the number of swabs, needles, scissors are correct.
- Get specific instructions from anesthetists for postoperative care.
- All information is to be recorded in case paper.
- Complete operative notes to be ensured.
- Proper care in postanesthetic recovery involves critical care required by the patients until they are conscious and stable.

Minimum criteria of patient to be discharged from recovery room includes:
- Patient is conscious and oriented.
- Respiratory function is adequate.
- Pulse and BP are within normal limits.
- There is no persistent bleeding from the site of operation.
- Satisfactory analgesics have been given.

POSTOPERATIVE CARE (FIG. 49.4)

Postoperative care focuses on early recovery and prevention of complications.
- **Circulatory problems**
  - Allow early mobilization when it is possible.
  - Record pulse and BP regularly.
- **Respiratory complications**
  - Observe, rate and depth of respirations.
  - Change position of patient every 2–3 hour to avoid bed sores.

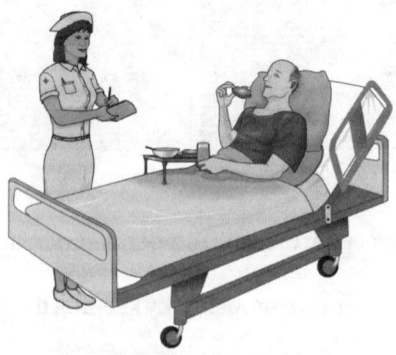

Fig. 49.4: Postoperative care.

- Recording of sputum.
- Provide adequate anesthesia.

❖ **Fluid balance**
- Keep a proper record of fluids.
- Measure quantity of urine.
- Listen to the complaints of patient sympathetically.

CHAPTER 50

Surgical Instruments

Surgical instruments are tools specifically designed and utilized by healthcare professionals during surgical procedures. These instruments are crucial for performing precise and delicate tasks, facilitating surgical maneuvers, and ensuring the safety and success of surgical interventions.

Instrument	Uses
Ramsey's sponge holding forceps	It is used to hold and manipulate surgical sponges/gauzes/cotton during procedures
Mayo towel clip	It is used to secure towels, drapes, or other sterile coverings
Doyen's towel clip	

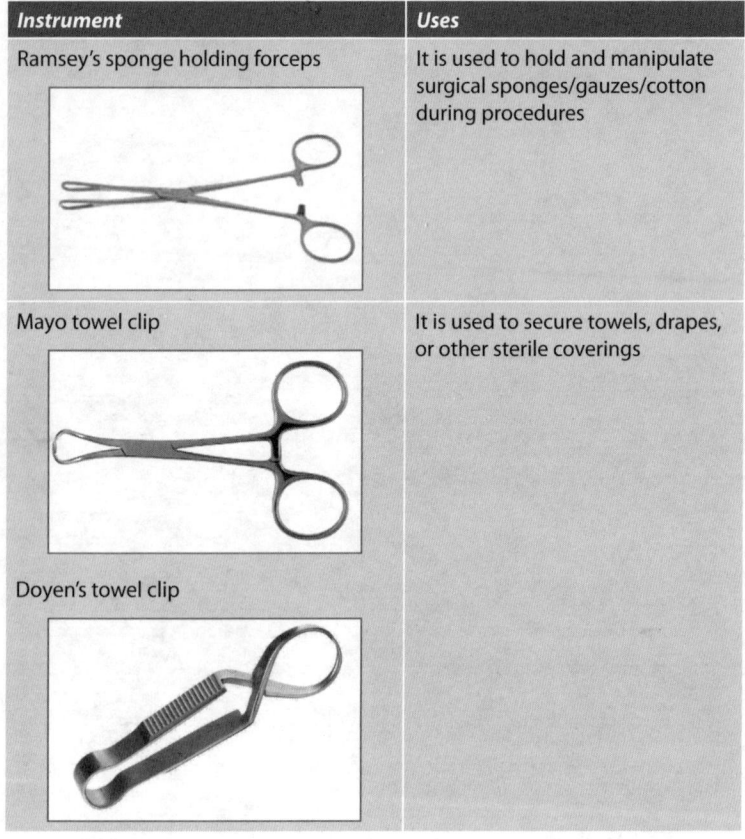

Surgical Instruments

Artery forceps 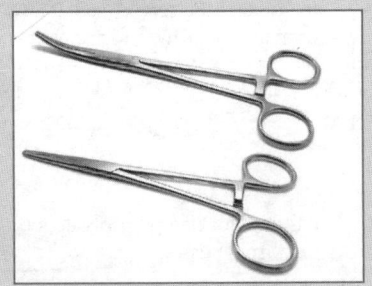	Also known as hemostatic forceps or surgical forceps, they are commonly used to clamp and occlude blood vessels during surgical procedures
Allis forceps 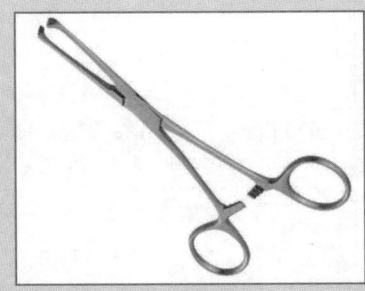	It is used to hold or grasp fascia and soft tissues such as breast or bowel tissue
Bab cock 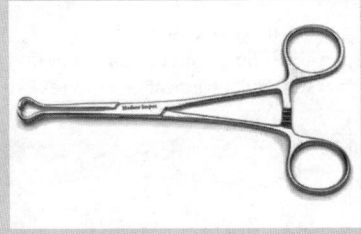	It is used to grasp delicate tissues during surgical procedures
Adson thumb forceps 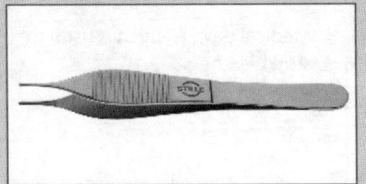	It is used to grasp, hold, and move tissue

Surgical Instruments

Vulsellum 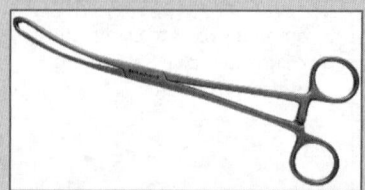	It is used to grip the cervical lips, to visualize the cervix and it is also used in vaginal hysterectomy
Right angle artery forceps 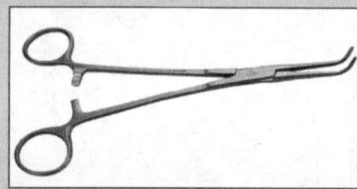	It is used for clamping, dissection, or grasping tissue
Kocher's forceps 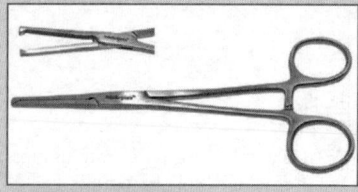	It is used to grasp heavy tissue or clamp large blood vessels to control bleeding
Bard parker handle 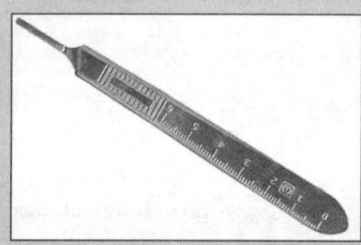	It is used for tissue separation, dissection, puncture or cut during surgery or surgical procedures
Cautery 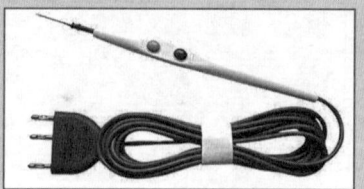	Medical device which is used to stop bleeding

Surgical Instruments

Cheatle forceps 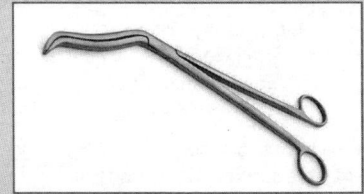	It is used to remove sterilized instruments from boilers and formalin cabinets
Doyen's retractor 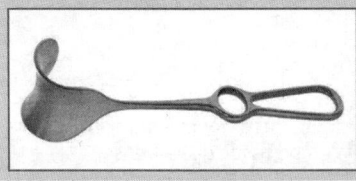	It used to retract organs. It is commonly used in abdominal OB/GYN procedures such as abdominal hysterectomies, cesarean section deliveries, and procedures for ectopic pregnancies
Deaver's retractor 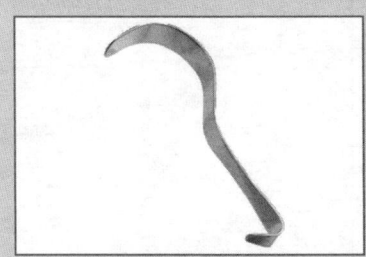	It is used to hold back the abdominal wall during abdominal or thoracic procedures. It may also be used to move or hold organs away from the surgical site
Cat's paw 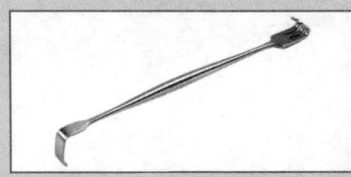	Senn-Mueller retractor commonly known as a "cat's paw" is a double ended small retractor for skin retraction in small and delicate wound
Langenbeck retractor 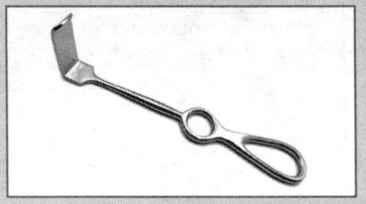	It is used to retract the superficial structures such as skin and subcutaneous tissues

Surgical Instruments

Instrument	Use
Morris double ended retractor 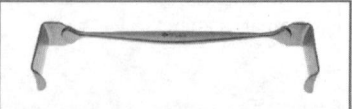	It is used to widen incision edges or wound borders during a broad range of surgical procedures, especially those involving the thoracoabdominal area
Needle holder (Mayo Hager Needle holder) 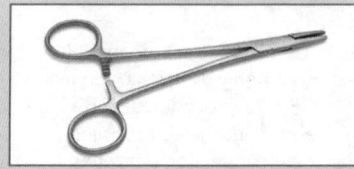	It is used to secure needles during the suturing of incisions
Scalpel blade 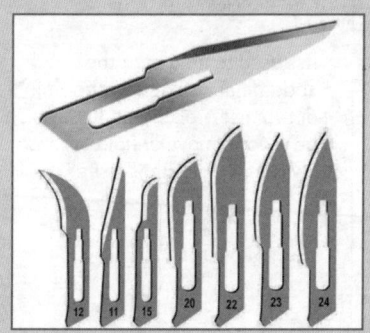	It is used for making skin incisions and tissue dissections
Iris scissors 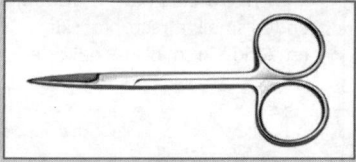	It is used to dissect the delicate tissues of the eye during ocular surgeries
Lister bandage scissors 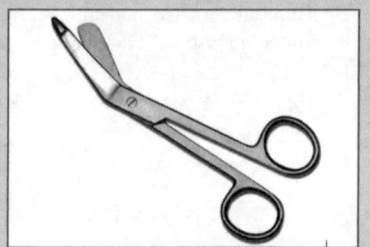	It is used to size bandages and dressings to be wrapped around the incision or wound

Surgical Instruments

Metzenbaum scissors 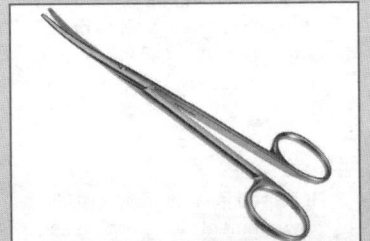	It is used for cutting delicate tissue and blunt dissection
Braun-Stadler Episiotomy scissors 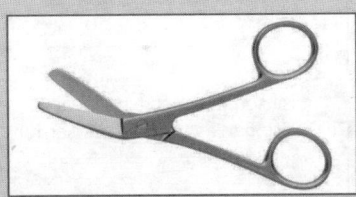	It is used to perform episiotomies during labor and delivery
Self-retaining retractor 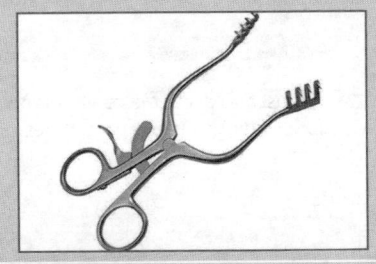	Commonly used in mastoid surgery to keep the blades apart and in place while spreading the edges of the incision and holding other tissue in place
Nasal speculum 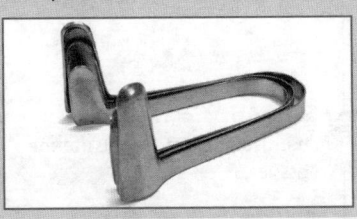	It is used to visualize nasal cavity
Aneurysm needle 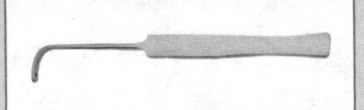	It is used for passing ligatures around vessels or aneurysms

Surgical Instruments

Instrument	Description
Trocar 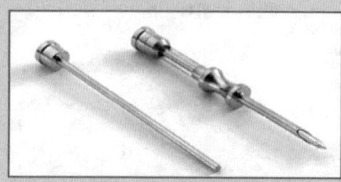	It is used during laparoscopic procedures and other minimally invasive surgery (MIS) to make small, puncture like incisions in outer tissue layers
Dissecting forceps 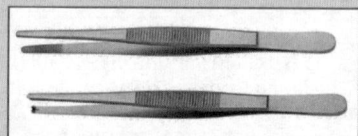	It is used in laboratory and clinical environments for grasping and holding
Tracheal dilator 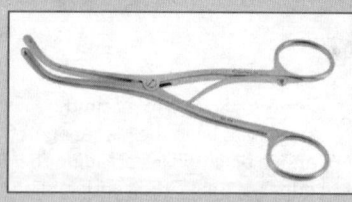	It is used to widen a tracheal incision to assist in tube insertion and placement
Uterine dilator 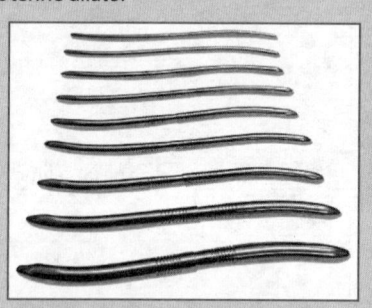	It is used to dilate the cervix, uterus for examinations and procedures
Uterine curette 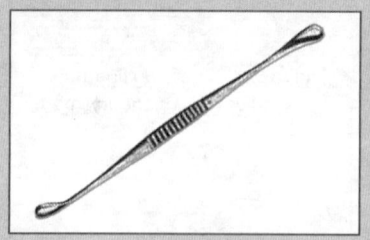	It is used to remove the uterine tissue

Surgical Instruments

Uterine sound 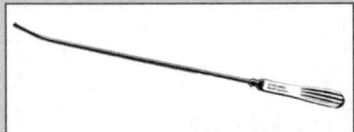	It is used to gauge the depth and position of the uterine cavity
Kelly's forceps 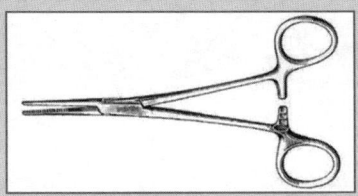	It is used for clamping large blood vessels or manipulating heavy tissue
Ovum forceps 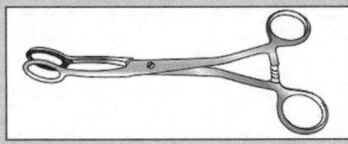	It is used to remove placental fragments inside the uterus
Magill forceps 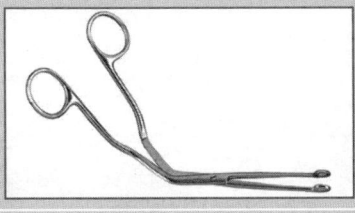	It is used to guide a tracheal tube into the larynx or a nasogastric tube into the esophagus under direct vision
Jolls thyroid retractor 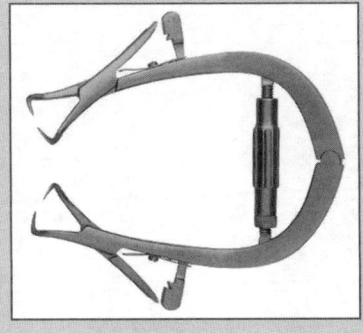	It is used in thyroid surgery to retract the organs

Surgical Instruments

Army navy retractor

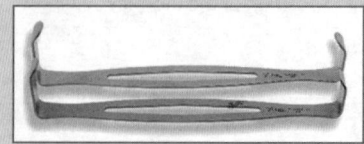

It is used to retract shallow or superficial incisions in abdominal surgeries

Index

Page numbers followed by *f* refer to figure, *fc* refer to flowchart, and *t* refer to table.

A

Abdomen 165, 323
   area, uncover 185
   auscultation for 165*f*
Abdominal examination 378
Abdominal girth, measurement of 380*f*
Abdominal palpation 380
Abdominal paracentesis 354
   procedure 355*f*
Abdominal route 375
Abduction 134, 135*f*
Abortion 374
Abstinence 374
Accommodation, loss of 311
Activities 175
Adduction 135*f*
Administer medication 264
Administer vaccine 272
Administering inhalation medication,
      methods of 268
Administering oxygen, process of 234
Admission 124
   process 125, 125*fc*
   purposes 124
   to discharge 124*fc*
Adson thumb forceps 395
Aerosol spray 267
Agents, surface-active 365
Air
   cushion 71
   hunger 30
   mattress 102, 103*f*
Airbeds 71
Alcohol 309
   swab 273, 279
Algor mortis 296
Alimentary system 20
Allergic reaction 253
Allergic testing 272

Allis forceps 395
Alpha-blockers 116
Ambu bag 236
Amenorrhea, period of 379
Aminophylline
   effects of 222
   suppository 222
Anaerobic exercise 133
Anal care 215
Aneroid sphygmomanometer 36*f*
Anesthetic suppository 222
Aneurysm needle 399
Ankle 142
Anoxemia 30
Anoxia 30
Antecubital fossa 231
Antenatal care 377
   articles required 377
Anticholinergics 116, 269
Antidote 302, 302*t*
   mechanical 302
   physiological 302
   types of 301
   universal 303
Antiscorpion antivenin 303
Antiseptic
   cleanser 266
   solution 212
Antisnake antivenin 302
Anxiety 27, 388
Aorta dissection 28
Apathy 388
Apgar score 318*t*
   interpretation of 318
Apical bronchi drainage 247, 247*f*
Apical pulse, auscultation of 28
Apnea 29
Appetite, loss of 199
Army navy retractor 402
Arsenic 301

Index

Arterial fibrillation 27
Artery forceps 209, 395
Articles
   care of 68
   preparation of 38
   required 180
Asepsis 79
Aspirin 301
Atelectasis 242
Atropine
   hypodermically 313
   sulfate 302
Auditory thermometers 18
Auscultation 159, 159f, 164, 165

B

B complex 311
Bab cock 395
Babinski reflex 325
Baby bath 317
Back 324
   straight 131
   using dominant hand 212
Back care 189, 195
   after care 198
   contraindications 195
   steps of procedure 196
Back lying position 108
   steps of procedure 108
Back rest 100, 100f
   uses 100
Bandage 143, 266
   adhesive spot 273
   circular 144f
   foot 148, 149f
   four-tailed 151f, 152
   hip 150, 151f
   many-tailed 151f, 152
   patterns used in 144
   principles of 143
   purposes 143
   recurrent 147, 147f
   shoulder 150, 150f
   special 151
   tailed 151
Bard parker handle 396
Barium
   meal 351
   studies 352f
Barium enema 353, 354f
   procedure 353f

Barium swallow 351
   procedure 352f
Basal body temperature method 374
Bath thermometer 217
Bathing 317
Bed
   amputation 97, 97f
   open 89
   ridden patient, case of 93
   stump 97
   unoccupied 89
Bed bath 183, 184f
   steps of procedure 184
Bed cradle 101, 101f
   uses 101
Bed making 88
   general rules for 88
   types of 88
Bedpan 68, 213, 215f, 220
   assisting with 213
   placing of 214f
Bedridden patients, case of 227
Bend knees 130
Bhang
   management 312
   symptoms 311
Bicycle ergometer 341
   test 342f
Biopsy 224
Birth control vaccine 374
Bisacodyl suppository 222
Bite, area of 304f
Bladder 40, 388
Bleeding
   control 143
   signs of 289
Blinking 326
Blistering 192
Blood
   components 253
   culture bottles 232, 232f
   process of transferring 253
Blood pressure 35
   assessment of 37, 39
   measurement 38f, 40t
   monitoring 36
Blood product 254
   inspect 256
Blood sample
   collection 231f, 232
   container 230f

Index

Blood transfusion 253
    complications 253
    steps of procedure 255
    types of 253
Blot's respiration 30
Body
    heat, conversion of 13
    part of 143
    vital signs 10f
Body mechanics 130
    principles of 131
Body temperature 10, 10f, 14
    maintenance of 315, 315t
    regulation of 12f, 23
Bowel 13, 388
    cleanser medication 219
    evacuation of 223
    gauge pieces in 201
Brachial artery 356
Bradycardia 26
Bradypnea 29
Brain injury
    minor 291
    moderate 291
    severe 291
Braun-Stadler episiotomy scissors 399
Breast 320, 387
    examination 387f
Breastfeeding 316, 317f
Breath, deep 223
Breathing difficulty, nursing care of 30
Breech presentation 383
Bromocriptine mesylate 303
Bronchi
    anterior 248
    lateral 248f
    superior 248
Bronchiectasis 243
Bronchitis 242
Bronchodilators 269
Bronchoscopy 336, 336f
Bruises 161f
BUBBLE HE acronym 387t
Burn 155f
    dressing 154
        steps of procedure 155
Buscopan 116

C

Calcium
    chloride 302
    folinate 303
    gluconate gel 302
Camphor 306f, 312
    management 312
    symptoms 312
Cannabis indica 311
Carbohydrate diet 311
Carbolic acid 301
Carbon monoxide 301
Cardiac bed 96, 96f
Cardiac catheterization 344, 345f
Cardiac position 106
Cardiac table 101, 101f
    uses 102
Cardiovascular system 339
Cat's paw 397
Catheter 212
    inflated balloon of 211f
    types of 208f
Catheterized patients 225
Celsius scales 16, 17
Centchroman nonhormonal pill 372
Cerebral angiography 355, 356f
    before procedure 356
    during procedure 356
Cerebrospinal fluid 224
Cervical
    mucus method 374
    OS 370
Charas 311
Cheatle forceps 397
Chemical antidote 301
Chemical dot 18
Chemical methods 363
Chest 323
    anterior 164
    posterior 164
    trauma to 244
    X-ray, imaging in 327f
Chest circumference 319, 320f
    measuring 170, 171f
Chest physiotherapy 242, 242f, 249
    contraindications 243
    indications 243
    techniques of 244
Cheyne-Strokes respiration 30
Chhaya 372
Chronic illness 234
Chronic obstructive pulmonary disease 242, 243
Circulatory system 20

Index

Clark's rule 261
Clean chewing surface 202
Clean tray containing 209
Cleaning, purposes of 68
Client
　health problems 10
　observation of 24
　preparation of 38
Clinical thermometer, assessing temperature with 32
Clove-Hitch restraint 120
Coitus interruptus 374
Cold application 46, 61
　classification of 47, 47*f*
　contraindications 48, 48*t*
　indications 48
　principles of 47
Cold compress 61
　steps of procedure 61
Cold pack 65
　steps of procedure 66
Collaborative care 194
Coma 300
Combined pills 371
Comfort devices 99
　types 99
Communication 1
　7C's of effective 5, 5*f*
　barriers of 9
　interpersonal 2
　levels of 2
　nonverbal 5
　process 3
　　elements of 3*f*, 4
　public 3
　small-group 2
　term 1
　types of 4
Concentration 261
Condom 362
　advantage of male 362
　application of
　　female 363
　　male 362
　disadvantages of male 362
　insertion of
　　female 364*f*
　　male 363*f*
　removal of female 364*f*

Conduct postnatal assessment 386
Confused conversation 293
Connecting suction catheter, method of 252*f*
Conscious patient, oral care of 199, 200*f*
Consciousness
　assessing level of 290
　level of 290
Constipation, treatment of 219
Contraception 360
Contraceptive methods 360, 361*fc*
　chemical of 365*f*
Convulsions 313
Copper T 380A, insertion of 367
Corrosive acids 306, 306*f*
Corticosteroids 269
Cotton ball 280
Coughing reflex 326
Creams 266
Cresol 301
Critical thinking
　fundamental principles of 172
　use of 173
Cuff 40
　placement of 40*f*
　size 39
Culture 225
　analysis 227
　media 233
Cumbersome 143
Cupped hand 245*f*
Cupping 198*f*
Cyanosis 30
Cyproheptadine 303
Cystic fibrosis 242, 243

D

Dancing reflex 325
Dandruff, cleansing hair of 186
Dantrolene 303
Data
　analyzing of 175
　biographic 156
　collection of 175
　documentation of 175
　organization of 175
　recording of 175
　validation of 175

Index

Dead body
  care of 296
  draping of 298f
Death 300
Deaver's retractor 397
Decerebrate posturing 294, 294f
Deep palpation 160f
Deep vein thrombosis 113
Delivery
  method, high flow 234
  type of 385
Dentures, care of 202
Dermal fillers 272
Dermis, medication into 273
Desferrioxamine 303
Device preparation 269
Dextrose 302
Dhatura 311
  management 311
  plant 306
  symptoms 311
Diagnostic label 176
Diagnostic testing 272
Diaphragm 360
Diarrhea, starch to check 217
Dichloro-diphenyl-trichloroethane 310
  management 310
  symptoms 310
Digital thermometer, assessing
  temperature with 34
Digital weighing scales 167, 167f
Digitalis toxicity 27
Digoxin specific antibody fragments
  fab 303
Dimercaptosuccinic acid 303
Direct percussion 160f
Dirty mouth causes 199
Discharge 127
  articles required 128
  preliminary assessment 127
  procedure 128
  process 128fc
  reasons for 127
Disease
  condition 29
  severe 300
  symptomatic treatment of 263
Disinfectants 301
Disinfecting solution 16

Disposable
  gloves 266
  paper thermometer 17, 17f
  wipes 269
Distilled water 209
Divergent spica 146
Doctor's order sheet 126
Document procedure 289, 351
Doing ROM exercises, methods of 133
Doll's eye 326
Dorsal recumbent position 108
Dorsiflexion 136f
Doyen's retractor 397
Doyen's towel clip 394
Drainage 192
Draw sheets 213
Dressing 143, 152, 266
Dropper 263
Drug calculation
  conversions 260
  formula 260
Drug dose calculations 257
Dry powder inhalers 269
Dry warm compress 51
Dry well 185
Dutch cap 360
Dynamic nature 173
Dyspnea 30

E

Ear 162, 163f, 287, 322
  articles required 287
  cartilage 320
  drops 282
    instillation of 283f
  irrigation of 287, 288f
  purposes 287
  steps of procedure 287
Echocardiography 343, 344f
Education 157, 194
Effleurage 196, 197f
Elastic band passes 237
Elbow 139, 139f
  divergent spica of 146f
  restraint 119
Electric cradle 53, 53f
Electric heating pads 52, 52f
Electric steam inhaler 240f
Electric steamer 238, 240

Index

Electrocardiogram
    components of 340, 340*t*
    procedure 339*f*
    waveform, normal 340*f*
Electrodes, placement of 341*f*
Electronic thermometer 16, 16*f*
Electrophysiologic testing 348
    procedure 348
Electrophysiology study 348*f*
Emergency assessment 174
Emollient 201
Emotions 388
Enamel ware 68
Encourage mobility 194
Enema 216
    anesthetic 217
    carminative 217
    cleansing 217
    coffee 217
    cold 217
    evacuant 217
    fleet 218
    hypertonic 217
    insertion of 216
    oxytocic 217
    packet of 220
    prepacked 220*f*
    proctoclysis 219
    sedative 217
    shelling 217
    steps of procedure 218
    types of 216, 216*f*
Episiotomy 388
Evidence-based practice 172
Exercise 26, 131, 194
    aerobic 132
    classification of 132, 132*fc*
    isokinetic 133
    isometric 133
    isotonic 133
    stress testing, types 341
Exophthalmos 162*f*
Expiratory reserve volume 335
Extremities 323
Eye 162, 285, 322
    abnormalities 162*f*
    articles required 285
    discharge from 162*f*
    drops 282, 283*f*
    irrigation of 286*f*
    open spontaneously 290
    opening 290
        response 291
    steps of procedure 286

F

Face 163
    mask, simple 235, 237*f*
    presentation 383
    tent 235
Face-to-face interaction 2
Facial expressions 2
Fahrenheit scales 16, 17
Family
    history 158
    members 122
    pedigree symbols and chart 158*f*
    planning 360
    tree 158
Fastigium 21
Febrile reactions 253
Feet 142
    movements of 135
    tying of 298*f*
Fencing reflex 325
Fertility regulating methods 360
Fetal back 381
Fetal heart sounds, listen to 383, 383*f*
Fetal small parts 381
Fetoscope 383, 383*f*
Fetus, head of 380
Fever 20
    constant 21
    continuous 21
    intermittent 21
    inverse 21
    irregular 21
    nursing care in 23
    quotidian 21
    relapsing 21
    remittent 21
    subside 21
    type of 21, 22*f*
Figure-of-eight 145, 145*f*
Finger restraint 120
First aid
    management 300
    measures 304
Flange hits cervix 371
Flex knee 185

Index

Flow meter 236
Fluid balance 393
Flumazenil 302
Fluoroscopy 356
Fly agaric mushroom 306*f*
Focus assessment 174
Fomepizole 303
Fontanelle 322
Footboard 102, 103*f*
Forceps, dissecting 209, 400
Forearm 139, 139*f*, 231
Fowler's position 106, 107*f*, 236, 246
    steps of procedure 107
Friction 197, 197*f*
    and shear 190
Fried's formula 260
Fundal grip 380
Fundal height, measurement of 378, 380*f*
Fundal palpation 380
Furniture 77
    use 77*f*
Furosemide 258

G

Gag reflex 325
Ganja 311
Gardenol 310
Gas poisons 304*f*
Gastric gavage 178
Gastrointestinal endoscopy, lower 350, 350*f*
Gastrointestinal system 349
Gauze pads 273
Gauze pieces 236
Genital care 206*f*
    female 204, 205*f*
    male 205, 206*f*
Genitalia 323
    female 321
    male 321
Gestational age at birth, assessment of 320, 320*t*
Glasgow coma scale 290, 291
Glassware 73
Gloves 70, 84
    don 273
Glucagon 302
Glucose, nutrient enema of 217
Glycerin suppository 221

Goal-oriented tasks 172
Gossypol 371
Gown 84
    doffing of 85, 85*f*
    donning of 85, 85*f*
Grab bars 121
Graphic rating scale 115, 116*f*
Great vessels
    oxygen concentration of 346*f*
    pressure in 346*f*

H

Hacking 197, 198*f*
Hair
    care of 186
    texture 320
Hair wash 186, 187*f*
    articles required 186
    procedure 187
    purposes 186
Hand 140, 140*f*
    sanitizer, alcohol-based 266, 279
Hand bandage 148
    triangular 148*f*
Hand wrist splints 104, 105*f*
    uses 105
Handheld peak flow meter 269
Handling pills 264
Handwashing
    articles required 79
    five moments of 80*f*
    indications of 79
    steps of procedure 79
    technique 79
Head 162
    and face 322
    and neck 162
    capeline bandages of 147, 148*f*
    injury, grading of 295
Head circumference 319
    measuring 170, 171*f*, 320*f*
Head to toe examination 161, 322
    general appearance 161
    preprocedure steps 161
Health
    and illness pattern 157
    and palliative treatment 263
    assessment 156
    team members, critical for 385
Healthcare professional 281

Index

Healthy newborn 314*f*
Heart
   catheterization, right 345
   chambers of 345, 346*f*
   conditions, parameters of 347*t*
   parameters of 346
Heat cradles 53
Heat loss, ways of 13
Heat production, ways of 11
Heat to body, application of 51
Height 167
   and weight 166
Hemoglobin, oxygen saturation of 42
Hemolytic transfusion reaction, acute 253
Hemoptysis 243
Hemorrhage 27, 113
Hip 141, 141*f*
History collection, components of 156
Homan's sign 388
   assessment of 388*f*
Hormonal contraceptives 371
   types of 372*f*
Hormonal therapies, administration of 275
Hormones 365
Hospital
   admission 124
   discharge 124
   enamel ware 69*f*
   glassware 73*f*
Hot application 46, 48
   classification of 47, 47*f*
   contraindications 48, 48*t*
   indications 48
   principles of 47
Hot compress 50
   application of 50*f*
   types 50
Hot water
   bag 49*f*, 71
   bottles 48, 72
   filling of 49*f*
   use of 14
Humidifier 236
   with distilled water 236
Hydration 191
Hydrocortisone 222
Hyoscine butylbromide 116
Hyperextension 134, 134*f*
Hyperpnea 29
Hyperpyrexia 23
Hyperthermia 23
Hypothalamus 11*f*
Hypoxemia 30, 234
Hypoxia 30, 234

I

Ibuprofen 116
Ice bags 62
Ice cap 62, 71
   application of 62*f*
   steps of procedure 63
Idarucizumab 303
Immobility 190
   and inactivity, impact of 131
Immunization 316, 317*f*
Impacted cerumen 163*f*
Incontinence 191
Index finger length 223
Indwelling catheterization 209, 212
Infantometer 169*f*
   infant using 168
Infections 242
Infrared
   lamp 53, 53*f*
   rays 53
Infusion pump 260
Inhalational medication administration 268
Inhaler 268, 269
   types of 268
   with spacer, parts of 270*f*
   without spacer 270*f*
Injection, site of 276*f*
Insomnia 388
Inspiratory reserve volume 335
Instillation 281
   steps of procedure 282
Instrument
   sharp 72
   stainless steel 72, 72*f*
   surgical 394
Insulin dosage 261
Intermittent catheterization 208
Intradermal injection 272
   administration 272
      steps of procedure 273
Intramuscular injection 278
   administration 278, 280*f*
   needle used for 278
   site for 279*f*

Index

Intrauterine contraceptive device 365
Intrauterine device
    copper releasing 366
    insertion of
        copper releasing 368*f*
        hormone releasing 369
        levonorgestrel 370*f*
    third-generation 369
    types of copper releasing 367*f*
Intravasal thread 375
Intravenous
    drip rates, calculation of 259
    fluid flow rate 261
    pyelography 358
        procedure 358*f*
Iodine 308
    management 308
    signs 308
    symptoms 308
Iris scissors 398
Irrigation 285
Irritability 388
Izal 301

J

Jacket restraint 119
Joint
    bandaging 149, 149*f*
    movement of 143
Jolls thyroid retractor 401
Jugular vein distension 164*f*

K

Kangaroo mother care 315
Kelly's forceps 401
Kerosene poisoning 310
    management 311
    symptoms 310
Kidney 13
    trays 69
Kitchen and pantry 78
Knee 141, 142*f*
Knee-chest position 106, 111, 111*f*
    steps of procedure 112
Kocher's forceps 396
Kussmaul's respiration 30

L

Langenbeck retractor 397
Laparoscopic application 376
Lateral position 110
L-carnitine 303
Left lower lobe 248
    drainage 248*f*
    lateral bronchi of 248
Left occiput anterior 383
Left sacrum
    anterior 384
    posterior 384
Left upper lobe 247
    lower part of 247
Leopold's maneuvers 379, 380
Levin's tube 179
Light palpation 160*f*
Linen 74
    care of 74
    types of 74*f*
Lingula 247*f*
Lip 163
Lipid emulsion 302
Lippes loop 365
    insertion of 366
    types of 366*f*
Liquid
    medication 263, 264
    metal 15
Lister bandage scissors 398
Lithotomy position 106, 110, 111*f*
    steps of procedure 111
Livor mortis 296
Lobes, middle 246
Lochia 388
Lotions 266
Low flow delivery method 236
Low pyrexia 21
Lower extremity 39, 166, 166*f*
Lower limbs
    movement 214
    restricted 214*f*
    unrestricted 214*f*
Lower lobe 246, 248
    drainage, right 248*f*
    right 248
Lubricant solution 217
Lump 161*f*
Lung 13, 163
    capacities 335*f*, 336
    scan 330
    ventilation of 31
    volume 335, 335*f*, 335*t*
        spirogram of 335*f*

Index

Lying position, lateral 110*f*
Lyses 21
Lysol 301

M

Mackintosh 69
   place 187
Macule 161*f*
Magill forceps 401
Maneuver
   first 380
   fourth 382
   second 380, 381
   third 381, 382
Manometer 40
Mantoux test 333
   method 333
   procedure 334*f*
Marital status 157
Mask
   doffing of 84
   donning of 84
   non-re-breather 235, 236
   sterile 84, 84*f*
   tracheostomy 236
   venturi 235
Massage 116, 196
Mattress 75
Mayo Hager needle holder 398
Mayo towel clip 394
Measuring tape 168*f*
Medical devices 191
   use of 191
Medical fomentation 54
   application of 56*f*
Medical handwashing 79
   steps of 81*f*
Medical termination of pregnancy kit 373*f*
Medication 27
   administration of 349, 351
   canister 269
   cup 263
   forms 266
   in inhalation, types of 269
   package 281
   subcutaneous route 277*f*
   using techniques 267
Menstrual cycle regulation 373*f*
Menstrual induction 373
Menstrual regulation 372
Mercuric sulfide 306*f*
Mercury 15
Mercury poisoning 308
   management 308
   symptoms 308
Mercury sphygmomanometer 36*f*
   parts of 37*f*
Metered-dose inhaler 268, 269
   with spacer 270
   without spacer 270
Methylprednisolone 258
Methylthioninium chloride 302
Metoprolol 257
Metzenbaum scissors 399
Mid-arm circumference, measuring 170, 171*f*
Middle lobe drainage, right 247*f*
Midstream urine, collection of 225*f*
Mifepristone 373
Mobility and immobility 130
Moist warm compress 50
Moisture 191
   evaporation of 14
   management 194
Mood swings 388
Moro reflex 324
Morphine 116
Morris double ended retractor 398
Motion, circular 231, 279
Motor response 291
Mouth 163, 323
   infections, treat 199
Movements, level of limitations in 213
Mucolytics 269
Mucous membranes 266
Mucus plugs 242
Mummy restraint 119
Muscular skeletal system 20
Mushrooms 312
   management 313
   symptoms 312
Myelography 357
   procedure 357*f*
Myocardial infarction 27

N

Nasal
   articles required 288
   drops, instillation of 284*f*

Index

prongs 236
purposes 288
septum deviation 163f
speculum 399
steps of procedure 289
structures 162
Nasal cannula 235
   high flow 235
Nasal irrigation 289f
   device 289
Nasogastric tube
   distance of 182f
   feeding 178
   insertion and feeding 178
   placement 178f
National Programme for Family
      Planning 360
Natural family planning methods 374
Nebulizers 268
Neck 137, 137f, 163, 323
Needle 73
   holder 398
Nelson's inhaler 238, 239f
Nervous system 20
Neurological system 355
Neuromuscular disorders 243
Newborn
   assessment 318
   care of 314
   normal 321
Non-skit slippers 122
Nonsteroidal anti-inflammatory drugs
      116
Nonverbal communication 5
   eye contact 5
   facial expression 5
   gait 5
   gesture 5
   physical appearance 5
   posture 5
   silence 5
   sound 5
   touch 5
   types of 5
Normal suction pressure 251
Nose 162, 323
   drops 283
Numeric pain rating scale 115
Nurse
   record 126

   responsibility 32
   role of 389
   tasks of 7
Nurse-patient relationship 1, 6
Nursing assessments, lack of 156
Nursing care, essential functions of 156
Nursing process 172, 177f
   assessment 173
   characteristics of 173, 173f
   diagnosis 175
   evaluation 177
   implementation 177
   planning 176
   purposes 172, 174
   sequential steps of 172f
Nursing work, fundamental of 88
Nutritional support 194

O

Obstetrical history 159
Occupied bed 91, 92f
Octreotide acetate 303
Ointments 266
Once-a-month pill 371
Open bed 89f
Opium 309
   management 309
   symptoms 309
Oral abortifacient 373
Oral cavity clean 199
Oral digital pacifier thermometer 18
Oral hygiene 199
   steps of procedure 200, 201
Oral medication administration 262
   route of 262, 262f
   steps of procedure 263
Oral medications, forms of 263
Oral pills 371
Oral suctioning 250, 251
   after care 252
   steps of procedure 252
Oral temperature 18f
Organ system 132
   inactivity on 132t
Organization's protocol 122
Organophosphorus
   compounds 307
   insecticides 306f
Orthopnea 29, 30
Ovum forceps 401

Oxygen
  administration of 237
  concentration 345
  delivery devices 235*t*
  delivery system, types of 234, 235*f*
  inhalation 31
  levels in blood, increase 234
  source of 234, 236
  therapy 234
Oxygen mask
  method, administration of 236
  simple 236
Oxygen saturation
  in tissue, increase 234
  measuring of 44*f*
Oxygenation 234

P

Pain 26, 114, 192, 289
  acute 26, 114
  assessment 114
    tools 115
  characteristics of 115
  chronic 26, 114
  localize to 293
  management 116
  neuropathic 114
  pethidine for 313
  physiological 114
  rating scale 115*f*
  somatic 114
  types 114
  visceral 114
  withdraws to 293
  worst 115
Palmar reflex 326
Palpate 162
Palpation 159, 160, 161, 163, 165, 166
  lateral 380, 381
Paper thermometers, single-use 17
Paradoxical pulse 28
Parasites, destroy 217
Parenteral dosage 261
Pawlik's grip 381
Peg solution 303
Pelvic grip
  deep 382
  first 382
  second 382
  superficial 382

Pelvic organs, surgery of 113
Pelvic palpation 382
Pentazocine 116
Percussion 159, 160, 164, 165, 244, 245*f*
Perineal care 203, 215
  indications 203
  steps of procedure 204
Personal hygiene, maintenance of 24
Petrissage 197, 197*f*
Phenobarbitone luminol 310
  management 310
  symptoms 310
Phentolamine 303
Physical examination 159
Physical restraints, types of 119
Physostigmine 303
Phytomenadione 303
Pill, male 371
Pillows 75, 100, 100*f*
  uses 100
Plantar creases 321
Plantar flexion 136*f*
Pneumonia 243
Poison 300, 301
  absorbed 305
  classification of 300, 300*t*
  common 306
  management of 300, 301
  unabsorbed 304
Poisonous substances, types of 306*f*
Polyethylene glycol 303
Polypnea 29
Poor nutrition 191
Popliteal artery 40*f*
Portable unit 251
  suction 251*f*
Positron emission tomography scan 331, 331*f*
Postauricular lymph nodes enlargement 163*f*
Postcoital pill 371
Postconceptional methods 372
Postnatal care 385
  steps of procedure 386
Postoperative bed 94, 94*f*
Postpartum
  blues, presence of 388
  care 385
Postural drainage 244, 244*f*
  positions in 246

Index

Potassium
    chloride 258
    iodide 303
Povidone-iodine 233
Powder 267
Pralidoxime 303
Premature baby 321
Prepacked enema, insertion of 221*f*
Prescription order 263
Pressure 345
    diastolic 35
    points, care of 189
    points, common sites of 189
    pulse 35
    redistribution 194
    systolic 35
Pressure sore
    care of 190
    causes of 190
    prevention of 193
    stages of 193, 193*f*
Pressure ulcers 192
    signs of 191, 192
    symptoms of 191, 192
Proctoclysis 219
Procyclidine injection 302
Progesterone only pill 371
Progestogen 365
Prone position 106, 108, 108*f*, 190, 246
    steps of procedure 109
Proper sterile technique 275
Protamine sulphate 303
Prothrombin complex concentrate 302
Psychological support 30
Ptosis 162*f*
Pulmonary angiography 331, 332*f*
Pulmonary function test 334, 334*f*
Pulse 25, 31
    aptitude 27
    assessment, common sites for 25, 26*f*
    beats per minute, number of 25
    bigeminal 27
    bouncing 27
    characteristics of 25
    Corrigan 27
    dicrotic 27
    oximeter 43*f*, 44*f*
        parts of 44*f*
    palpation of 166*f*
    rate 26
    thready 27
    weak 27
    wiry 27
Pulse oximetry 42
    steps of procedure 43
Pulsus alternans 27
Puncture proof container 231, 233
Pus formation 203
Pyrexia
    high 23
    moderate 21
Pyridoxine 303

Q

Quality nursing, foundation for 156

R

Radiant warmer 316
Rale 30
Ramsey's sponge holding forceps 394
Range of motion exercises 133
Recent surgery 244
Rectal area, inspect 223
Rectal tube, inserting tip of 219*f*
Reflexes 324, 324*t*
    stepping 325
    sucking 324
Renal system 358
Residual volume 335
Respiration 28, 32
    artificial 311
    characteristics of 28
    normal 29
    variations abnormal 29
Respiratory complications 392
Respiratory conditions, severe 268
Respiratory distress, severe 244
Respiratory system 20, 327
Restraint 117
    and safety devices 117
    application of 118
    types of 118
    use of 118
Rhythm 27, 29
    circulation 14
Ribs, fractured 244
Right angle artery forceps 396
Right middle lobe, lower part of 247

Index

Right sacrum
   anterior 384
   posterior 384
Rigor mortis 296
Rinse mouth 271
Room, ventilation of 30
Rooting reflex 324
Rotatory movements 381
Routine examination 227
Rubber
   tubes 71
   ware 69, 70f

S

Safety belts 120
Safety device 117, 121
Salem tube 179
Saline
   normal 266
   physiological 218
Saliva, stimulate flow of 199
Salivary glands, prevent infection of 199
Sandbags 104, 104f
   uses 104
Sandostatin 303
Scalp, hair distribution on 320
Scalpel blade 398
Scanty urine 311
Scarred tympanic membrane 17
Scrotum 207
Secure dressing 154f
Self-administer subcutaneous injections 275
Self-retaining retractor 399
Semi-Fowler's position 107f
Sensation, reduced 190
Sensitivity testing 272
Sensory impairment 41
Sepsis 203
Septic reaction 253
Sexually transmitted diseases, transmission of 362
Shock 113
Shoulder 137, 138f
Side lying position 110, 110f, 189, 246
   steps of procedure 110
Sim's position 106, 109, 109f
   steps of procedure 109
Sinus arrhythmia 27
Sitting position 246

Sitz bath 59, 60f
   steps of procedure 59
Skills, assessment 174
Skin 13
   assessment, regular 193
   breakdown 192
   care 194, 317
   dermis layer of 272
   flora 82
   pinching 276f
   problems 161f
   pruritic 161f
   rashes 161f
   rejuvenation treatments 272
   texture 320
      changes 192
   turgor, decrease 161f
Skin-to-skin contact 315
Small bowl 209
Small staff meeting 2
Sneezing 326
Sodium
   bicarbonate 302
   carbonate 307
   nitrite 302
   phosphate 218
   thiosulphate 302
Sounds, incomprehensible 293
Specimen collection 224
   steps of procedure 225
Speech 4
Spermatozoa 375
Sphygmomanometer 36
   digital 37f
Spica 146
   of thumb 146f
Spine 324
Spiral bandage
   reversed 145, 145f
   simple 144f
Sputum
   colour of 332
   cups 69
   examination 332
Squeeze off water 188
Stadiometer 169, 169f
Stadiums 21
Staggering gait 311
Stains, types of 76t
Startle reflex 324

Index

Steam inhalation 238, 240
    care procedure for 241
    steps of procedure 239, 240
    types 238
Sterile cotton balls 273
Sterile dressing, applying 154f
Sterile gauze 280
    pieces 209
Sterile gloves
    doffing of 87, 87f
    donning of 86, 86f
Sterile kidney tray 209
Sterile soak 58
    steps of procedure 58
Sterile syringe 209
Sterile technique, maintaining 349, 351
Sterile towel 209
Sterile water 252
Sterilization, female 375
Steroid suppository 222
Stertorous respiration 30
Stethoscope 41
Stool sample 227f
    container 226f
Stool specimen, routine and culture 226
Stridor 30
Subcutaneous implants 372
Subcutaneous injection
    administration 275
    steps of procedure 276
Succimer 303
Suction catheter 250f, 252
Sugammadex 302
Sulfuric acid 306f
Supine position 108, 189
    pressure points in 189f
    with bed tilted 246
    with head elevated 246
    with pillow 246
Suppositories, types of 221
Suppository 221, 223, 223f
    insertion of 223f
    steps of procedure 222
Supraorbital notch 292f
Surgical fomentation 56
    steps of procedure 57
Surgical handwashing 82
    steps of 82f
        procedure 83
Suspension-based lotion 267

Sutures 322
Swallowing reflex 325
Sweating, stage of 25
Swelling 192
    prevent 143
Swollen lymph nodes 164f
Symptothermal method 374
Syringe 73, 211
    plunger of 231, 233
Systolic pressure, measuring 41

T

Tachycardia 26
Tachypnea 29
Talkativeness 311
Tamsulosin 116
Tape and ruler 167
Tapotement 197, 198f
T-bandage 151, 151f
    double 151, 151f
Temperature 31
    assessment of 14
    by axilla 19, 19f
    by ear 20
    by mouth 18, 18f
    by rectum 19, 19f
    common sites 18
    controlling center 11f
    core 11
    degree of 14
    maintaining 315
    sensitive strips 18, 18f
    subnormal 23
    surface 11
    through ear 20f
    types of 11
    variations, normal 14
Tenaculum, remove 369
Tension 28
Tepid sponging 63
    steps of procedure 64
Therapeutic communication
    elements of 6
    phases of 7
    techniques 8
Therapeutic positions 106
    types 106
Thermometer 16
    clinical 14, 15, 33t
    digital 34t

disinfection of 16, 16*t*
glass 14
lotion 15
oral and rectal 15*f*
types of 14
Thiamine 302
Thiopentone 222
Thoracentesis 338, 338*f*
Thoracoscopy 337, 337*f*
procedure 337
Thorax 163
Throat swab 224
specimen for culture 227
steps of procedure 228
specimen, collecting 228*f*
Thumb
forceps 201
grip of white rod 369
Tidal volume 335
Tissue 269
Toes 142, 142*f*
tying of 298*f*
Toilet tissues 217
Tongue depressor 201, 227
Tonic neck reflex 325
Topical medication 266
administration 265
steps of procedure 266
types of 265*f*
Tourniquet 231, 304
Toxic
exposure 302
substances 302*t*
Tracheal dilator 400
Transdermal patch 267
Transfusion, types of 254*t*
Trapeze 121
bar 102, 103*f*
uses 102
Trapezius squeeze 292*f*
Treadmill 341
test 342*f*
Trendelenburg's position 106, 112, 112*f*, 246
steps of procedure 113
Trocar 400
Trochanter roll 102, 104*f*
uses 104
Trunk 138, 138*f*
Tube feeding, administering 180
Tubectomy 375
Tuberculosis, active 244
Tubes, types of 179
Tympanic membrane thermometer 17, 17*f*

U

Umbilical cord, care of 317
Unconscious patient, oral care of 200, 201*f*
Upper extremities 166, 166*f*
Upper gastrointestinal endoscopy 349
procedure 349*f*
Upper lobes 246
anterior part of 247, 247*f*
right 247
Urinals 68
Urinary catheter, insertion of 211*f*, 212*f*
Urinary catheterization 208
steps of procedure 210
types 208
Urinary system 20
Urine
collection 225
sites of 203
specimen 224, 226
Uterine
cavity 370
curette 400
dilator 400
fundus 369, 371
sound 401
Uterus 387
height of 379
palpation of 387*f*

V

Vaginal diaphragm 361, 361*f*
insertion of 361
removal of 362
Vaginal opening 203
Vaginal rings 372
Vaginal sponge 363, 364*f*
Vas clips 375
Vas valve 375
Vasectomy male 375
Vaseline 217
Verbal communication 4
oral 4
written 4

Verbal response 291, 292
Vibration 116, 197, 198*f*, 244, 245*f*
Visual analogue scale 115, 116*f*
Vital signs 10, 166
    assessment of 10
    monitoring 349, 351
Vitamin K1 303
Vulsellum 396

W

Wall mount suction 251*f*
Wall unit 251
Ward inventory 78
Warmth 192
Wash chest thoroughly 185
Wash leg 185
Washing soda 307
Water
    clean 269
    hammer 27
    mattress 102, 103*f*
        uses 102

Weighing machine 166
Weight of infant, measuring 169, 170*f*
Wet sheet pack 65
Wheeze 30
Withdraw finger 223
Withdrawing needle 231*f*
Words, inappropriate 293
Wound 154*f*
    cleaning of 154*f*
    debris, removing 155*f*
Wound dressing 152
    steps of procedure 153
Wound swab
    collecting 229*f*
    for culture 228
        steps of procedure 229
Wrist 140, 140*f*

Z

Zinc sulphate 305